# HIV Infection Treatment: Progress and Challenges

# HIV Infection Treatment: Progress and Challenges

Editor: Spencer Brooks

MURPHY & MOORE
www.murphy-moorepublishing.com

www.murphy-moorepublishing.com

MURPHY & MOORE

**Cataloging-in-Publication Data**

HIV infection treatment : progress and challenges / edited by Spencer Brooks.
p. cm.
Includes bibliographical references and index.
ISBN 978-1-63987-306-7
1. HIV infections--Treatment. 2. AIDS (Disease)--Treatment. 3. Sexually transmitted diseases--Treatment. I. Brooks, Spencer.
RC606.6 .H58 2022
616.979 2--dc23



Murphy & Moore Publishing,
1 Rockefeller Plaza,
New York City, NY 10020, USA

ISBN 978-1-63987-306-7 (Hardback)

# Contents

# Preface

HIV infection is treated through antiretroviral therapy (ART). It is also known as highly active antiretroviral therapy (HAART). It helps in the management of the disease by reducing the viral load to very low levels. This helps in controlling the transmission of infection to other people. It works by preventing the virus from replicating within the body of the infected person. This in turn reduces the damage to the immune system. It also helps in decreasing the chances of catching an opportunistic infection. Through highly active antiretroviral treatment, the transmission of virus from mother to child can also be prevented. This book brings forth some of the most innovative concepts and elucidates the unexplored aspects of highly active antiretroviral treatment. It explores all the clinical complications of these medications in the present day scenario. The book is appropriate for students seeking detailed information in this area as well as for experts.

This book has been the outcome of endless efforts put in by authors and researchers on various issues and topics within the field. The book is a comprehensive collection of significant researches that are addressed in a variety of chapters. It will surely enhance the knowledge of the field among readers across the globe.

It gives us an immense pleasure to thank our researchers and authors for their efforts to submit their piece of writing before the deadlines. Finally in the end, I would like to thank my family and colleagues who have been a great source of inspiration and support.

**Editor**

# 1

# Endothelial Dysfunction in HIV

Vani Subbarao[1], David Lowe[2,3],
Reza Aghamohammadzadeh[4,5] and Robert J. Wilkinson[2,3,6]
[1]*Madwaleni Hospital, Elliotdale, Eastern Cape*
[2]*Clinical Infectious Disease Research Initiative,*
*Institute of Infectious Diseases and Molecular Medicine, University of Cape Town*
[3]*Wellcome Trust Centre for Research in Clinical Tropical Medicine,*
*Department of Medicine, Imperial College London*
[4]*British Heart Foundation Clinical Research Fellow*
[5]*NIHR Manchester Biomedical Research Centre Clinical Research Fellow*
[6]*Division of Mycobacterial Research, MRC National Institute for Medical Research, The Ridgeway, Mill Hill, London*
[1,2]*South Africa*
[3,4,5,6]*UK*

## 1. Introduction

The UNAIDS global report estimated that the number of people living with HIV/AIDS by the end of 2009 was 33 million. By 2008, the global funding for HIV/AIDS had climbed to $15.6 billion (Kates *et al.*, 2009) and by 2009, WHO estimated that 5.2 million were on ART in low and middle income countries (WHO, 2010).

Over 30 years of the AIDS epidemic and since the introduction of highly active antiretroviral therapy (ART) in 1996, the management of HIV-1 infection has gradually moved from treatment of opportunistic infections towards regular monitoring and maintenance of a suppressed viral load. As expected, this has lead to dramatic improvements in morbidity and mortality from HIV-1. Whilst the median life expectancy following diagnosis with HIV-1 prior to the advent of ART was 7 years, it has now reached 35 years in the developed world (Lohse *et al.*, 2007). Consequently there has been a parallel growth in the complications that arise from chronic infection with HIV-1 and its treatments.

Atherosclerotic and ischemic cardiovascular disease, which once predominantly afflicted the elderly, is now increasing in prevalence in HIV-1 infected persons. In the pre-ART era, the cardiac manifestations of HIV-1 were mainly HIV cardiomyopathy and pulmonary hypertension. The first documented case reports of acute myocardial infarction in HIV-1 infected patients were described in 1998 (Bozzette *et al.*, 2003). Supporting these findings were autopsy reports which demonstrated that HIV-1 infected patients without traditional cardiac risk factors also had unexpectedly higher rates of atherosclerosis, with endothelial lymphocytic infiltration, compared with controls (Joshi *et al.*, 1987). The current incidence of coronary artery disease in the HIV-1 infected population is at least three-fold higher than the general population (Vittecoq *et al.*, 2003) even in the absence of traditional risk factors, suggesting that HIV-1 is an independent risk factor for vascular disease.

The pathogenesis of endothelial dysfunction in HIV-1 infection is still being studied. However, several mechanisms have been postulated: HIV-induced endothelial cell injury, activation of endothelial cells by pro-inflammatory cytokines and mediators, and toxicity from ART which may itself have direct and indirect actions. This review will first examine endothelial dysfunction in non-HIV infected people and then explore the determinants of this process in HIV-infected patients. We will cover the most recent studies which suggest an interaction between HIV proteins and endothelium, recent developments in the link between the pro-inflammatory cascade and endothelial dysfunction and the effect of ART on both these mechanisms.

## 2. Background: The endothelium in non-HIV infected patients

From our knowledge of coronary artery disease in non-HIV infected subjects, we know that the earliest hallmark of vascular abnormalities is endothelial dysfunction. The endothelium is part of the barrier between the vessel wall and the circulation. It serves many purposes including regulation of muscle tone, lipid metabolism, thrombogenesis and vessel permeability (Kharbanda R, 2005). The healthy endothelium is not readily permeable, is anti-adhesive and able to relax vascular smooth muscle. This latter ability is governed by an intricate balance between vasodilatory (e.g. nitric oxide and prostacycline) and vasoconstrictive (predominantly endothelin-1, ET-1) substances that are released by the endothelial cells (Kharbanda R, 2005). Under normal conditions, the vascular endothelium is left in a predominantly dilated state; indeed, endothelial dysfunction is defined as impaired nitric oxide synthesis and vascular reactivity. However, the terminology is also used to describe the associated pro-inflammatory and pro-thrombogenic state.

### 2.1 Vasodilatation and vasoconstriction

In healthy endothelium, nitric oxide is produced from the precursor L-arginine via the constitutively expressed enzyme, endothelial nitric oxide synthase (e-NOS), which is activated in response to physical stimuli, such as shear stress (Kharbanda R, 2005). In addition to its vasodilatory action, the anti-thrombotic effects of nitric oxide are two-fold, inhibiting both leukocyte aggregation and platelet activation.

Factors such as smoking, dyslipidemia, diabetes, aging and sedentary lifestyle have all been shown to reduce NO synthesis and therefore impair endothelial function.

Endothelial cells also produce vasoconstrictive substances, one of the most potent being ET-1. Endothelin-1 acts via 2 receptor subtypes, Endothelin-A and Endothelin-B (ET-A and ET-B), which are expressed in varying quantities. Endogenous levels of ET-1 act via ET-A to induce coronary vasoconstriction but also serve to increase smooth muscle proliferation and induce cytokine production *in vitro* (Kharbanda R, 2005). Selective antagonism of ET-A receptors has been shown to improve endothelial function (Verhaar *et al.*, 1998).

In a healthy vessel, blood flow is laminar and shear stresses of the blood flow are maximal at the vessel wall. Following shear stress, endothelial cells elongate and align to the direction of blood flow (Lowe, 2003).

Work by Virchow, von Rotitansky and Ross (Ross *et al.*, 1977) first generated the hypothesis that endothelial damage was characterized by a loss of the normal orientation of endothelial cells in the direction of flow resulting in low-flow and low-shear circulation of blood cells in contact with the vessel wall. As this mechanical change reduces the release of nitric oxide, vasoreactivity is impaired: this explains why the earliest stages of endothelial dysfunction are characterized by a reduced ability of vessels to vasodilate. Subsequently, there is an accumulation of platelets, fibrin and monocytes over the injured endothelium; these then release substances (such as platelet derived growth factor, PDGF, and tissue growth factor B, TGF-B) which stimulate smooth muscle proliferation and connective tissue production. Recruited macrophages absorb circulating lipids (such as low density lipoprotein and cholesterol) and are converted to foam cells, which perpetuate a cycle of reduced laminar flow, haemostasis and inflammation (Lowe, 2003).

## 2.2 Haemostasis

Haemostasis, characterized by activation of the coagulation pathway and fibrin formation, is well described in atherosclerosis. The endothelium synthesizes and releases fibronectin, von Willebrand factor (vWF) and thrombospondin in response to any pro-haemorrhagic stimuli (Kharbanda R, 2005). vWF acts as a 'glue' linking platelets to the endothelial matrix. There is a subsequent production of fibrin, which then crosslink the mesh creating a haemostatic seal. Complete vascular occlusion by the matrix is usually prevented by endothelial synthesis and activation of specific anti-thrombotic compounds such as protein C, anti-thrombin and tPA (tissue plasminogen activator) which mediate endogenous fibrinolysis. Pro-coagulant activity is also modulated by nitric oxide which inhibits platelet aggregation and cell-cell adhesion activity.

Haemostasis and thrombosis are central to the progression of atherosclerosis and acute arterial occlusion; several studies have looked at the role of pro-coagulant factors in arterial disease and it is suggested that there may be an imbalance of haemostatic factors in the development of atherosclerosis (Signorelli *et al.*, 2007). High plasma levels of fibrinogen have been found in patients with peripheral atherosclerosis and are prognostic predictors for the development of myocardial infarction and cardiac arrest in patients with stable intermittent claudication (Thor *et al.*, 2002). In addition, previous studies have shown that patients with established coronary artery disease were more likely to develop ischemia, as indicated by dobutamine stress echo testing, if they had a hypercoaguable state, which comprised increased levels of fibrinogen and factor VIII (De Lorenzo *et al.*, 2003).

## 2.3 The effect of inflammation in the non HIV infected-endothelium

Because atherosclerosis is typified by the cycle of haemostasis, lipid accumulation and inflammation, it is considered an inflammatory disease. Factors such as smoking and hyperlipidemia are, in effect, chronically stimulating the endothelium which in turn changes the endothelial architecture and creates a permanent state of endothelial inflammation.

In recent years the importance of inflammation in the development of endothelial changes has been increasingly recognized. C-reactive protein (CRP), an acute phase protein synthesized by the liver, is a sensitive marker of inflammation. Increased levels of CRP have been demonstrated in patients with type 2 diabetes and are believed to occur in response to chronic intra-arterial inflammation (Tan *et al.*, 2002). Several studies have shown that the CRP level is closely correlated with the extent of endothelial dysfunction and this marker has been found to be increased in patients who have developed atherosclerosis. CRP was shown to be a strong predictor of cardiovascular events in a large prospective study involving 28,000 women (Ridker *et al.*, 2002). The CRP appears not only to be an indicator of inflammatory disease, but can also directly amplify the inflammatory response via activation of the complement cascade, tissue damage and activation of endothelial cells (Signorelli *et al.*, 2007). Indeed systemic inflammation of any cause, including autoimmune diseases such as rheumatoid arthritis and systemic lupus erythematosus, may initially drive the process of endothelial damage leading to a greater risk of cardiovascular disease (Turesson *et al.*, 2008). It is hypothesized that HIV as a chronic inflammatory disease gives rise to atherosclerosis in a similar way.

## 2.4 Cytokines and endothelial dysfunction

Cytokines are polypeptide chemical messengers that play critical roles in the inflammatory cascade, following endothelial injury. Cytokines are able to act at low concentrations and over a range of time-scales; they act through paracrine, autocrine or endocrine routes (Signorelli *et al.*, 2007). Cytokines, including Interleukin-1 (IL-1), interleukin-6 (IL-6), tumour necrosis factor alpha, Interferon-gamma (IFNγ) and monocyte-chemotactic protein-1 (MCP-1) are proinflammatory. IL-6 may be directly responsible for the production of CRP (Signorelli *et al.*, 2007). IL-2, IFNγ and TNF-α appear to be responsible for induction of adhesion molecules and chemokines in the vascular wall (Signorelli *et al.*, 2007) and there is mounting evidence that IL-6 works in concert with TNF-α and other cytokines to activate endothelial cells and enhance leukocyte adhesion (Mu *et al.*, 2007).

The role of cytokines in endothelial dysfunction has mostly been studied in the obese population, those with established atherosclerosis and in diabetic patients. CRP has been shown to induce macrophage colony stimulating factor (M-CSF) release from mononuclear phagocytes, promoting a positive feedback loop with further proliferation of the macrophages which infiltrate the inflammatory plaque (Devaraj *et al.*, 2009). Type 1 helper T cells (Th1) secrete TNF-α and IFNγ which can stimulate macrophagic internalization of modified lipoproteins leading to foam cell formation. TNF-α achieves this via up-regulation of receptors on the macrophage for uptake of modified lipoproteins (Hsu *et al.*, 2000) and IFNγ reduces cholesterol efflux (Wang *et al.*, 2002). The activated macrophages continue to release cytokines which increase the inflammatory response and seem to modulate smooth muscle architecture. Increased TNF levels are also believed to directly inhibit nitric oxide mediated coronary vasodilatation (Zhang *et al.*, 2006).

Clinical findings support the *in vitro* evidence. Elevated levels of TNF-α have been reported in association with myocardial ischemia and may contribute to irreversible myocardial tissue injury (Zhang *et al.*, 2002). Similarly, a recent meta-analysis demonstrated an odds ratio of 3.34 for myocardial infarction or coronary death per two standard deviation increase in long-term average IL-6 level (Danesh *et al.*, 2008).

## 2.5 Adhesion molecules

Endothelial inflammation induces over-expression of intercellular and vascular cell adhesion molecules (ICAM-1, VCAM-1), P-selectin and E-selectin, all of which attract monocytes and neutrophils to the area (Goldberg, 2009) and hence contribute to plaque formation. ICAM-1 and VCAM-1 mediate adhesion of inflammatory cells at the vascular endothelium. Monocytes then migrate into the sub-endothelial space of the vascular wall and subsequently differentiate into macrophages (Goldberg, 2009).

*In vivo*, P-selectin is not expressed on normal endothelium; its expression on diseased endothelium can occur in response to a number of insults including an oxidized form of internalized low density lipoprotein (oxLDL) (Johnson-Tidey *et al.*, 1994). In a study using rabbits fed only on an atherogenic diet, P-selectin was expressed after one week and infiltration of macrophages with lipoprotein occurred after two weeks (Sakai *et al.*, 1997). Mice with homozygous knockout for the P-selectin gene showed a reduction in the atherosclerotic lesion size within the endothelium compared to wild-type mice (Collins *et al.*,

2000). Similarly E-selectin is found in increased concentration on atherosclerotic endothelial cells and appears to be induced by TNF and IL-1 alpha (Galkina *et al.*, 2007; Stocker *et al.*, 2000). Combined deficiency of P-selectin and E-selectin in mice elicited an 80% protective effect in the early stages of atherosclerosis (Dong *et al.*, 1998).

Likewise, there are several reports showing increased expression of VCAM-1 on aortic endothelium in response to cholesterol accumulation within the intima (Truskey *et al.*, 1999). Furthermore, treatment of human umbilical vein endothelial cells with TNF-α up-regulated VCAM-1 and ICAM-1 expression *in vitro* (Ramana *et al.*, 2004), implying that adhesion molecule expression can be cytokine dependent.

## 3. The effect of HIV-1 infection on endothelial dysfunction

In recent years, reports have shown that HIV-infected patients have a greater risk of developing coronary artery disease compared to HIV-uninfected patients of the same age (Vittecoq *et al.*, 2003).

In the absence of anti-retrovirals, chronic inflammation, hypercoagulability, cell adhesion and platelet activation appear to drive the pathogenesis behind endothelial dysfunction in HIV-infected individuals (Francisci *et al.*, 2009).

### 3.1 Measuring atherosclerosis and endothelial dysfunction in HIV-1

Surrogate measures of atherosclerosis include carotid artery intima-media thickness (C-IMT), which directly correlates with the extent of atherosclerosis; other techniques, such as brachial artery flow mediated dilatation, can also be used and these evaluate endothelial dysfunction.

#### 3.1.1 Carotid intima-media thickness

Several studies have used C-IMT as a marker to assess sub-clinical atherosclerosis in HIV-infected patients. C-IMT is a non-invasive technique using high resolution B-mode ultrasonography and is a reliable predictor of myocardial infarction and stroke after adjustment for other risk factors (O'Leary *et al.*, 1999). C-IMT can be measured over time and has therefore been used as a primary endpoint for treatment success in clinical trials with cardioprotective drugs.

C-IMT appears to be the most sensitive indicator of subclinical atherosclerosis (Hsue *et al.*, 2010b). In a study evaluating methods for assessment of atherosclerosis in HIV-1 infection, C-IMT was compared with coronary artery calcium, measured by computerized tomography (CAC) (Hsue *et al.*, 2010b). Older age, duration of HIV-1 infection, low nadir CD4 count and hypertension in HIV-1 infected patients were shown to be associated with significantly higher C-IMT compared to controls. In contrast, the CAC was only increased in older HIV-infected patients (Hsue *et al.*, 2010b).

Hsue *et al* demonstrated that HIV-infected patients (whether or not they were on antiretroviral treatment) have a higher baseline mean C-IMT compared to age and sex-matched controls (Hsue *et al.*, 2004). In addition, the rate of progression of C-IMT was several fold higher than in HIV-uninfected subjects. In the same study, nadir CD4 T cell count less than 200 cells/microlitre was implicated as a compounding risk factor for increased C-IMT. Similar results have been replicated elsewhere - a case control study of 77 HIV-infected men in the Netherlands showed that they had a 10.8% greater C-IMT compared with controls (van Vonderen *et al.*, 2009).

However, these findings are not universal. In an earlier study comparing well-matched cohorts (for age, sex and cardiovascular risk factors) of HIV-infected patients and non-HIV infected controls, there was no statistically significant difference in the C-IMT as a static measure of atherosclerosis (Currier *et al.*, 2005). One reason for the discrepancy in results may be the lack of uniform approach to C-IMT measurements. Whereas some studies measure C-IMT at the carotid bifurcation, most examine the common carotid. It is believed that the bifurcation may be more susceptible to inflammation and injury therefore could manifest early atherosclerosis (Hsue *et al.*, 2010a).

### 3.1.2 Brachial artery flow-mediated dilatation

The hallmark of endothelial dysfunction is impaired endothelial dependent vasodilation. This can be non-invasively measured using a technique called brachial artery flow mediated vasodilation (FMD). The technique provokes the release of nitric oxide resulting in vasodilation following transient forearm ischemia and can be quantified as a measure of vasomotor function. FMD measures endothelial dysfunction in response to shear stresswhereas C-IMT measures structural defects and reflects more long term exposure to atherogenic factors (Ho *et al.*, 2009).

Studies have previously shown that HIV-1 infected patients have impaired endothelial function as assessed by FMD when compared to non-infected controls (Solages *et al.*, 2006). The severity of impairment may be related to the level of viral replication.

### 3.2 Pathogenesis

The molecular mechanisms by which HIV-1 induces endothelial dysfunction have yet to be fully elucidated but several theories have been proposed and are currently being researched (Monsuez *et al.*, 2009):

1. Direct endothelial injury from the HIV-1 virus and the component proteins of HIV-1
2. HIV-induced chronic inflammation
3. HIV-induced dyslipidaemia and metabolic syndrome
4. Direct endothelial injury from antiretroviral therapy
5. ART-induced dyslipidaemia and metabolic syndrome

It is likely to be the combination of viraemia, elevated inflammatory markers and adhesion molecules, a pro-atherogenic lipid profile and the effects of ART, which heighten the risk of cardiovascular disease in HIV-infected persons.

### 3.2.1 The effects of HIV viral load

It is likely that the increased viral load provides a permanent "on-switch" which constantly activates the endothelium: this may be via direct toxic insult, the concomitant inflammatory response in HIV infection, or both. One study demonstrated a 4-fold greater cardiovascular mortality in patients with higher viral loads (defined by at least 5 $Log_{10}$ copies/ml) which was independent of CD4 count – this study suggested that the viral load was a surrogate marker for endothelial activation and IL-6 release (Marin *et al.*, 2009). A study conducted in Argentina showed that patients with detectable HIV-1 viraemia had significantly higher levels of von Willebrand Factor (vWF) which implies endothelial activation and therefore may predict future cardiovascular risk (de Larranaga *et al.*, 2003). Although some studies have shown no relationship between peak viral load and cardiovascular risk (Friis-Moller *et al.*, 2007), there is now a general consensus on the association between viral load, chronic inflammatory activity and endothelial dysfunction. Moreover, recent results confirm that HIV viraemia is a significant predictor of acute myocardial infarction irrespective of CD4 cell count (Triant *et al.*, 2010).

The strategies for the management of antiretroviral therapy (SMART) longitudinal study demonstrated that patients who were initially assigned to intermittent ART therapy had increased cardiovascular events compared to the constant treatment arm which is believed to be due to 'rebound viraemia' after stopping treatment (El-Sadr *et al.*, 2006). Similarly, fluctuations in viral load during ART correlate with adverse changes in flow mediated dilatation (Torriani *et al.*, 2008).

### 3.2.2 The effect of the component proteins within the HIV virion

One of the genes within the HIV virion, "env", encodes a single protein called Gp160. When Gp160 is synthesized, carbohydrate molecules are attached to it and the complex is turned into a glycoprotein (Wilson *et al.*, 2008). The glycoprotein migrates to the cell surface envelope where it is cleaved into a trimeric complex comprised of a transmembrane protein (Gp41) and a surface glycoprotein (Gp120) which is embedded in the lipid bilayer. The Gp120 facilitates viral entry through interaction with the CD4 receptor and co-receptors on the receiving cell, which are either CXCR4 or CCR5.

Studies have shown that during this interaction there may be some damage to the endothelium, which itself expresses CD4 receptors and co-receptors (Ullrich *et al.*, 2000). Contact between Gp120/Gp160 and the CXCR4 co-receptor initiates the apoptotic cascade in umbilical vein endothelium (Huang *et al.*, 2001). Another study showed that Gp120 significantly increased the expression of human endothelial intercellular adhesion molecules (ICAM-1) at both m-RNA and protein levels, although it did not alter expression of VCAM-1 and E-selectin (Ren *et al.*, 2002). Furthermore, Gp120 has been shown to significantly reduce eNOS expression and endothelium dependent vasorelaxation in porcine and coronary arteries pre-treated with TNF-α; the authors also demonstrated that the combination of Gp120 and TNF-α substantially up-regulated ICAM-1 expression in these arteries (Jiang *et al.*, 2010). In a different study the same authors showed that the HIV viral proteins Tat and Nef could also inhibit eNOS expression in endothelial cells. Tat additionally appears to induce expression of several adhesion molecules on endothelium. These results suggest that several viral proteins potentially contribute to the vascular complications seen in HIV-infected patients (Duffy *et al.*, 2009).

### 3.2.3 HIV induced inflammatory cascade and adhesion markers

Another mechanism by which HIV-1 may contribute to endothelial dysfunction is via systemic inflammation. We know from non-HIV infected patients that inflammation plays an important role in endothelial dysfunction and atherosclerosis. As we have mentioned previously, raised CRP has been implicated in the pathogenesis of atherosclerosis in HIV uninfected individuals. Similarly, higher levels of CRP have been found in HIV-infected patients compared to controls and this has been shown to predict cardiovascular mortality and morbidity even after accounting for viral load and CD4 count (Hsue *et al.*, 2004). Levels of CRP do appear to reduce following ART initiation, but not back to normal levels - data from the AIDS clinical trial group (ACTG 5095) showed that CRP levels did not normalize after 96 weeks of treatment (Shikuma *et al.*, 2011).

The CRP is not the only marker of inflammation in HIV-1 infection; HIV-1 appears to be associated with a generalized inflammatory activation of the vascular wall. Proinflammatory markers and adhesion molecules that are implicated in the pathogenesis of cardiovascular disease in non-HIV individuals are similarly studied in the context of HIV-1. TNF-α, for example, is expressed in large quantities by macrophages in HIV-infected individuals (Herbein *et al.*, 1994). Studies by the Tanga Aids Working Group in Tanzania showed a significant increase in many proinflammatory cytokines in HIV-1 infected people and these displayed a positive correlation with HIV-1 RNA levels, suggesting that HIV-1 replication itself may cause a pathological cytokine response (Haissman *et al.*, 2009). The plasma levels of IL-6 are also higher in HIV-infected patients and are directly associated with the HIV-1 viral load (de Larranaga *et al.*, 2003).

Of note, a study which examined the cardiovascular characteristics of a group of HIV-1 positive "elite controllers" (Deeks *et al.*, 2007) (so called as they can maintain undetectable viral loads in the absence of ART), demonstrated raised CRP levels even in these patients (Hsue *et al.*, 2009a). Elite controllers are likely to exhibit a state of viral replication which is not detected by current assays; this low level of replication may be sufficient to increase T-cell specific responses with subsequent IL-6 and CRP release. Likewise, patients who are clinically well on long term ART may still have a low level of replication which is not detectable but which may be driving an atherogenic response.

Not only does the increase in pro-inflammatory cytokines correlate with HIV-1 plasma viral load, but also with pro-thrombotic molecules such as vWF. Platelet activation is increased in HIV-1, resulting in increased thrombogenesis (Aukrust *et al.*, 2000). Several studies have shown increased circulating levels of the endothelial adhesion markers VCAM-1 and ICAM-1 as well as selectins in HIV-infected patients and this may also correlate with disease progression (Galea *et al.*, 1997). Moreover, raised levels of vWF, ICAM-1 and VCAM-1 have been associated with raised D-dimer levels, which are fibrin-degradation products produced when fibrinolysis occurs following coagulation (Wolf *et al.*, 2002). The significance of this association may be that endothelial activation correlates with activation of the coagulation cascade and therefore increased thrombogenic potential. Consistently, these biomarkers closely correlate with HIV-1 plasma viraemia corroborating the interplay between inflammatory biomarkers, HIV-1 viral load and endothelial dysfunction (figure 1.).

In keeping with these results, another study which looked specifically at risk factors for increased cardiovascular mortality demonstrated that levels of D-dimer and VCAM-1 in HIV-infected patients positively correlated with cardiovascular risk; the D-dimer was identified as an independent risk factor for cardiovascular disease in addition to the traditional risk factors of hypercholesterolaemia and smoking (Ford *et al.*, 2010). These findings may suggest a role for biomarkers in future risk stratification in HIV-infected patients.

### 3.2.4 AntiRetroviral Therapy (ART) and endothelial dysfunction

There are currently 6 classes of antiretrovirals that have been approved for use. These are the nucleoside reverse transcriptase inhibitors (NRTIs), the non-nucleoside reverse transcriptase inhibitors (NNRTIs), protease inhibitors (PIs), fusion inhibitors, CCR5-antagonists and integrase inhibitors. Recommended initial regimens usually include combinations of two NRTIs and one NNRTI, or two NRTIs and one PI.

Antiretroviral therapy appears to be somewhat of a 'double edged sword' in terms of cardiovascular effects. Treatment with ART reduces viral load and the concentration of inflammatory markers that are likely to perpetuate cardiovascular risk. However, this may be offset by direct toxic effects of ART on endothelium and ART-induced metabolic syndrome. It seems likely that the effects of ART on endothelial dysfunction may depend on nadir CD4 count and peak viral load prior to ART, the type of antiretroviral given and other contributing 'classical' cardiovascular risk factors.

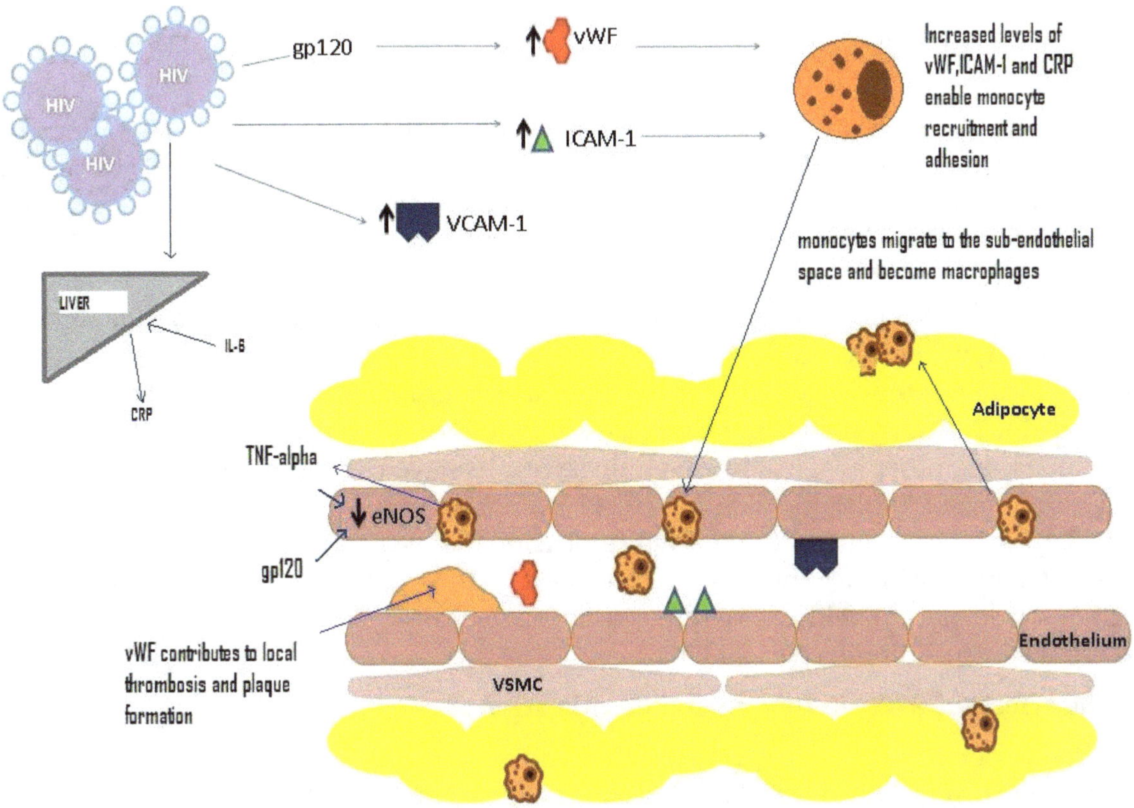


Fig. 1. The key processes involved in plaque formation in anti-retroviral naïve, HIV-1 infected patients. The HIV-1 virus leads to increased levels of adhesion molecules, ICAM-1 and VCAM-1 and increased levels of vWF. Heightened plasma levels of IL-6 contribute to C-reactive protein synthesis from the liver. The adhesion molecules and CRP promote monocyte recruitment to the area. Monocytes migrate to the sub-endothelial tissue and mature into macrophages. Macrophages contribute to foam cell formation and release TNF-α. TNF-α and gp120 inhibit eNOS expression and endothelium dependent vasorelaxtion. The net result is a proliferation of macrophages, foam cell formation and atheromatous plaques with associated haemostasis exacerbated by increased vWF levels.

#### 3.2.4.1 The effects of ART on viral load and cardiovascular disease

It is well established that HIV-1 viraemia and proinflammatory markers are intrinsically linked. Therefore one would presume that by reducing the viral load, ART should also arrest inflammatory processes. The SMART (Lundgren *et al.*, 2008) study showed that interrupted ART was associated with a higher risk of cardiovascular events implying that viral replication and inflammation following treatment cessation is linked with cardiovascular disease. A similar interruption study demonstrated a significant increase in the pro-inflammatory markers IL-6 and D-dimer and an associated increase in cardiovascular mortality in the ART sparing arm compared to those who continued therapy (Kuller, 2008).

#### 3.2.4.2 The effect of ART on inflammatory markers and endothelial dysfunction

Various biological markers of endothelial dysfunction have been shown to increase in HIV-1 infected patients. A longitudinal study comparing biomarkers in HIV-infected patients at ART initiation to two months and then 14 months into treatment demonstrated a normalization or significant reduction in levels of E-selectin, ICAM-1, VCAM-1 and CRP at the two month interval. These changes persisted up to 14 months except for E-selectin which did not change (Kristoffersen *et al.*, 2009). Similar findings have been reported in other cohort studies, showing significant reductions in both vWF and VCAM-1 levels after six months following initiation of ART, with no demonstrable difference between PI and NNRTI containing regimes (Francisci *et al.*, 2009). In another study the levels of VCAM-1 and vWF correlated positively with viral load in the ART-naïve group; following five months of treatment with a regimen which included either a PI or an NNRTI, there was a significant reduction in levels of VCAM-1 and vWF suggesting a marked reduction in endothelial activation following ART (Wolf *et al.*, 2002).

In recent years, the NRTI, abacavir, has been linked with increased cardiovascular risk in certain observational studies (Sabin *et al.*, 2008). The SMART study has also suggested that the use of abacavir is independently associated with a significant increase in plasma levels of CRP and IL-6 (Lundgren *et al.*, 2008), implying that abacavir itself has pro-inflammatory effects compared to other NRTIs. However, these results have not been uniformly replicated in other randomized trials. Indeed the HEAT study, which compared efficacy between abacavir/lamivudine/kaletra and tenofovir/emtricitabine/kaletra regimens, retrospectively showed that there was a decline of CRP, IL-6 and VCAM-1 in both regimens along with viral load reduction. Neither regime was specifically associated with increased cardiovascular events (Smith *et al.*, 2009).

#### 3.2.4.3 The effects of ART on flow mediated dilatation

It seems logical that by reducing systemic inflammation in HIV-1 infected patients, there would be a concurrent improvement in brachial flow mediated dilatation. This concept was demonstrated in a pilot trial which examined the effects of the anti-inflammatory nuclear factor kappaB-inhibitor, salsalate, on HIV-1 infected patients who were not on ART: a significant improvement in FMD was witnessed after 8 weeks of salsalate therapy (Gupta *et al.*, 2008). Since ART also reduces systemic inflammation it might be expected to improve flow mediated dilatation (FMD).

Indeed, a study which examined the effects of ART (two NRTIs and one NNRTI, two NRTIs and one PI or one PI and one NNRTI) on FMD, viral load and lipid profile showed that after 24 weeks of treatment there was an increase in brachial artery FMD in all 3 ART regimens. This occurred despite an associated increase in total cholesterol and low density lipoprotein levels in all participants, suggesting that decreased inflammation with ART may have a protective effect on the endothelium (Torriani *et al.*, 2008).

However, in another study vascular dilatation in HIV-1 infected patients on ART was significantly impaired compared with ART naïve patients (with no demonstrated difference between PI and NRTI containing regimens) (Andrade *et al.*, 2008). Another study comparing 37 HIV-1 infected patients receiving ART against age and diabetes matched non-HIV-1 infected patients showed that the FMD was equally reduced between the HIV-1 infected patients virally controlled on ART and HIV-1 negative diabetic patients (van Wijk *et al.*, 2006). Again, certain antiretrovirals may be particularly implicated: in HIV-1 infected patients treated with abacavir and achieving virological suppression, a significant reduction in FMD was observed compared to those receiving abacavir-sparing regimes (Hsue *et al.*, 2009b).

#### 3.2.4.4 The effects of ART on vasomotor activity and endothelial cells

Impairment of FMD demonstrates the macro-structural alterations elicited by ART. However, ART also leads to direct microvascular changes. ART can provide a direct insult and subsequent cell death through mitochondrial DNA damage and necrotic pathways, a theory that was demonstrated on human endothelial cells treated with ritonavir *in vitro*

(Zhong *et al.*, 2002). *In vitro* cytotoxic effects have also been exhibited by zidovudine (AZT) and indinavir, both damaging intercellular gaps between adjacent endothelial cells (Fiala *et al.*, 2004) thus providing a platform for the inflammatory cascade.

There may be a causal relationship between the toxic effects of ART and impaired vasomotor reactivity. Ritonavir has been shown to reduce endothelial NO synthase (eNOS) mRNA and protein levels in cultured human coronary endothelial cells (Fu *et al.*, 2005). Similarly, administration of combination antiretrovirals, which included zidovudine and indinavir in the regimento rats have been shown to increase levels of endothelin-1, a marker of endothelial injury and inducer of vasoconstriction (Jiang *et al.*, 2006).

As with other chronic insults, ART-induced endothelial dysfunction may progress to established vascular disease over time. A study by Jiang *et al* showed that short term treatment (five days) of mice with AZT resulted in a reduction in endothelium-dependent vessel relaxation; however after two weeks of treatment the authors showed a significant increase in injury-induced vascular smooth muscle proliferation and neo-intimal hyperplasia (Jiang *et al.*, 2010). In the same study the authors demonstrated that this increase in neo-intimal hyperplasia correlated with an increase in vascular cell adhesion molecule staining, providing a link between ART and induction of cell adhesion molecules.

## 4. The metabolic profile of chronic HIV infection and ART and its impact on cardiovascular risk

Both HIV and antiretrovirals may also induce endothelial damage via modification of 'classical' vascular insults, especially blood lipids and glucose.

HIV-1 is a known risk factor for hypertriglyceridaemia, elevated low density lipoprotein cholesterol, depressed levels of high density lipoprotein cholesterol and insulin resistance (Oh *et al.*, 2007). In treatment naïve patients, higher HIV-1 RNA levels independently associate with very low density lipoprotein (VLDL) and triglyceride levels. In patients with low CD4 cell counts there is also a higher risk of insulin resistance (El-Sadr *et al.*, 2005). Thus, the metabolic changes that are often attributed to ART may be difficult to interpret because of established abnormalities already present due to infection alone. Nevertheless, it is generally accepted that the PIs and NRTIs are associated with metabolic side effects such as lipodystrophy, and shift the lipid profile to a proatherogenic pattern.

The ongoing Data Collection on Adverse Events of Anti-HIV drugs (D:A:D) study showed that the relative risk of a myocardial infarction (MI) associated with cumulative PI use was 1.16 per year of exposure (whereas NNRTIs did not appreciably increase the risk of an MI) (Friis-Moller *et al.*, 2007). However, there appears to be a metabolic difference between various types of PIs. In the CASTLE study, patients treated with lopinavir/ritonavir had significantly raised fasting total cholesterol and triglyceride levels compared to patients given atazanavir/ritonavir (Molina *et al.*, 2010). Other studies have now demonstrated that boosted lopinavir appears to elicit a worse lipid profile compared to other PI-containing regimens (Molina *et al.*, 2010; Mills *et al.*, 2009).

The data supporting the role of NRTIs in generating metabolic abnormalities is mainly found in studies which used them in combination with a PI. Again, certain drugs are particularly implicated. The ACTG 5052 study compared efficacy in HIV-infected patients between abacavir/lamivudine and tenofovir/emtricitabine given with efavirenz or ritonavir-boosted atazanavir for 96 weeks. At week 48, fasting lipid levels had significantly increased in the arm receiving abacavir/lamivudine.

The use of NNRTIs may also be associated with adverse lipid effects - recent data from the ACTG 5095 study showed that a regime containing efavirenz significantly increased lipid levels above the baseline values and above those seen in 'NRTI only' combinations (Shikuma *et al.*, 2007) 96 weeks after treatment initiation.

## 5. Assessment and management of patients with increased cardiovascular risk

Given that HIV-1 itself is an independent risk factor for cardiovascular disease, there is an increasing need to apply a cardiovascular risk stratification score in HIV-1 infected patients. A cross-sectional study of HIV-1 infected patients in a Spanish outpatient setting demonstrated that the traditionally used Framingham risk calculation score identified a higher proportion of HIV-1 infected men with a moderate cardiovascular risk compared to other available risk stratification tools (Knobel *et al.*, 2007). However, this tool may not be equally applicable to all populations - for example, in a study which examined the predicted cardiovascular risk in an HIV-1 infected Thai population, the Framingham calculation over estimated the risk of cardiovascular disease compared to other cardiovascular risk equations (Edwards-Jackson *et al.*, 2011).

When managing cardiovascular risk in the HIV-1 infected patient, one must advise in the same way as HIV-1 uninfected individuals; for example, addressing lifestyle factors as well as measuring lipid levels, blood pressure and signs of glucose intolerance. However, trials of non-drug therapies and dietary advice alone may not be sufficient to control HIV and ART associated dyslipidaemia.

After addressing lifestyle measures it may then be prudent to review the current antiretroviral therapy. Firstly, it may be possible to switch within the class - for example, changing from nelfinavir to atazanavir can reduce the total cholesterol and triglyceride level sufficiently (Calza *et al.*, 2005; Oh *et al.*, 2007). Another strategy, if the patient is on a PI, is to switch them to another class providing there is established viral suppression and a compatible viral resistance profile (Dube *et al.*, 2003).

In terms of lipid-lowering pharmacotherapy, the Adult ACTG (Dube *et al.*, 2003) have provided some guidance in approaching HIV-patients with dyslipidemia and raised cardiovascular risk. There are few changes in management compared to the general population and the use of statins (hydroxyl-methyl-glutaryl coenzyme A reductase inhibitors) as a therapy is widely advocated in patients with established isolated hypercholesterolemia (elevated total and LDL-cholesterol and triglyceride level less than 5mmol/l).

The advantages of using a statin are two-fold; firstly, statins reduce the levels of cholesterol, which is implicated in endothelial dysfunction and atheroma formation. Secondly, there is increasing evidence that statins also exhibit anti-inflammatory effects (Jain *et al.*, 2005). Recently a double-blinded cross-over trial (8 weeks of high dose 80mg atorvastatin versus placebo in HIV-1 infected ART naïve patients) showed a significant reduction in immune activation with statin therapy, as measured by a fall in activated CD8+ T cells, without any affect on HIV-1 RNA viral load (Ganesan *et al.*, 2011). This further supports the use of statins in HIV-1 infected patients even without established lipid abnormalities. Lowering of oxidized LDL-cholesterol and total LDL cholesterol with 40mg pravastatin has also been shown to improve endothelial dysfunction, as measured by FMD, in patients on a PI-containing ART regime (Hurlimann *et al.*, 2006).

However, some caution must be exercised when using statins as there may be significant interactions with PIs. The concentration of pravastatin has been shown to markedly increase when used with boosted darunavir, although its levels are decreased with all other PIs. Therefore, whilst there is a potential increase in the side effect profile of all statins, pravastatin is usually considered the safest to use with PIs other than darunavir (Seker, 2007).

Statins are not the only lipid-lowering drug available; the combination of a statin and a fibrate should be considered (albeit with close monitoring due to the exaggerated side effect profile) when the triglyceride level is above 5mmol/l and may be the best approach to achieve lipid targets in these patients. Ezetimibe is a newer agent that acts by reducing intestinal cholesterol absorption and has been shown to be better tolerated but equally efficacious compared to statins in HIV-infected patients with hypercholesterolaemia (Negredo *et al.*, 2006). Ezetimibe may be used when statins are not tolerated or as an adjunct to other anti-lipid agents in severe lipid disturbance.

In non-HIV-1 infected patients, the beneficial effects of aspirin have largely been attributed to its action on thromboxane synthesis and platelet aggregation; however, there is also evidence suggesting that aspirin improves endothelial dysfunction through endothelium dependent vasodilatation (Husain *et al.*, 1998). Current guidelines, as outlined by the U.S Preventative Services Task Force, recommend the use of aspirin in male patients between 45-79 years old when the benefits of a reduction in risk of mycocardial infarction, taking into account overall cardiovascular risk, outweighs the potential risks associated with aspirin therapy (Calonge N, 2009). Spanish researchers applied these standards to their HIV-infected cohort and found that aspirin would be indicated in 30.8% of their male patients (Tornero *et al.*, 2010). Moreover, salsalate, a compound which exists within the same class as aspirin, has been shown to significantly improve flow mediated dilatation in HIV-infected patients after 8 weeks (as discussed above), perhaps suggesting a role for these agents in reducing endothelial dysfunction (Gupta *et al.*, 2008). Whether or not aspirin should be considered as primary prevention in HIV-infected patients is still debatable and certainly it should not be seen as a replacement for timely ART.

## 6. Conclusions

As the HIV-1 infected population grows, management of patients is increasingly focused on chronic care issues such as cardiovascular comorbidity and metabolic disturbances including lipodystrophy and glucose intolerance. In recent years, there has been increasing recognition that endothelial dysfunction plays a pivotal role in atherosclerosis in HIV-1 infected patients, and that HIV-1 may be as important as other more "traditional" risk factors for accelerated coronary artery disease. The pathology is complex and multifactorial; the HIV-1 virus and its component proteins are likely to perpetuate a cycle of chronic inflammation, haemostasis and endothelial activation. The role of ART is even less well understood, with the benefits of viral suppression being offset by the toxic and metabolic effects of ART itself (figure 2).

However, what is certain is that early detection and appropriate management of HIV-1 and its complications is imperative in attempting to reduce the devastating global impact that HIV-1 has had within the last 30 years. Effective viral suppression, establishing coronary risk and modifying behavioral risk factors may provide the best initial approach to endothelial dysfunction. Following this, the option to switch antiretroviral drugs and treat the patient with pharmacotherapeutic agents aiming to optimize lipids, glucose and blood pressure may then be effective.

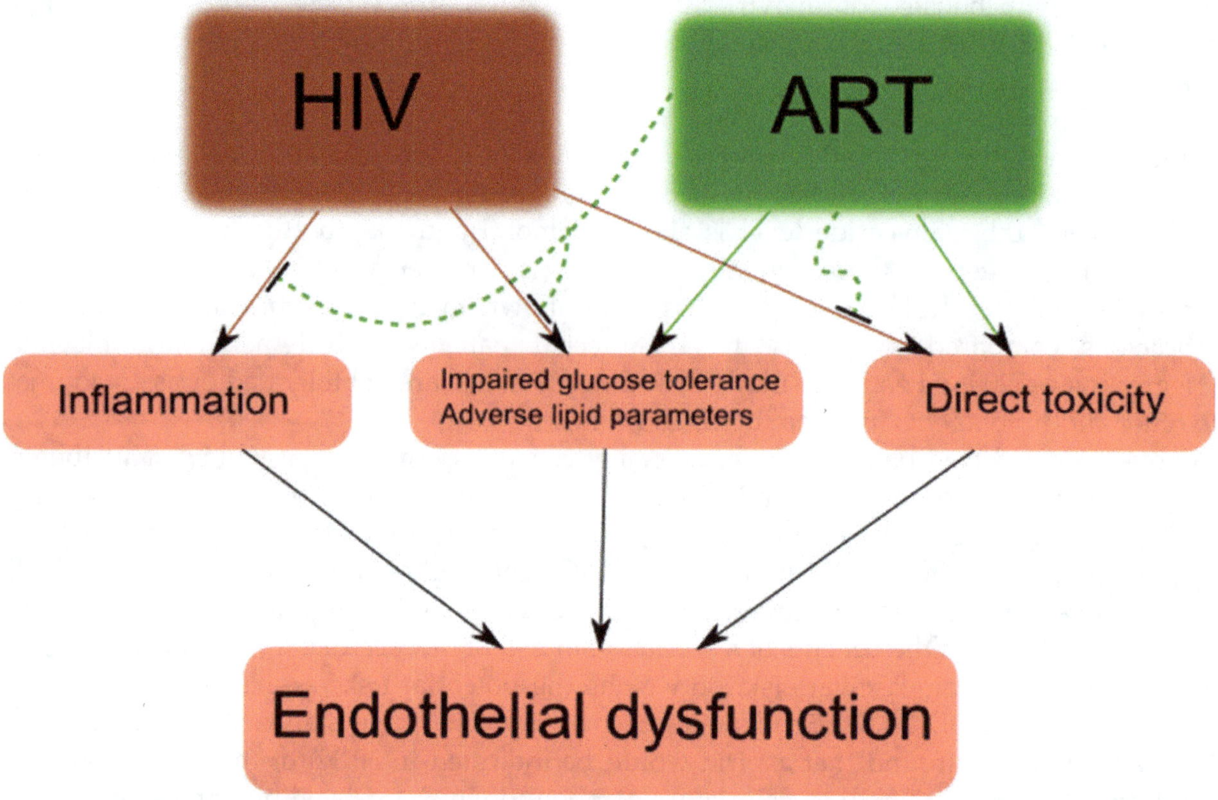


Fig. 2. Interplay between HIV, ART and endothelial dysfunction. Schematic diagram explaining how endothelial dysfunction is potentially caused through the effects of HIV itself and the effects of ART. Treatment naïve individuals can develop endothelial dysfunction as a consequence of direct toxicity of the virus, HIV-induced metabolic disturbances and associated chronic inflammation. ART acts to reduce these phenomena but can itself be toxic to endothelium and induce dyslipidaemia and glucose intolerance. ART = antiretroviral therapy.

## 7. References

Andrade AC, Ladeia AM, Netto EM, Mascarenhas A, Cotter B, Benson CA, *et al.* (2008). Cross-sectional study of endothelial function in HIV-infected patients in Brazil. *AIDS Res Hum Retroviruses* 24(1): 27-33.

Aukrust P, Bjornsen S, Lunden B, Otterdal K, Ng EC, Ameln W, *et al.* (2000). Persistently elevated levels of von Willebrand factor antigen in HIV infection. Downregulation during highly active antiretroviral therapy. *Thromb Haemost* 84(2): 183-187.

Bozzette SA, Ake CF, Tam HK, Chang SW, Louis TA (2003). Cardiovascular and cerebrovascular events in patients treated for human immunodeficiency virus infection. *N Engl J Med* 348(8): 702-710.

Calonge N PD, DeWitt TG, Gordis L, Gregory KD, Harris R, Isham G, LeFevre ML, Loveland-Cherry C, Marion LN, Moyer VA, Ockene JK, Sawaya GF, Siu AL, Teutsch SM, Yawn BP. (2009). Aspirin for the prevention of cardiovascular disease: U.S. Preventive Services Task Force recommendation statement. *Ann Intern Med* 150(6): 396-404.

Calza L, Manfredi R, Colangeli V, Tampellini L, Sebastiani T, Pocaterra D, *et al.* (2005). Substitution of nevirapine or efavirenz for protease inhibitor versus lipid-lowering therapy for the management of dyslipidaemia. *AIDS* 19(10): 1051-1058.

Collins RG, Velji R, Guevara NV, Hicks MJ, Chan L, Beaudet AL (2000). P-Selectin or intercellular adhesion molecule (ICAM)-1 deficiency substantially protects against atherosclerosis in apolipoprotein E-deficient mice. *J Exp Med* 191(1): 189-194.

Currier JS, Kendall MA, Zackin R, Henry WK, Alston-Smith B, Torriani FJ, *et al.* (2005). Carotid artery intima-media thickness and HIV infection: traditional risk factors overshadow impact of protease inhibitor exposure. *AIDS* 19(9): 927-933.

Danesh J, Kaptoge S, Mann AG, Sarwar N, Wood A, Angleman SB, *et al.* (2008). Long-term interleukin-6 levels and subsequent risk of coronary heart disease: two new prospective studies and a systematic review. *PLoS Med* 5(4): e78.

de Larranaga GF, Petroni A, Deluchi G, Alonso BS, Benetucci JA (2003). Viral load and disease progression as responsible for endothelial activation and/or injury in human immunodeficiency virus-1-infected patients. *Blood Coagul Fibrinolysis* 14(1): 15-18.

De Lorenzo F, Xiao H, Scully M, Kadziola Z, Kakkar VV (2003). Pre-thrombotic state and impaired fibrinolytic potential in coronary heart disease patients with left ventricular dysfunction. *Blood Coagul Fibrinolysis* 14(1): 67-75.

Deeks SG, Walker BD (2007). Human immunodeficiency virus controllers: mechanisms of durable virus control in the absence of antiretroviral therapy. *Immunity* 27(3): 406-416.

Devaraj S, Yun JM, Duncan-Staley C, Jialal I (2009). C-reactive protein induces M-CSF release and macrophage proliferation. *J Leukoc Biol* 85(2): 262-267.

Dong ZM, Chapman SM, Brown AA, Frenette PS, Hynes RO, Wagner DD (1998). The combined role of P- and E-selectins in atherosclerosis. *J Clin Invest* 102(1): 145-152.

Dube MP, Stein JH, Aberg JA, Fichtenbaum CJ, Gerber JG, Tashima KT, *et al.* (2003). Guidelines for the evaluation and management of dyslipidemia in human immunodeficiency virus (HIV)-infected adults receiving antiretroviral therapy: recommendations of the HIV Medical Association of the Infectious Disease Society of America and the Adult AIDS Clinical Trials Group. *Clin Infect Dis* 37(5): 613-627.

Duffy P, Wang X, Lin PH, Yao Q, Chen C (2009). HIV Nef protein causes endothelial dysfunction in porcine pulmonary arteries and human pulmonary artery endothelial cells. *J Surg Res* 156(2): 257-264.

Edwards-Jackson N, Kerr S, Tieu H, Ananworanich J, Hammer S, Ruxrungtham K, *et al.* (2011). Cardiovascular risk assessment in persons with HIV infection in the developing world: comparing three risk equations in a cohort of HIV-infected Thais. *HIV Med.* doi: 10.1111/j.1468-1293.2011.00916.x

El-Sadr WM, Lundgren JD, Neaton JD, Gordin F, Abrams D, Arduino RC, *et al.* (2006). CD4+ count-guided interruption of antiretroviral treatment. *N Engl J Med* 355(22): 2283-2296.

El-Sadr WM, Mullin CM, Carr A, Gibert C, Rappoport C, Visnegarwala F, *et al.* (2005). Effects of HIV disease on lipid, glucose and insulin levels: results from a large antiretroviral-naive cohort. *HIV Med* 6(2): 114-121.

Fiala M, Murphy T, MacDougall J, Yang W, Luque A, Iruela-Arispe L, *et al.* (2004). HAART drugs induce mitochondrial damage and intercellular gaps and gp120 causes apoptosis. *Cardiovasc Toxicol* 4(4): 327-337.

Ford ES, Greenwald JH, Richterman AG, Rupert A, Dutcher L, Badralmaa Y, *et al.* (2010). Traditional risk factors and D-dimer predict incident cardiovascular disease events in chronic HIV infection. *AIDS* 24(10): 1509-1517.

Francisci D, Giannini S, Baldelli F, Leone M, Belfiori B, Guglielmini G, *et al.* (2009). HIV type 1 infection, and not short-term HAART, induces endothelial dysfunction. *AIDS* 23(5): 589-596.

Friis-Moller N, Reiss P, Sabin CA, Weber R, Monforte A, El-Sadr W, *et al.* (2007). Class of antiretroviral drugs and the risk of myocardial infarction. *N Engl J Med* 356(17): 1723-1735.

Fu W, Chai H, Yao Q, Chen C (2005). Effects of HIV protease inhibitor ritonavir on vasomotor function and endothelial nitric oxide synthase expression. *J Acquir Immune Defic Syndr* 39(2): 152-158.

Galea P, Vermot-Desroches C, Le Contel C, Wijdenes J, Chermann JC (1997). Circulating cell adhesion molecules in HIV1-infected patients as indicator markers for AIDS progression. *Res Immunol* 148(2): 109-117.

Galkina E, Ley K (2007). Vascular adhesion molecules in atherosclerosis. *Arterioscler Thromb Vasc Biol* 27(11): 2292-2301.

Ganesan A, Crum-Cianflone N, Higgins J, Qin J, Rehm C, Metcalf J, *et al.* (2011). High dose atorvastatin decreases cellular markers of immune activation without affecting HIV-1 RNA levels: results of a double-blind randomized placebo controlled clinical trial. *J Infect Dis* 203(6): 756-764.

Goldberg RB (2009). Cytokine and cytokine-like inflammation markers, endothelial dysfunction, and imbalanced coagulation in development of diabetes and its complications. *J Clin Endocrinol Metab* 94(9): 3171-3182.

Gupta SK, Johnson RM, Saha C, Mather KJ, Greenwald ML, Waltz JS, *et al.* (2008). Improvement in HIV-related endothelial dysfunction using the anti-inflammatory agent salsalate: a pilot study. *AIDS* 22(5): 653-655.

Haissman JM, Vestergaard LS, Sembuche S, Erikstrup C, Mmbando B, Mtullu S, *et al.* (2009). Plasma cytokine levels in Tanzanian HIV-1-infected adults and the effect of antiretroviral treatment. *J Acquir Immune Defic Syndr* 52(4): 493-497.

Herbein G, Keshav S, Collin M, Montaner LJ, Gordon S (1994). HIV-1 induces tumour necrosis factor and IL-1 gene expression in primary human macrophages independent of productive infection. *Clin Exp Immunol* 95(3): 442-449.

Ho JE, Hsue PY (2009). Cardiovascular manifestations of HIV infection. *Heart* 95(14): 1193-1202.

Hsu HY, Twu YC (2000). Tumor necrosis factor-alpha -mediated protein kinases in regulation of scavenger receptor and foam cell formation on macrophage. *J Biol Chem* 275(52): 41035-41048.

Hsue P, Hunt P, Schnell A, Wu Y, Ho J, Hoh R, *et al.* (2010a). Rapid Progression of Atherosclerosis at the Carotid Bifurcation Is Linked to Inflammation in HIV-infected Patients. *Seventeenth Conference on Retroviruses and Opportunistic Infections (CROI)*; Abstract 125

Hsue P, Ordovas K, Lee T, Schnell A, Ho JE, Selby V, *et al.* (2010b). Abstract 10273: Markedly Increased Carotid Intima-Media Thickness in the Absence of Coronary Calcium Among HIV-Infected Individuals. *Circulation* 122(21-MeetingAbstracts): A10273.

Hsue PY, Hunt PW, Schnell A, Kalapus SC, Hoh R, Ganz P, *et al.* (2009a). Role of viral replication, antiretroviral therapy, and immunodeficiency in HIV-associated atherosclerosis. *AIDS* 23(9): 1059-1067.

Hsue PY, Hunt PW, Wu Y, Schnell A, Ho JE, Hatano H, *et al.* (2009b). Association of abacavir and impaired endothelial function in treated and suppressed HIV-infected patients. *AIDS* 23(15): 2021-2027.

Hsue PY, Lo JC, Franklin A, Bolger AF, Martin JN, Deeks SG, *et al.* (2004). Progression of atherosclerosis as assessed by carotid intima-media thickness in patients with HIV infection. *Circulation* 109(13): 1603-1608.

Huang MB, Khan M, Garcia-Barrio M, Powell M, Bond VC (2001). Apoptotic effects in primary human umbilical vein endothelial cell cultures caused by exposure to virion-associated and cell membrane-associated HIV-1 gp120. *J Acquir Immune Defic Syndr* 27(3): 213-221.

Hurlimann D, Chenevard R, Ruschitzka F, Flepp M, Enseleit F, Bechir M, *et al.* (2006). Effects of statins on endothelial function and lipid profile in HIV infected persons receiving protease inhibitor-containing anti-retroviral combination therapy: a randomised double blind crossover trial. *Heart* 92(1): 110-112.

Husain S, Andrews NP, Mulcahy D, Panza JA, Quyyumi AA (1998). Aspirin improves endothelial dysfunction in atherosclerosis. *Circulation* 97(8): 716-720.

Jain MK, Ridker PM (2005). Anti-inflammatory effects of statins: clinical evidence and basic mechanisms. *Nat Rev Drug Discov* 4(12): 977-987.

Jiang B, Hebert VY, Zavecz JH, Dugas TR (2006). Antiretrovirals induce direct endothelial dysfunction *in vivo*. *J Acquir Immune Defic Syndr* 42(4): 391-395.

Jiang B, Khandelwal AR, Rogers LK, Hebert VY, Kleinedler JJ, Zavecz JH, *et al.* (2010). Antiretrovirals induce endothelial dysfunction via an oxidant-dependent pathway and promote neointimal hyperplasia. *Toxicol Sci* 117(2): 524-536.

Johnson-Tidey RR, McGregor JL, Taylor PR, Poston RN (1994). Increase in the adhesion molecule P-selectin in endothelium overlying atherosclerotic plaques. Coexpression with intercellular adhesion molecule-1. *Am J Pathol* 144(5): 952-961.

Joshi VV, Pawel B, Connor E, Sharer L, Oleske JM, Morrison S, *et al.* (1987). Arteriopathy in children with acquired immune deficiency syndrome. *Pediatr Pathol* 7(3): 261-275.

Kates J, Lief E, Avila C (2009). '*Financing the Response to AIDS in Low- and Middle- Income Countries: International Assistance from the G8, European Commission and Other Donor Governments in 2008*'. . UNAIDS. Available from
http://www.kff.org/hivaids/7347.cfm (Access date June 2011)

Kharbanda R MR (2005). The Atherosclerosis Time-Line and the Role of the Endothelium. *Current Medicinal Chemistry - Immunology, Endocrine & Metabolic Agents* 5: 47-52.

Knobel H, Jerico C, Montero M, Sorli ML, Velat M, Guelar A, *et al.* (2007). Global cardiovascular risk in patients with HIV infection: concordance and differences in estimates according to three risk equations (Framingham, SCORE, and PROCAM). *AIDS Patient Care STDS* 21(7): 452-457.

Kristoffersen US, Kofoed K, Kronborg G, Giger AK, Kjaer A, Lebech AM (2009). Reduction in circulating markers of endothelial dysfunction in HIV-infected patients during antiretroviral therapy. *HIV Med* 10(2): 79-87.

Kuller L (2008). Elevated Levels of Interleukin-6 and D-dimer Are Associated with an Increased Risk of Death in Patients with HIV. *Fifteenth Conference on Retroviruses and Opportunistic Infections (CROI)*; Abstract 139.

Kumar PN, Rodriguez-French A, Thompson MA, Tashima KT, Averitt D, Wannamaker PG, *et al.* (2006). A prospective, 96-week study of the impact of Trizivir, Combivir/nelfinavir, and lamivudine/stavudine/nelfinavir on lipids, metabolic parameters and efficacy in antiretroviral-naive patients: effect of sex and ethnicity. *HIV Med* 7(2): 85-98.

Lohse N, Hansen AB, Pedersen G, Kronborg G, Gerstoft J, Sorensen HT, *et al.* (2007). Survival of persons with and without HIV infection in Denmark, 1995-2005. *Ann Intern Med* 146(2): 87-95.

Lowe GD (2003). Virchow's triad revisited: abnormal flow. *Pathophysiol Haemost Thromb* 33(5-6): 455-457.

Lundgren J, Neuhaus J, Babiker A, Cooper D, Duprez D, El-Sadr W, *et al.* (2008). Use of nucleoside reverse transcriptase inhibitors and risk of myocardial infarction in HIV-infected patients. *AIDS* 22(14): F17-24.

Marin B, Thiebaut R, Bucher HC, Rondeau V, Costagliola D, Dorrucci M, *et al.* (2009). Non-AIDS-defining deaths and immunodeficiency in the era of combination antiretroviral therapy. *AIDS* 23(13): 1743-1753.

Molina JM, Andrade-Villanueva J, Echevarria J, Chetchotisakd P, Corral J, David N, *et al.* (2010). Once-daily atazanavir/ritonavir compared with twice-daily lopinavir/ritonavir, each in combination with tenofovir and emtricitabine, for management of antiretroviral-naive HIV-1-infected patients: 96-week efficacy and safety results of the CASTLE study. *J Acquir Immune Defic Syndr* 53(3): 323-332.

Mills AM, Nelson M, Jayaweera D, *et al.* (2009). Once-daily darunavir/ritonavir vs. lopinavir/ritonavir in treatment-naïve, HIV-1-infected patients: 96-week analysis. *AIDS* 23(13): 1679–1688.

Monsuez JJ, Charniot JC, Escaut L, Teicher E, Wyplosz B, Couzigou C, *et al.* (2009). HIV-associated vascular diseases: structural and functional changes, clinical implications. *Int J Cardiol* 133(3): 293-306.

Mu H, Chai H, Lin PH, Yao Q, Chen C (2007). Current update on HIV-associated vascular disease and endothelial dysfunction. *World J Surg* 31(4): 632-643.

Negredo E, Molto J, Puig J, Cinquegrana D, Bonjoch A, Perez-Alvarez N, *et al.* (2006). Ezetimibe, a promising lipid-lowering agent for the treatment of dyslipidaemia in HIV-infected patients with poor response to statins. *AIDS* 20(17): 2159-2164.

Oh J, Hegele RA (2007). HIV-associated dyslipidaemia: pathogenesis and treatment. *Lancet Infect Dis* 7(12): 787-796.

O'Leary DH, Polak JF, Kronmal RA, *et al.* (1999). Carotid-artery intima media thickness as a risk factor for myocardial infarction and stroke in older adults. For the Cardiovascular Health Study Collaborative Research Group. *N Engl J Med* 340(1):14–22.

Ramana KV, Bhatnagar A, Srivastava SK (2004). Inhibition of aldose reductase attenuates TNF-alpha-induced expression of adhesion molecules in endothelial cells. *FASEB J* 18(11): 1209-1218.

Ren Z, Yao Q, Chen C (2002). HIV-1 envelope glycoprotein 120 increases intercellular adhesion molecule-1 expression by human endothelial cells. *Lab Invest* 82(3): 245-255.

Ridker PM, Rifai N, Rose L, Buring JE, Cook NR (2002). Comparison of C-reactive protein and low-density lipoprotein cholesterol levels in the prediction of first cardiovascular events. *N Engl J Med* 347(20): 1557-1565.

Ross R, Glomset J, Harker L (1977). Response to injury and atherogenesis. *Am J Pathol* 86(3): 675-684.

Sabin CA, Worm SW, Weber R, Reiss P, El-Sadr W, Dabis F, *et al.* (2008). Use of nucleoside reverse transcriptase inhibitors and risk of myocardial infarction in HIV-infected patients enrolled in the D:A:D study: a multi-cohort collaboration. *Lancet* 371(9622): 1417-1426.

Sakai A, Kume N, Nishi E, Tanoue K, Miyasaka M, Kita T (1997). P-selectin and vascular cell adhesion molecule-1 are focally expressed in aortas of hypercholesterolemic rabbits before intimal accumulation of macrophages and T lymphocytes. *Arterioscler Thromb Vasc Biol* 17(2): 310-316.

Sax PE, Tierney C, Collier AC, Fischl MA, Mollan K, Peeples L, *et al.* (2009). Abacavir-lamivudine versus tenofovir-emtricitabine for initial HIV-1 therapy. *N Engl J Med* 361(23): 2230-2240.

Seker V (2007). Pharmacokinetic drug-drug interaction between the new HIV-protease inhibitor darunavir (TMC114) and the lipid lowering agent pravastatin. *8th International work-shop on pharmacology of HIV therapy*; Abstract 54.

Shikuma CM, Ribaudo HJ, Zheng Y, Gulick RM, Meyer WA, Tashima KT, *et al.* (2011). Change in High-Sensitivity C-Reactive Protein Levels Following Initiation of Efavirenz-Based Antiretroviral Regimens in HIV-Infected Individuals. *AIDS Res Hum Retroviruses* 27(5): 461-468.

Shikuma CM, Yang Y, Glesby MJ, Meyer WA, 3rd, Tashima KT, Ribaudo HJ, *et al.* (2007). Metabolic effects of protease inhibitor-sparing antiretroviral regimens given as initial treatment of HIV-1 Infection (AIDS Clinical Trials Group Study A5095). *J Acquir Immune Defic Syndr* 44(5): 540-550.

Signorelli SS, Mazzarino MC, Spandidos DA, Malaponte G (2007). Proinflammatory circulating molecules in peripheral arterial disease. *Int J Mol Med* 20(3): 279-286.

Smith KY, Patel P, Fine D, Bellos N, Sloan L, Lackey P, *et al.* (2009). Randomized, double-blind, placebo-matched, multicenter trial of abacavir/lamivudine or tenofovir/emtricitabine with lopinavir/ritonavir for initial HIV treatment. *AIDS* 23(12): 1547-1556.

Solages A, Vita JA, Thornton DJ, Murray J, Heeren T, Craven DE, *et al.* (2006). Endothelial function in HIV-infected persons. *Clin Infect Dis* 42(9): 1325-1332.

Stocker CJ, Sugars KL, Harari OA, Landis RC, Morley BJ, Haskard DO (2000). TNF-alpha, IL-4, and IFN-gamma regulate differential expression of P- and E-selectin expression by porcine aortic endothelial cells. *J Immunol* 164(6): 3309-3315.

Tan KC, Chow WS, Tam SC, Ai VH, Lam CH, Lam KS (2002). Atorvastatin lowers C-reactive protein and improves endothelium-dependent vasodilation in type 2 diabetes mellitus. *J Clin Endocrinol Metab* 87(2): 563-568.

Thor M, Yu A, Swedenborg J (2002). Markers of inflammation and hypercoagulability in diabetic and nondiabetic patients with lower extremity ischemia. *Thromb Res* 105(5): 379-383.

Tornero C, Ventura A, Mafe M (2010). Aspirin Is Indicated for Primary Prevention of Cardiovascular Events in HIV-Infected Patients. *J Acquir Immune Defic Syndr* 54(5): 560

Torriani FJ, Komarow L, Parker RA, Cotter BR, Currier JS, Dube MP, *et al.* (2008). Endothelial function in human immunodeficiency virus-infected antiretroviral-naive subjects before and after starting potent antiretroviral therapy: The ACTG (AIDS Clinical Trials Group) Study 5152s. *J Am Coll Cardiol* 52(7): 569-576.

Triant VA, Regan S, Lee H, Sax PE, Meigs JB, Grinspoon SK (2010). Association of Immunologic and Virologic Factors With Myocardial Infarction Rates in a US Healthcare System. *J Acquir Immune Defic Syndr* 55(5):615-619

Truskey GA, Herrmann RA, Kait J, Barber KM (1999). Focal increases in vascular cell adhesion molecule-1 and intimal macrophages at atherosclerosis-susceptible sites in the rabbit aorta after short-term cholesterol feeding. *Arterioscler Thromb Vasc Biol* 19(2): 393-401.

Turesson C, Jacobsson LT, Matteson EL (2008). Cardiovascular co-morbidity in rheumatic diseases. *Vasc Health Risk Manag* 4(3): 605-614.

Ullrich CK, Groopman JE, Ganju RK (2000). HIV-1 gp120- and gp160-induced apoptosis in cultured endothelial cells is mediated by caspases. *Blood* 96(4): 1438-1442.

van Vonderen MG, Smulders YM, Stehouwer CD, Danner SA, Gundy CM, Vos F, *et al.* (2009). Carotid intima-media thickness and arterial stiffness in HIV-infected patients: the role of HIV, antiretroviral therapy, and lipodystrophy. *J Acquir Immune Defic Syndr* 50(2): 153-161.

van Wijk JP, de Koning EJ, Cabezas MC, Joven J, op't Roodt J, Rabelink TJ, *et al.* (2006). Functional and structural markers of atherosclerosis in human immunodeficiency virus-infected patients. *J Am Coll Cardiol* 47(6): 1117-1123.

Verhaar MC, Strachan FE, Newby DE, Cruden NL, Koomans HA, Rabelink TJ, *et al.* (1998). Endothelin-A receptor antagonist-mediated vasodilatation is attenuated by inhibition of nitric oxide synthesis and by endothelin-B receptor blockade. *Circulation* 97(8): 752-756.

Vittecoq D, Escaut L, Chironi G, Teicher E, Monsuez JJ, Andrejak M, *et al.* (2003). Coronary heart disease in HIV-infected patients in the highly active antiretroviral treatment era. *AIDS* 17 Suppl 1: S70-76.

Wang XQ, Panousis CG, Alfaro ML, Evans GF, Zuckerman SH (2002). Interferon-gamma-mediated downregulation of cholesterol efflux and ABC1 expression is by the Stat1 pathway. *Arterioscler Thromb Vasc Biol* 22(5): e5-9.

WHO (2010). *World Health Organisation: Towards universal access:scaling up priority HIV/AIDS interventions in the health sector. Progress report* Available from http://www.who.int/hiv/pub/2010progressreport/en (Access date June 2011)

Wilson D, Cotton M, Bekker L, Meyers T, Venter F, Maartens G (2008). *Oxford Handbook of HIV Medicine.* 2nd edn. Oxford University Press: Cape Town, South Africa.

Wolf K, Tsakiris DA, Weber R, Erb P, Battegay M (2002). Antiretroviral therapy reduces markers of endothelial and coagulation activation in patients infected with human immunodeficiency virus type 1. *J Infect Dis* 185(4): 456-462.

Zhang C, Hein TW, Wang W, Ren Y, Shipley RD, Kuo L (2006). Activation of JNK and xanthine oxidase by TNF-alpha impairs nitric oxide-mediated dilation of coronary arterioles. *J Mol Cell Cardiol* 40(2): 247-257.

Zhang DX, Yi FX, Zou AP, Li PL (2002). Role of ceramide in TNF-alpha-induced impairment of endothelium-dependent vasorelaxation in coronary arteries. *Am J Physiol Heart Circ Physiol* 283(5): H1785-1794.

Zhong DS, Lu XH, Conklin BS, Lin PH, Lumsden AB, Yao Q, *et al.* (2002). HIV protease inhibitor ritonavir induces cytotoxicity of human endothelial cells. *Arterioscler Thromb Vasc Biol* 22(10): 1560-1566.

# 2

# Spondylodiscitis and HIV – Diagnosis and Treatment Strategies

Jan Siewe, Kourosh Zarghooni and Rolf Sobottke
*Department for Orthopaedic and Trauma Surgery, University of Cologne, Germany*

## 1. Introduction

### 1.1 Spinal infections

#### 1.1.1 History

Infection of the spine is a disease with a long, well-documented history. Excavations of human skeletons from an archaeological site from the Iron Age showed likely cases of individual spinal infection (Tayles & Buckley, 2004). Tuberculosis of the spine is often described as Pott's disease; the pattern of the disease was reported by Percivall Pott in the year 1779 (Sir D'Arcy Power, 1923). A case series of 102 patients with pyogenic spinal osteomyelitis was reported in the year 1936 (Kulowski, 1936).

#### 1.1.2 Anatomical distribution

Spinal infections can affect several anatomical structures and are described as spondylitis, discitis, spondylodiscitis, pyogenic facet arthropathy, epidural infections, meningitis, polyradiculopathy, and myelitis (Tali, 2004). When the diagnosis is ascertained, often radiological inflammatory signs both in the vertebra and the disc can be observed. The point of origin of the bacterial inflammation in the spine cannot be determined. Therefore spondylitis and spondylodiscitis are often used synonymously.

#### 1.1.3 Epidemiology

Spondylodiscitis remains rare, but an increasing incidence of vertebral infections has been observed due to increasingly susceptible populations as well as the availability of more effective diagnostic tools (Gouliouris et al., 2010). In addition, a number of causative factors are collaborating in this increase, including the HIV-epidemic, especially in Sub-Saharan Africa, the large number of intravenous drug abusers, the currently widely-used aspiration and catheter techniques, and the recurrence of tuberculosis in industrialized nations. In general, patients in an immunocompromised state have a higher risk of contracting spondylodiscitis.

#### 1.1.4 Clinical course

Initially, the clinical course is characterized by nonspecific back pain. Therefore a delay in diagnosis by several months is commonly seen. The patients are often treated for degenerative diseases of the spine, and this misguided therapy interferes with early accurate diagnosis. Pain can occur at rest as well as during movement. Eventually, patients will show the systemic signs of fever and weight loss. (Frangen et al., 2006; Tali, 2004)

### 1.2 Spinal infections and HIV

HIV positive patients are more susceptible to other opportunistic infections (Nichols et al., 1989) some of which may affect the musculoskeletal system. However, the occurrence of osteoarticular infections in patients with HIV appears comparatively low, although, the prevalence increases when patients with a history of intravenous drug abuse are included in the group. In that case, infections of the spine becomes more prevalent (Busch et al., 2007). Furthermore, in patients with HIV infection, the lethality of musculoskeletal infectious diseases has been reported at about 20% (Vassilopoulos et al., 1997). The incidence of spinal infections is significantly higher in patients with HIV infection than in HIV negative patients. This predilection persists even when intravenous drug users are eliminated from analysis (Weinstein et al., 2005).

## 2. Diagnosis

### 2.1 Infection pathway

Generally for spinal infections, the aetiology must be differentiated into exogenous and endogenous sources. Pathogenic inoculation is usually endogenous. A focus of infection somewhere in the body results in haematogenous spread of the pathogen. Inoculation occurs within the bone marrow of the vertebral body, close to the endplates and near the anterior longitudinal ligament in particular. This pattern is based on the distinct vascularization of the subchondral bone and the paravertebral blood vessel supply (Müller et al., 2004; Wiley & Trueta, 1959). Frequently, the primary focus of infection is not detectable when the spinal infection is first identified. The exogenous pathway can be initiated iatrogenically or by injury. Infiltrations, spine surgery, as well as invasive diagnostic procedures can be causative agents (Frangen et al., 2006). In HIV positive patients, the endogenous pathway is of primary consideration (Sobottke et al., 2009). In addition, the treating physician should consider that involvement of the posterior spinal column is more common with tuberculous and fungal spondylitis (Gouliouris et al., 2010).

### 2.2 Pathogens

Generally, it is important to distinguish non-tuberculosis (non-specific) versus tuberculosis (specific) spondylodiscitis. Various pathogens have been associated with spondylodiscitis (bacterial, mycobacterial, fungal, and parasitic). Nevertheless, Staphylococcus aureus is the predominant agent causing the non-tuberculosis cases in 20-84% of cases. Tuberculosis is the most common cause of spinal infection worldwide, and accounts for 9%-46% of cases in developed countries. Skeletal system involvement occurs in 1%-3% of all tuberculosis infections. The spine is involved in approximately half of these cases (Gouliouris et al. 2010; Tuli, 2007). There is evidence suggesting that the frequency of vertebral tuberculosis in HIV positive patients is similar to the HIV-negative individuals. In a population of 2519 patients, only 1% of patients with vertebral osteomyelitis were HIV positive. Of these, vertebral tuberculosis developed in 31% (Grammatico et al., 2008). Other authors have reported spinal tuberculosis in about 35% of HIV positive patients with spondylodiscitis (Weinstein et al. 2005). Our own results identified spinal tuberculosis in 30% of HIV positive patients. Declaredly, 25% of the pathogens in this study could not be detected (Sobottke et al. 2009).

However, the reported mortality rate associated with tuberculosis is higher in HIV positive patients (39/100,000) than in HIV negative individuals (26/100,000) (World Health Organization, 2009).

### 2.3 Differential diagnosis

Differential diagnoses include erosive intervertebral osteochondrosis, vertebral fractures, ankylosing spondyloarthritis, avascular necrosis, haemophilia, chronic recurrent multifocal osteomyelitis, and Scheuermann's disease. Furthermore, the following conditions must also be considered as differential diagnosis: dialysis arthropathy, Charcot joint, rheumatoid arthritis, pseudarthrosis, and primary and secondary cancer lesions including vertebral lymphoma, multiple lymphoma, chordoma, and metastases (Tali et al. 2003). Pyelitis and pathologies of the kidney can also cause back pain. An accurate physical examination and detailed evaluation of the medical history is essential.

### 2.4 Physical examination

The inspection of the patient should focus on infected lesions (e.g. skin, intravenous drug abuse) as the origin of the spinal infection. Evaluation for neurological deficits is essential. Distinguishing symptoms of spinal infection include pain on heel strike or axial compression and percussion. If the patient is still able to stand, the relief posture might attract attention. Loading of the ventral column of the spine, inclination, and returning to a stand are often described as painful.

### 2.5 Laboratory examinations

Erythrocyte sedimentation rate (ESR) is a sensitive marker for infection, but lacks specificity. Over the course of this disease, the fall in ESR appears to be a good prognostic marker. However, an unchanged or rising ESR is more difficult to interpret, and it should be looked at in conjunction with other parameters such as C-reactive protein (CRP). In most reports, the ESR is elevated in over 90% of cases with a mean value ranging from 43 mm/h to 87 mm/h (Gouliouris et al., 2010; Carragee et al.; 1997a). Similarly, C-reactive protein (CRP) levels are increased in the large majority of cases with spondylodiscitis. CRP has been suggested as the preferred marker for monitoring response to treatment (Gouliouris et al., 2010; Hsieh et al.; 2004). The leucocyte count appears to be the least useful of the inflammatory markers. It is high in only one third to one half of affected patients. Especially immunocompromised and older (>60 years) patients can show normal white cell counts (Gouliouris et al., 2010; Carragee et al. 1997b). In patients with with HIV, the CD4 blood count is crucial in determining the clinical course of spondylodiscitis. Discitis and/or osteomyelitis occur in HIV positive patients with a mild-to-moderate decrease (>200 cells/ μL) in the CD4-T-cell count, and the infection responds to appropriate antibiotics. Patients with a more severe decline in CD4 count (50-200 cells/μL) are more prone to develop spinal tuberculosis, and patients with very low CD4 counts (<50 cells/μL) are more likely to develop epidural abscesses. The probability of mixed infections rises with a CD4 T-cell count less than 100 μL. A protocol for evaluating HIV positive patients who have a suspected spinal infection should be based on a CD4-T cell count, white blood cell count, erythrocyte sedimentation rate, and C-reactive protein level. In addition, blood cultures should be obtained in all patients (Sobottke et al., 2009; Weinstein & Eismont, 2005).

## 2.6 Radiology

### 2.6.1 X-ray

X-ray is the first procedure often recommended for people with back pain. For the diagnosis of vertebral osteomyelitis, plain radiographs have a sensitivity of 82%, a specificity of 57%, and an accuracy of 73% (Modic et al., 1985). In the early clinical stages of the disease, plain radiographs do not indicate spondylodiscitis and are non-specific. At this stage, only subtle changes such as endplate demineralization and/or irregularity may be noticed, or radiographs may be completely normal (Maiuri et al., 1997; Price et al., 1983, Sharif et al., 1989). Radiographically, the progression of infection is characterized by further destruction of the vertebral body affecting the opposite end plate, and eventual extension of inflammation through the anterior, lateral, and posterior surfaces. Although paravertebral soft tissue mass with displacement of the surrounding structures may be seen, soft tissue contrast resolution is poor. Identification of destruction of two neighbouring vertebral bodies extending from a narrowed intervertebral disc leads to the correct diagnosis (Jevtic, 2004; Sammak et al., 1999). However, even in later stages, signs of the disease on radiographs may be slight and may be difficult or impossible to distinguish from degenerative diseases.

### 2.6.2 MRI (magnetic resonance imaging)

Magnetic resonance imaging is the study of choice for the diagnosis of spinal infections. Common MRI findings in infectious spondylitis are hypointensity of the involved tissue on T1-weighted images, hyperintensity on T2-weighted images, destruction of two or more adjacent vertebral bodies with involvement of the intervening disc, and epidural and paraspinal extension and/or abscesses. In addition, MRI provides a diagnostic view of the paravertebral and spinal space (Chang et al., 2006; An et al., 1991; Modic et al. 1985). In HIV positive patients, the treating physician must deal with the specific type of infection (e.g. vertebral tuberculosis, Figure 1). The following parameters can help distinguish TB from pyogenic spondylitis. The most distinctive finding of TB spondylitis is a pattern of mainly bone destruction with relative preservation of the disc. The vertebral body shows focal and heterogeneous contrast enhancement. In addition, a well-defined paraspinal area of abnormal signal intensity is often detectable. On the sagittal views, an intraosseous rim enhancement of the vertebra may occur. In comparison, pyogenic spondylitis is characterized by a pattern of discitis (disc destruction) with mild to moderate peri-discal bone destruction. The vertebral body shows a relatively diffuse and homogenous contrast enhancement. Furthermore, an ill-defined paraspinal area of abnormal signal intensity with peri-discal rim enhancement provides a hint to the correct diagnosis (Chang et al., 2006). In any case, the use of contrast medium during the procedure is highly recommended. MRI is the gold standard diagnostic to detect spondylodiscitis. Nevertheless, in early stages it may show only subtle, non-specific subchondral changes to the endplate. This can lead to a misdiagnosis (e.g. Modic I, degenerative endplate change). If the clinical course raises suspicions of an infectious process of the spine, a second MRI after 2-3 weeks is highly recommended (Dunbar et al., 2010).

### 2.6.3 CT (computed tomography)

Generally, the radiologic diagnosis of spondylodiscitis is based on MRI findings. Nevertheless, valuable information may be provided by computed tomography. CT enables

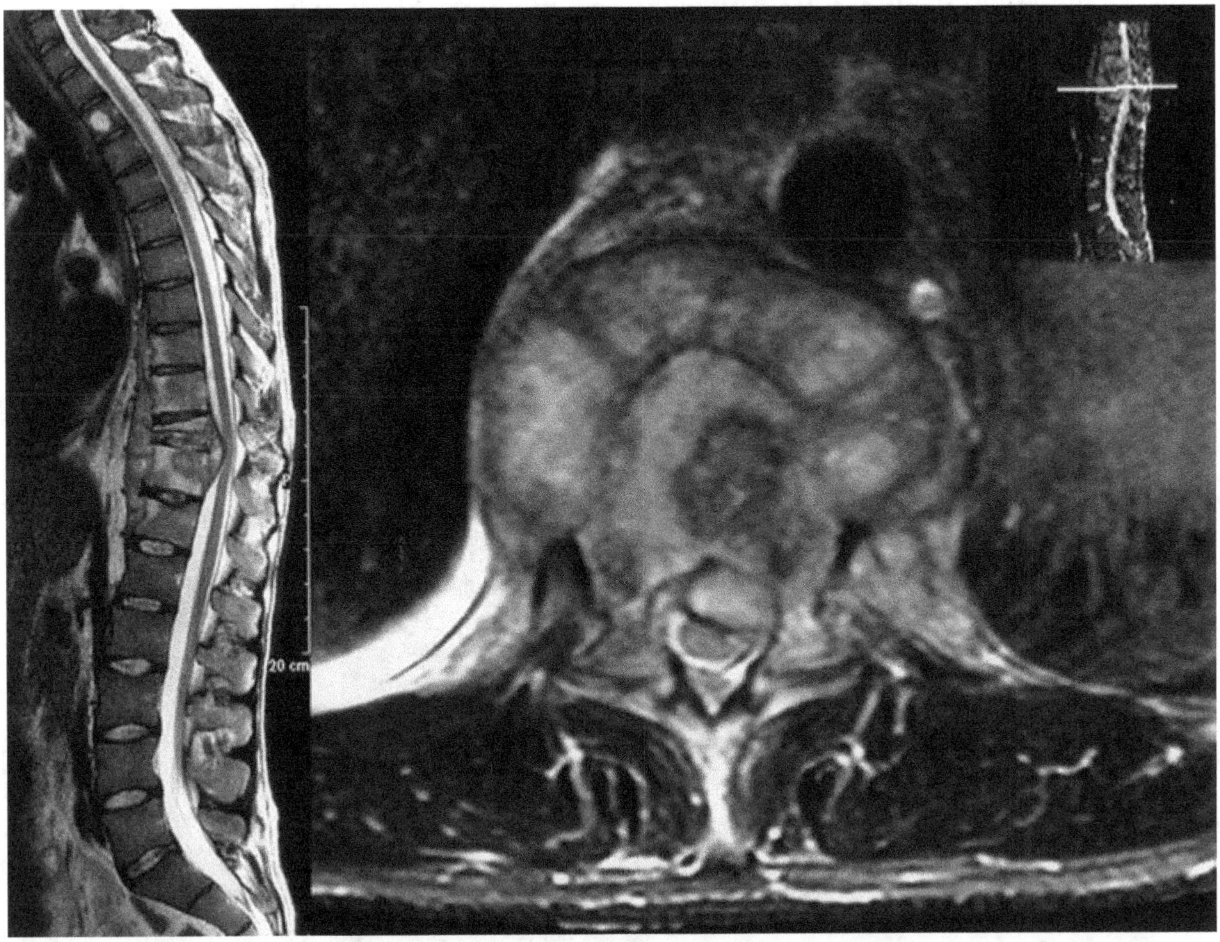

Fig. 1. Spondylodiscitis (Mycobacterium Xenopi). Sagittal and axial T2-weighted MRI with contrast medium.

accurate assessment of bone destruction (Figure 2). In addition, in combination with contrast medium, paravertebral abscesses with psoas involvement can be identified and treated by CT-guided aspiration or drainage (Maiuri et al., 1997; Golimbu et al., 1984). CT yields positive findings during the early stages of spondylitis, because the involved disc shows areas of hypodensity. Computed tomography also shows the disc flattening and the vertebral endplate destruction that are not visible on conventional radiographs in the early stages (Maiuri et al., 1997, as cited in Heithoff, 1982; La Berge et al., 1984; Price et al., 1983; Reininko et al., 1984)). CT scans provide slice imaging despite the presence of neurostimulators and cardiac pacemakers. A shorter imaging time (in comparison to MRI) is also more favourable for extremely ill or anxious patients.

### 2.6.4 Multiple phase scintigraphies

This procedure is not a first-line choice in the diagnostic pathway for spinal infections. Nevertheless, three-phase bone scintigraphy is sensitive for the diagnosis of osteomyelitis (Al-Sheikh et al., 1985). However, false-negative findings in haematogenous vertebral osteomyelitis have been reported (Schlaeffer et al., 1987). Even more limiting is the fact that multiple phase bone scintigraphy is unable to distinguish infectious processes from other causes of pathologic bone turnover (f.e. degenerative diseases or tumours).

### 2.6.5 Inflammation scintigraphy with labelled leukocytes or Tc-99m-labeled antibodies

Leukocyte scintigraphy is a supplement to multiphase scintigraphy. In this procedure, radioactively labelled native blood cells or (now, preferably) Tc-99m-labeled anti-granulocyte antibodies are used to detect inflammatory changes of the bone tissue. However, anti-granulocyte antibodies also label haematopoiesis occurring in the bone marrow, so that the spinal column exhibits physiological enrichment. Inflammation scintigraphy is therefore more suitable for the extremities.

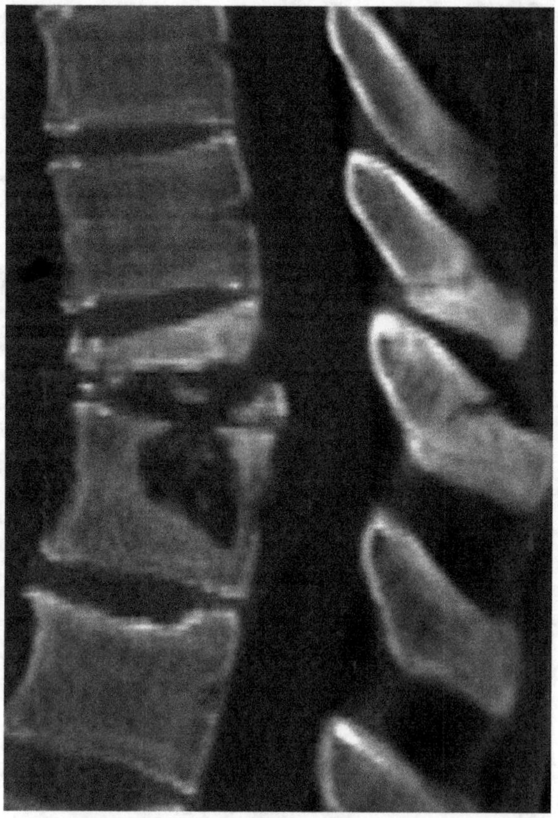

Fig. 2. Spondylodiscitis (Mycobacterium Xenopi). Sagittal computed tomography scan of the thoracic spine: the bony destruction can be accurately assessed.

### 2.6.6 Positron emission tomography with fluorine-18 fluorodeoxyglucose (F-18 FDG PET)

Imaging of the spine by F-18 FDG PET allows differentiation of degenerative processes of the vertebral endplates from spondylodiscitis (Figure 3). In addition, this technique implements a rapid imaging procedure with acceptable exposure to radiation (3.7 to 7.4 mSv), as well as good spatial resolution. However, distinguishing from malignant processes is challenging. The glucose metabolism of the inflammatory cells absorbs the F-18-FDG. Uptake depends on the activity level of glucose metabolism. Spinal infections show up as a "hot spot," because there is only marginal uptake of F-18-FDG in the healthy tissue of the bone marrow and spinal column (Schmitz et al., 2001; Stumpe et al., 2002). This diagnostic tool is generally not necessary. However, particularly when a definitive diagnosis cannot be established using standard procedures (e.g. MRI, laboratory), it can be very helpful in providing more information.

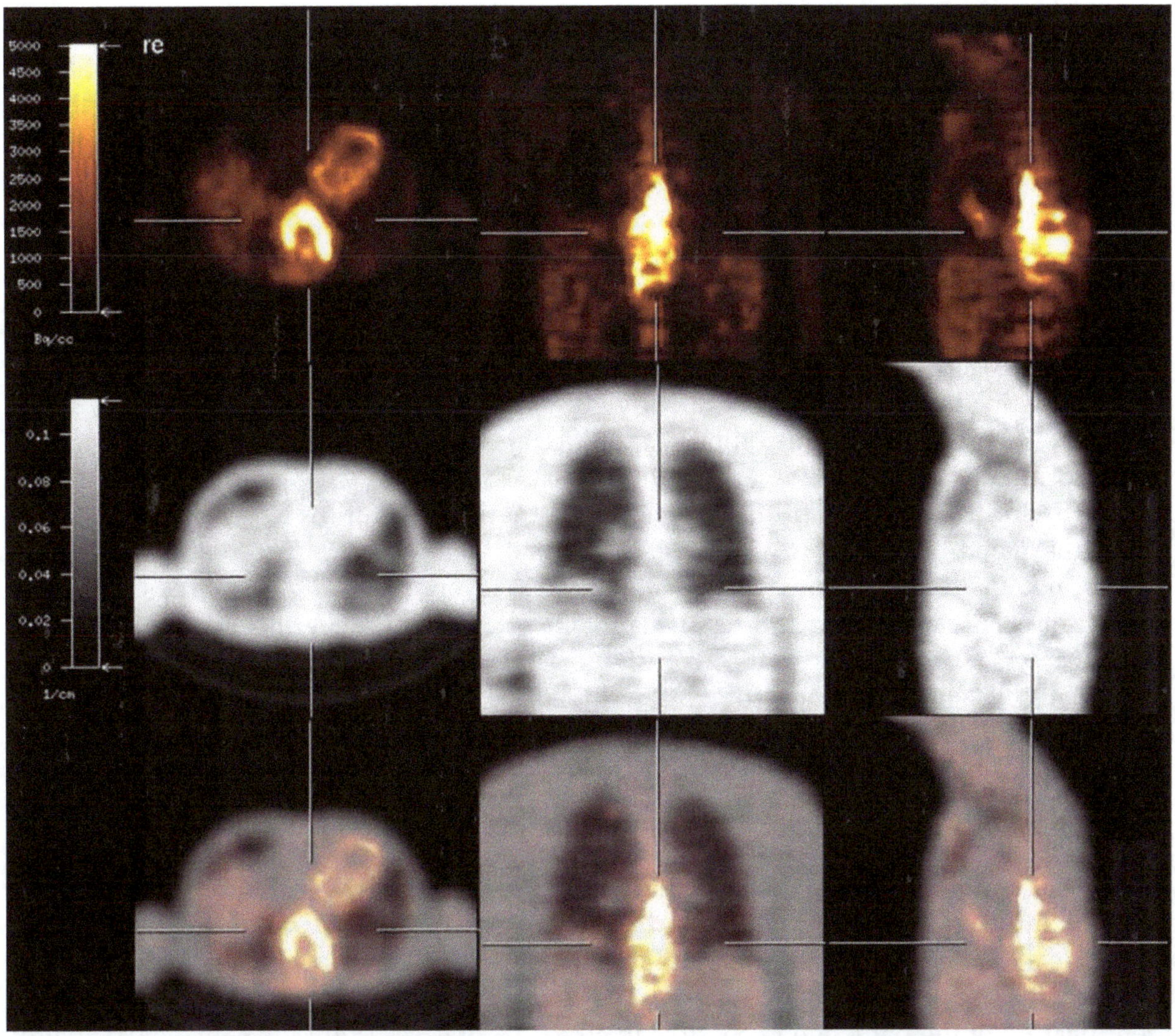

Fig. 3. Spondylodiscitis (Mycobacterium Xenopi). Positron Emission Tomography (PET) with 18-F-fluorodeoxyglucose as tracer (F18-FDG-PET) showing a pronounced increase in accumulation extending over several segments (approximately T9-T12) with a SUV (mean standard uptake value) maximum of 9.1.

### 2.7 Pathogen identification

Identification of the pathogen is crucial to the subsequent clinical course. One pillar of therapy is appropriate antibiotic treatment. This requires accurate diagnosis with identification of the pathogen as well as a spectrum of antibiotic resistance. Considering the diversity of potential pathogens in the HIV positive patients, this becomes even more vital. Furthermore, the increasing number of antibiotic-resistant pathogens necessitates precise determination of the causative agent. Empirical broad-spectrum antibiotic therapy is linked to increased rates of complications such as Clostridium difficile-associated diarrhoea as well as higher healthcare costs, and should be reserved for patients presenting with severe sepsis, once blood cultures have been taken (Gouliouris et al., 2010; Lilie et al., 2008). Identification of the pathogen is successful in up to 85% of patients with spondylodiscitis (Lucio et al., 2000). In our own collective of 20 HIV positive patients, pathogen identification was successful in 75 % of the cases (Sobottke et al., 2009). The main cause for failure of pathogen identification is previous use of systemic antibiotic treatment. If possible, antibiotic therapy should be initiated only after sample materials are obtained. In cases where the patient is already receiving antibiotic treatment and the health status is stable, the medication should be discontinued for at least 3 days prior to culture. In such cases, we believe that attempts to identify the pathogens are more likely to be successful.

### 2.7.1 Blood culture

Infections of the spine are generally monomicrobial, and often have a haematogenous source. Therefore, blood cultures are a simple and cost effective method for identifying bacterial pathogens of spinal infections. A positive culture can be expected in 40%-60% of clinically defined cases of pyogenic spondylodiscitis (Gouliouris et al., 2010; Sapico, 1996). However, the previous administration of systemic antibiotic therapy severely handicaps the ability to identify the causative agent. In such cases, temporary interruption of antibiotic administration is necessary prior to performing the blood culture. It is recommended to repeat the blood culture up to 3 times for definite identification.. The pathogen is often successfully identified, not only in the acute phase of fever or the presence of sepsis, but also in clinically bland cases of afebrile patients (Nolla et al., 2002). Nevertheless, there is a high incidence of infective endocarditis (26%) reported during enterococcal and streptococcal spondylodiscitis. Routine echocardiography should be performed when these pathogens are suspected (Mulleman et al., 2006).

### 2.7.2 Biopsy

Other alternatives for identifying the pathogen are use of a percutaneous punch under anaesthesia, and CT-guided fine needle aspiration. The latter can be performed while concomitantly placing a drain to reduce pressure on the abscess. In obtaining a histological diagnosis for cases of malignant disease, a percutaneous spinal biopsy is accurate. In cases of spondylodiscitis, however, the reported accuracy is more variable. Identification of the pathogen is possible in 40%-73% of cases (Rankine et al., 2004; Shaltot et al., 1982, Borowski et al, 1998). Nonetheless, spinal biopsy leads to a direct change in management for 35% of patients, and is still worthwhile even if the patient has already started on antibiotics. However, success of the procedure for identification of the pathogen is much greater prior to starting antibiotics (Rankine et al., 2004). If antibiotics have already been initiated, the treating physician should consider stopping this treatment for 2-3 days prior to the biopsy. If the first attempt to identify the pathogen by percutaneous biopsy fails, a second procedure should be considered. Friedman et al. identified microbiological growth in 50% of cases after disc space biopsy in patients with spontaneous spondylodiscitis. Repeat biopsies brought this rate up to 79% (Friedman et al. 2002). Even more promising is open surgical biopsy, if the first set of cultures is negative (Lew & Waldvogel, 2004).

### 2.7.3 Intraoperative sampling

The highest probability for probe acquisition enabling identification of the pathogen is surgical sampling (Figure 4). Open bone biopsies can yield the microbial aetiology of spondylodiscitis in almost 100% of cases (Jimenz-Mejias et al., 1999). In this case, it is recommended to obtain at least 2 probes for histological and microbiological examination (Lucio et al., 2000).

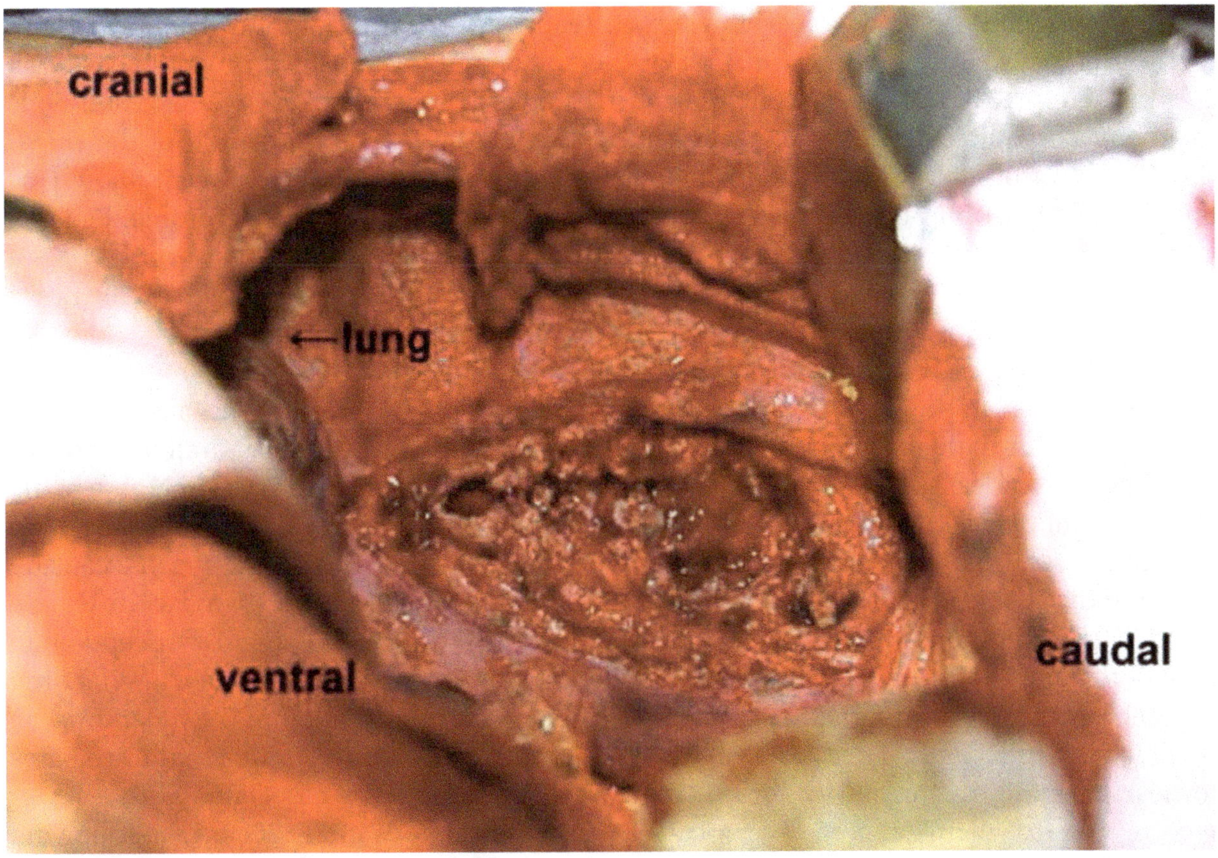


Fig. 4. Spondylodiscitis (Mycobacterium Xenopi). Intraoperative findings after thoracotomy, after opening of the abscess cavity, and accomplished vertebrectomy of T10.

### 2.7.4 Histology

In addition to culture, histologic examination of the specimen is helpful. It allows discrimination between pyogenic or granulomatous origin of disease. Additional stains, such as Ziehl-Neelsen for mycobacteria as well as periodic acid Schiff for fungi should be considered. To rule out a potential malignant process in the spine, which imitates the radiological signs of infectious disease, histological examination is essential. Therefore, histological and microbiological examination of the tissue are both recommended (Gouliouris et al., 2010; Turunc et al. 2007; Rankine et al., 2004, Buchelt et al., 1993; Frazier et al., 2009).

## 3. Treatment strategies

### 3.1 Basic information

At this time, no general treatment guidelines for spondylodiscitis are available. To date, no prospective, controlled, clinical trials have been published. Level of evidence for treatment recommendations does not exceed Level C (Grados et al., 2007; Sackett et al., 1996). With HIV, there is ambivalence among physicians, and often the decision to surgically treat HIV positive patients with spondylodiscitis is made based on the patients' general condition, the stage of HIV disease, and life expectancy of the patient. Apart from this, many surgeons fear complications after spinal surgery such as wound infections or delayed wound healing. Statements within the literature concerning postoperative complication rates in HIV positive patients are inconsistent. However, the aim of treatment is to eradicate the infection, restore and preserve the structure and function of the spine, and alleviate pain (Goulioutis et al. 2010). Therefore, the affected segments must be immobilized, and appropriate antibiotic treatment is required. If necessary, surgical debridement and decompression of the spinal canal must also be considered. As previously mentioned, antibiotic treatment should be initiated after identification of the pathogen and according to the resistance profile. Bed rest is recommended if the pain level does not allow mobilisation of the patient, or if there is a high risk of spinal instability (Quinones-Hinojosa et al., 2004). Since the advent of antibiotics, mortality from this disease has dropped from up to 56% to less than 5% (Goulioutis et al., 2010; Bauman et al., 1923; Sapico et al.; 1979). Guidelines regarding the route of administration for and/or duration of antibiotic treatment do not exist for spondylodiscitis patients with or without HIV infection. Intravenous administration of antibiotics for at least 2-4 weeks is recommended (Lew & Waldvogel, 2004; Sobottke et al., 2008) If antibiotic treatment without direct pathogen identification is required, the medication selected should be appropriate for the most common pathogens causing spondylodiscitis, i.e. Staphylococcus aureus and Escherichia coli, after blood cultures are taken. The intravenous phase can be shortened when the organism is highly susceptible to antimicrobials, and the patient has negative blood cultures, normal motor function, and no evidence of endocarditis (Grados et al., 2007). Furthermore, observation of the inflammatory parameters are recommended. The optimal duration for antibiotic administration remains unclear. Overall, treatment for more than 12 weeks appears to be associated with a lower recurrence rate when compared with that of 4-8 weeks (Grados et al., 2007). The following antibiotics diffuse extremely well to bone tissue: fluoroquinolones, clindamycin, rifampicin, fusidic acid, and metronidazole. Fair diffusion can be contributed by ß-lactams, glycopeptides, phosphomycin, and sulphonamides (Grados et al., 2007). In case of tuberculosis spondylodiscitis, anti-tubercular chemotherapy should be started after histological and microbiological evidence is obtained, and should be carried out for 18-24 months. Spondylodiscitis caused by fungus should be treated with appropriate antimycotic medication. In advanced cases, antimycotic drug therapy is thought to be ineffective. An overriding indication for surgery is recommended, in particular when spinal structures show progressive destruction (van Ooij et al., 2000).

### 3.2 Conservative treatment

In addition to antibiotic treatment, immobilization of the affected region of the spinal column is required. Reclining ortheses distribute stress over the unaffected segments and their joints. Thereby, release of the affected ventral column can be obtained. Wearing the orthesis, patients can be fully mobilized. In our study of HIV positive patients, only half of the conservatively-treated patients were supplied with a reclination brace, which was worn for an average of about 51 days. In addition, 4 of the patients undergoing surgery were also treated with such a reclination brace. The condition of 2 patients worsened under initial conservative treatment and so surgery was required (Sobottke et al., 2009). Generally, if conservative treatment yields no radiologically evident fusion reaction, continued destruction occurs, and/or there is no clinical improvement, surgery should be considered (Hsieh et al., 2004; Quinones-Hinojosa et al., 2004). When major defects exist in the ventral column, the lower lumbar column, or at the lumbosacral border, necessary fusion through non-operative measures can only be achieved by at least six weeks bed rest. Mobilisation of the patient is only recommended once osseous infiltration becomes visible (Sobottke et al., 2008, as cited in Eysel & Peters, 1997 & Cramer et al., 2003).

## 3.3 Surgical treatment

### 3.3.1 Drainage of abscesses

Large abscesses, particularly those persisting even after antibiotic treatment, must be eliminated. One alternative is drain placement (Figure 5), inserted during an open procedure or CT-guided. Especially when the general state of health of the patient is poor and precludes open surgery, drain placement should be considered. It has been shown as an adequate technique to treat abscesses outside of the spine e. g. ilio-psoas muscle or pleural cavity (Grados et al., 2007).

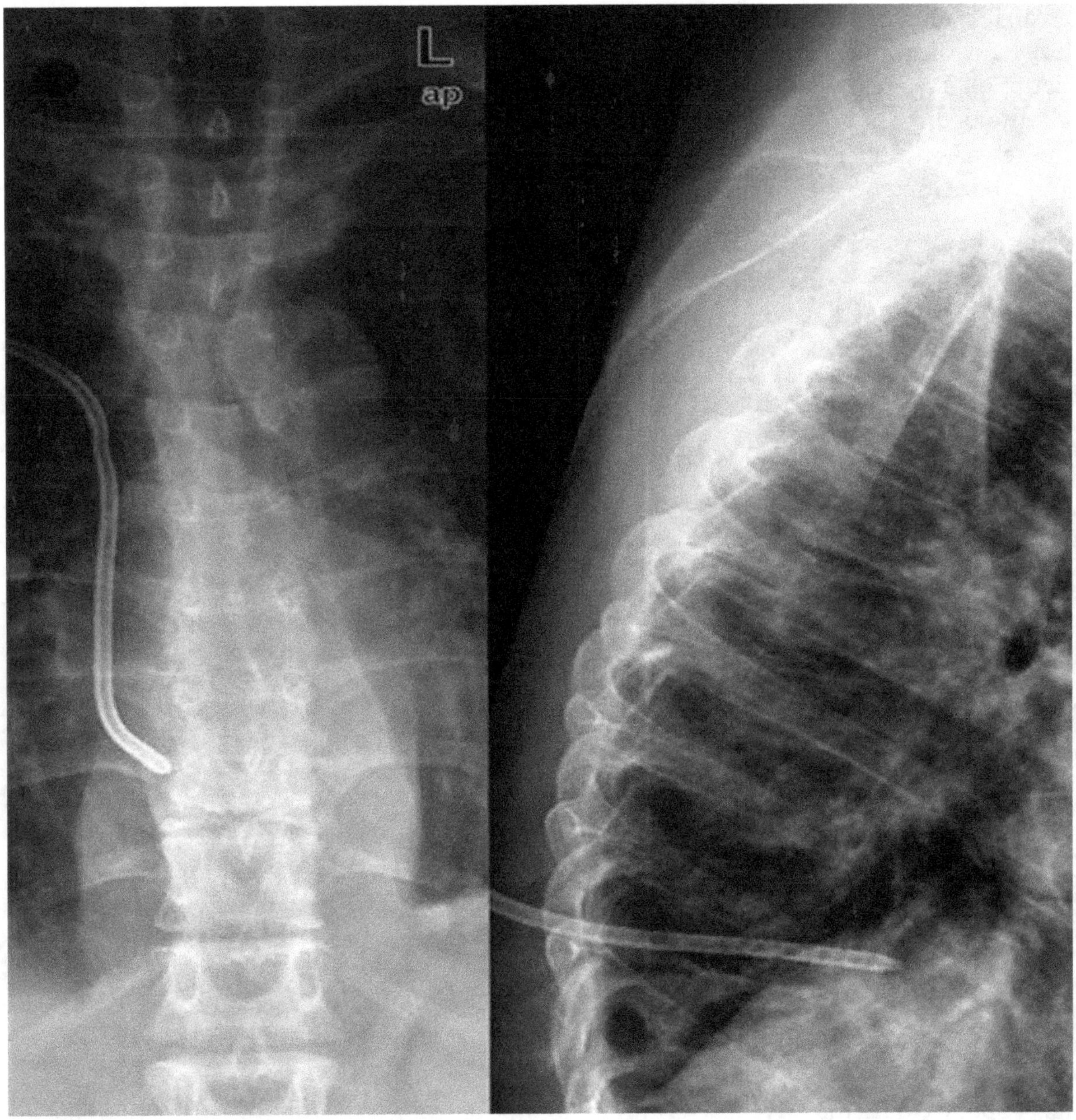


Fig. 5. Spondylodiscitis (Mycobacterium Xenopi). Control X-ray after CT-guided draining of the paravertebral abscess.

### 3.3.2 Surgery

Surgical intervention should be considered when there is no response to therapy and patient is experiencing persistent and high intensity pain. The surgical procedure is aimed to relieve compression of the spinal cord or to drain epidural or paravertebral abscesses and to improve spinal stability (Lew & Waldvogel, 2004). It includes excision of the infected spinal and paravertebral tissue, retrieval of the pathogen for identification, and stabilisation of the spine via fusion of the affected segments. Surgical alternatives include dorsal instrumentation with pedicle screw-based systems, either minimally invasive, if no spinal decompression is required, or using open technique in combination with spinal canal decompression. Ventral approaches can be performed combined with dorsal instrumentation or alone using a ventral stabilization system (Figure 6). This approach enables treatment of the frequently-involved ventral column. Extensive debridement must be carried out on both the affected intervertebral disc space and the vertebral endplates. Spinal fusion can be achieved using autologous bone interposition or with cage fusion (Figure 6). Treatment of the cervical spine may include ventral stabilization by plate, cage, or autologous bone interposition. Instrumentation via dorsal approach is usually unnecessary (Müller et al., 2004). Generally, no evidence-based guidelines regarding surgical treatments are available (Sobottke et al., 2008). Of course, the implantation of

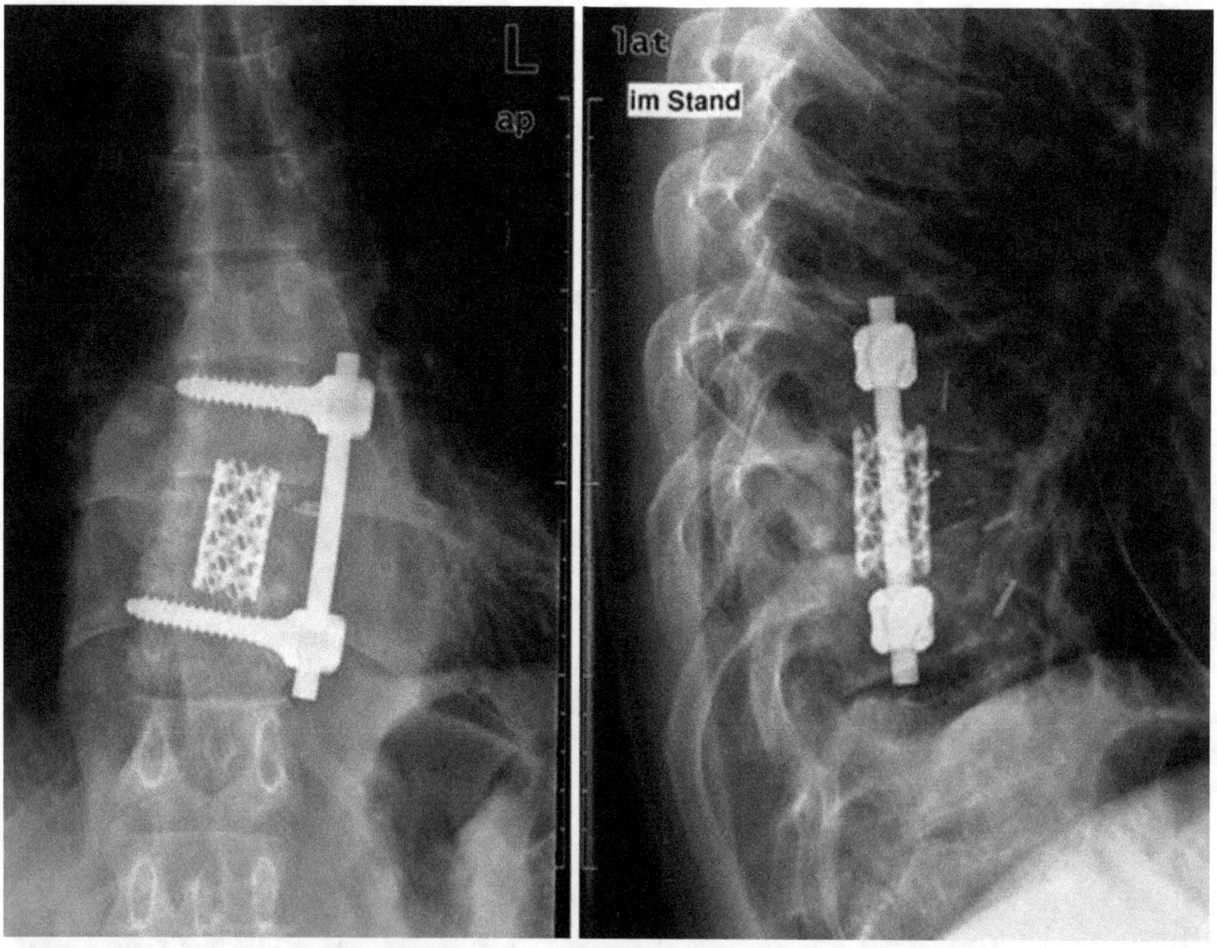


Fig. 6. Spondylodiscitis (Mycobacterium Xenopi). Control X-ray after debridement of the infected segment and ventral spondylodesis. It shows a properly inserted cage (titanium, Pyramesh, Medtronic) and an anterolateral monobar system (titanium, ART system, AMT).

fixation materials in an infected wound area can lead to microbial colonization of the metal surface and persistent infection. This risk is reduced by thorough debridement, with simultaneous application of an antibiotic carrier. Titanium implants do not appear to increase the rate of recurrence (Sobottke et al., 2008, as cited in Cramer et al., 2003 & Oga et al., 1993).

## 4. Outcome

Excluding the presence of HIV infection, the mortality of spondylodiscitis has been reported as less than 5%, ranging from 0-11%. Early mortality is related to uncontrolled sepsis (Gouliouris et al., 2010). Previous studies have suggested that the clinical presentation of spinal tuberculosis is similar in HIV positive and negative patients, and that good outcomes can be expected with regard to mycobacterial disease. However, in this study, all 7 patients responded to therapy and completed a 12-month course. One patient died 13 months after diagnosis, with cryptococceal meningitis and bacterial sepsis (Leibert et al., 1996). The mortality rate in our HIV- positive population is higher, with an inpatient mortality rate of 5% and an outpatient mortality rate of 20% (Sobottke et al., 2009). Weinstein et al. reported an inpatient mortality rate of 17% (Weinstein et al. 2005). A cohort of 39 HIV infected patients with spinal tuberculosis showed a 15% mortality rate within two years of surgery (Govender et al., 2001). The problem of postoperative complications in HIV positive patients has been widely discussed. A significantly higher frequency of postoperative infection with associated symptoms has been reported in HIV patients (Hoekman et al., 1991). In contrast, Horberg et al. did not detect higher perioperative complication rates, except for that of pneumonia (Horberg et al., 2006). Similarly, Govender et al. did not identify a higher incidence of wound healing disturbance in their population than that found in HIV-negative subjects. However, the ultimate outcome of surgery for HIV-infected patients depends on a number of factors, including the nature of the procedure (emergent or elective), coexisting medical problems, nutritional status, and the stage of the disease (Govender et al., 2001).

### 4.1 Surgery or conservative treatment for HIV-positive patients?

The purpose of our study was to determine the relevant clinical presentation and outcomes for HIV positive patients with spondylodiscitis as a function of treatment. We performed a national, multicentre, retrospective case series of HIV positive patients with spondylodiscitis presenting between 1991 und 2007, comparing operative intervention versus conservative therapy. All patients fulfilled the following inclusion criteria: age ≥18 years; compatible clinical history and imaging; HIV; spondylodiscitis; follow-up >6 months; with imaging and records available (Table 1). Infection was considered cured if patients showed no signs or symptoms of localized infection on clinical examination, in laboratory markers of inflammation, and on imaging. Relapse of infection was presumed for patients with recurrence of symptoms in association with rising inflammatory markers (WBC, CRP) and deteriorating MRI findings. Twenty patients were included in the study. The average age of the patients at the time of admission was 43.0 years. The gender ratio m:f was 2.3:1. On admission, 50% of the patients were in CDC stage C3. The CD4 T-cell count averaged 237.5/L. At the time of presentation with spondylodiscitis, HIV had been diagnosed for a mean 8.5 years. Radiologically, paravertebral abscesses were seen in 80.0%, epidural abscesses in 33.3%, and psoas abscesses in 13.3% of patients. The causative pathogen was identified in 75% of the cases (see Table 1). In 3 cases, mixed infections were present. Half of the patients underwent surgery. Wound infections or delay to healing were not observed. One patient died during inpatient admission. Eleven of the 19 patients completed an average follow-up of 13 months after discharge. Over the follow-up period, a further 3 patients died at an average of 45 months after discharge (Table 2).

| Gender | | Age on admission | CDC | CD4 T-cell count on admission | CD4/CD8-ratio | HIV-RNA | Pathogen |
|---|---|---|---|---|---|---|---|
| m | w | [years] | | [absolute/µl] | | [copies/ml] | |
| | | | | standard value: 435-1.600 | Stand. value: 0.6-2.8 | | |
| | 1 | 29 | C 1 | 500 | 0.4 | - | *Mycobacterium tuberculosis* |
| | 1 | 41 | C 3 | 330 | 0.9 | - | Sterile |
| | 1 | 21 | - | - | - | - | *Mycobacterium tuberculosis* |
| 1 | | 41 | - | - | - | - | *Staphylococcus aureus* |
| 1 | | 54 | C 2 | - | - | - | *Staphylococcus aureus* |
| | 1 | 48 | - | - | - | - | Sterile |
| | 1 | 33 | B 2 | 50 | 0.4 | 1800 | *Staphylococcus aureus, Pseudomonas aeruginosa* |
| 1 | | 67 | C 3 | 100 | 0.4 | <50 | Coagulase-negative Staphylococci |
| 1 | | 29 | C 3 | 220 | 0.3 | 130 | Sterile |
| 1 | | 28 | C 3 | 400 | 0.5 | <50 | M. xenopi |
| 1 | | 36 | A 2 | 430 | 0.3 | - | Sterile |
| 1 | | 40 | A 2 | - | - | - | *Staphylococcus aureus* |
| 1 | | 58 | C 3 | 98 | 0.1 | 1.920 | *Staphylococcus aureus* |
| 1 | | 49 | A 2 | 310 | 0.2 | <50 | *Mycobacterium tuberculosis* |
| 1 | | 42 | C 3 | 82 | 0.2 | <50 | *Staphylococcus aureus*,coagulase-negative Staphylococci |
| | 1 | 39 | A 3 | 157 | 0.3 | - | *Staphylococcus aureus* |
| 1 | | 51 | C 3 | 102 | 0.3 | 377 | *Staphylococcus aureus* |
| 1 | | 33 | C 3 | 129 | 0.1 | <50 | *Mycobacterium bovis, Klebsiella pneumoniae* |
| 1 | | 60 | C 3 | 355 | 0.4 | - | Sterile |
| 1 | | 61 | C 3 | 300 | 0.7 | <50 | *Mycobacterium tuberculosis* |

Table 1. Demographic and HIV related details.

| In-patient | | Outpatient after Discharge | |
|---|---|---|---|
| conservative | operative | conservative | operative |
| 2 progressive infections and sepsis | 1 respondylodesis (screw pull-out) | 1 persistent infection | 1 relapse (patient noncompliance |
| 1 decubital sacral ulcer (grade 4) | 1 pneumothorax (after central venous catheter) | 1 deep venous thrombosis | |

Table 2. Inpatient and outpatient outcome and complications (conservatively versus operatively treatment).

## 5. Conclusion

An increasing incidence of spondylodiscitis has been observed. Factors implicated and collaborating in this increase include the HIV epidemic, particularly that in Sub-Saharan Africa, the large numbers of intravenous drug abusers, the currently widely-used aspiration and catheter techniques, as well as the recurrence of tuberculosis in industrialized nations. In principle, patients of all ages can contract spondylitis, but it appears that 50 to 70 year-old patients are most likely to fall ill from it. The peak age of disease in HIV positive patients lies substantially earlier: 10% are under 30 years of age when they first contract spondylitis. The estimated number of patients who are seropositive for human immunodeficiency virus is about 50 billion people worldwide, and continues to increase. Potential pathogens responsible for spondylitis include bacteria, fungi, and parasites (e. g. hydatidosus). As a general rule, the infection is of bacterial origin. However, especially in immune deficient patients, the possibility of infection stemming from fungi or atypical mycobacteria should be taken into account. The probability of an infection by MOTT (Mycobacteria Other Than Tuberculosis) strongly depends on the CD4 T-cell count. Highly Active Anti-Retroviral Therapy (HAART) has accomplished rapid increases of the CD4 T-cell count, and thus caused a so-called "immune reconstitution syndrome," which has resulted in atypical, creeping disease processes and at times even to spontaneous complete recovery. Several years may elapse between the inception of symptoms and the final diagnosis of spondylodiscitis. Primary factors resulting in successful treatment of spondylodiscitis are early diagnosis and rapid onset of treatment to prevent progressive stages with serious complications. Immobilisation of the affected spine segments, antibiotic therapy, and, depending on the extent of the disease, debridement, decompression, and stabilisation are basic requirements for successful treatment leading to a complete recovery from spondylodiscitis. Emergent surgical intervention is required for spondylodiscitis on the development of neurological deficits and/or sepsis. Further indications for surgery are instability, impending or already existing deformities, intraspinal space-occupying lesions, an unclear origin with the suspicion of malignancy, and lack of response to conservative therapy. Relative indications for surgical treatment include uncontrollable pain symptoms and lack of patient compliance with conservative therapy. The occurrence of spondylodiscitis in HIV positive patients is accompanied by high mortality. We recorded a hospital mortality of 5% and a total mortality of 20%. The occurrence of spondylodiscitis in HIV positive patients is associated with a low CD4 T-cell count. The probability of mixed infections rises with a CD4 T-cell counts below 100/L, but there is no correlation between a low CD4 T-cell count and probability of infection by MOTT. Because increased surgical morbidity is not evident among HIV positive patients, HIV infection or AIDS should not interfere with the decision to perform operative stabilisation of the affected spinal segments. The existence of HIV infection or AIDS in a patient with spondylodiscitis should not influence the decision for or against conservative or operative therapy. However, these patients should be treated in a specialized hospital by an experienced team of consultants.

## 6. Further research

To date, no global data has been collected or published regarding the aetiopathology, clinical course, and/or treatment strategies for spinal infections in patients also afflicted with HIV. This information, however, is a prerequisite for an understanding of the disease and the development of a successful clinical pathway for treatment. We have developed and implemented an English-language registry, which can be accessed globally via internet at www.clinicalsurveys.net (Figure 7). With an individual account, any physician can document patients online. Participants will be remunerated for their effort. This registry was submitted as a project of the German Surgical Trial network (CHIR–NET), funded by the German Federal Ministry of Education and Research. Patient documentation in the registry is divided into the following sections: 1. Centre identification, 2. Identifier, 3. Opportunistic infection, 4. Antiviral therapy, 5. CDC Stage, 6. Diagnosis, 7. Radiology, 8. Symptoms, 9. Laboratory, 10. Microbiology, 11. Treatment , 12. Complications, 13. Outcome, 14. Remarks. In the "Treatment" section, antibiotic and surgical therapy is surveyed in depth. With the global, web-based registry spondHIVreg, we have introduced an instrument to survey HIV-positive patients with spondylodiscitis. All physicians involved in the treatment of these patients are invited to participate, thereby contributing to a better understanding of the disease and an improvement of its treatment.

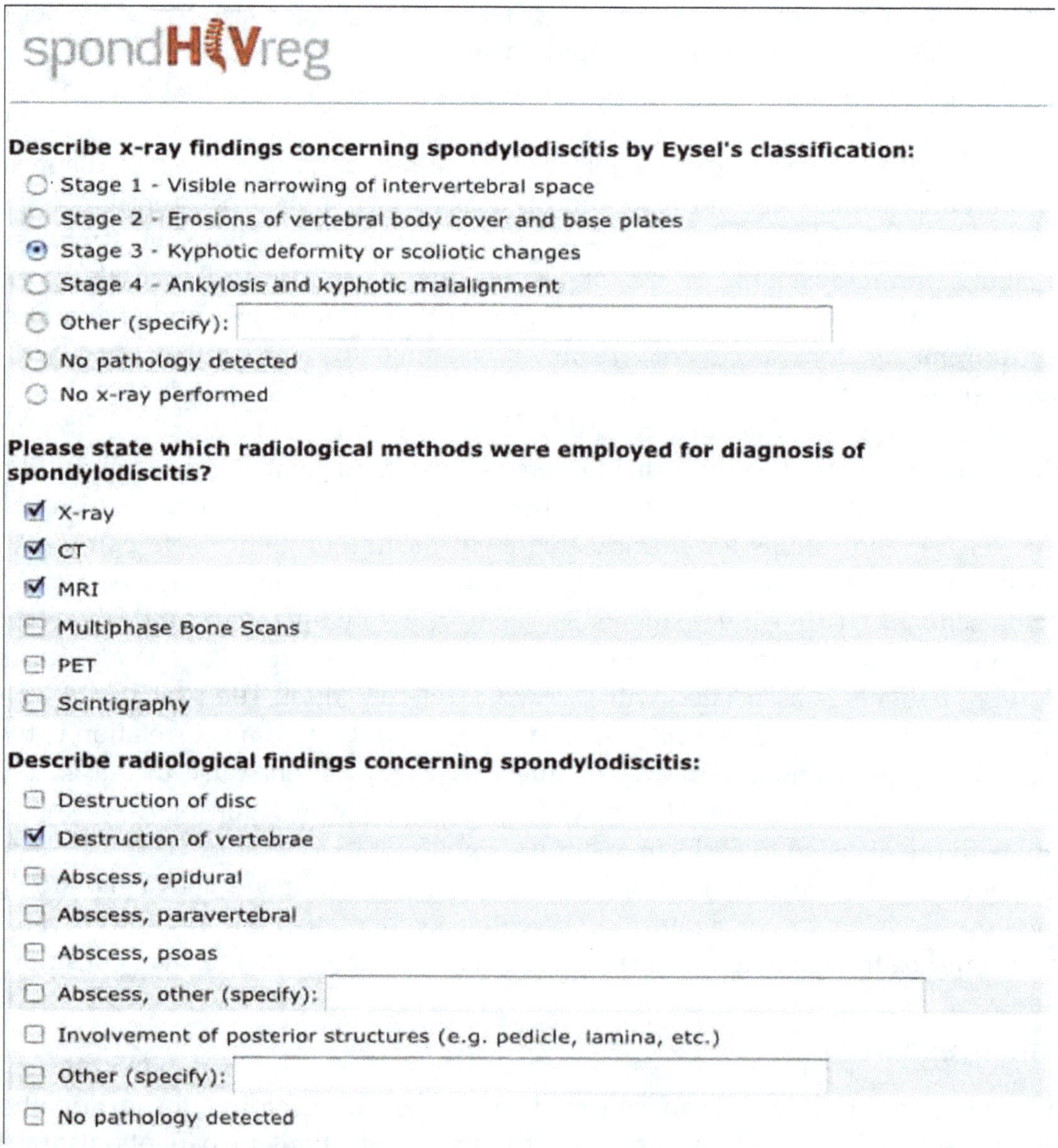
spondHIVreg

**Describe x-ray findings concerning spondylodiscitis by Eysel's classification:**

- ○ Stage 1 - Visible narrowing of intervertebral space
- ○ Stage 2 - Erosions of vertebral body cover and base plates
- ◉ Stage 3 - Kyphotic deformity or scoliotic changes
- ○ Stage 4 - Ankylosis and kyphotic malalignment
- ○ Other (specify):
- ○ No pathology detected
- ○ No x-ray performed

**Please state which radiological methods were employed for diagnosis of spondylodiscitis?**

- ☑ X-ray
- ☑ CT
- ☑ MRI
- ☐ Multiphase Bone Scans
- ☐ PET
- ☐ Scintigraphy

**Describe radiological findings concerning spondylodiscitis:**

- ☐ Destruction of disc
- ☑ Destruction of vertebrae
- ☐ Abscess, epidural
- ☐ Abscess, paravertebral
- ☐ Abscess, psoas
- ☐ Abscess, other (specify):
- ☐ Involvement of posterior structures (e.g. pedicle, lamina, etc.)
- ☐ Other (specify):
- ☐ No pathology detected

Fig. 7. Full page of the survey list of the global web-based registry SpondHIVreg.

## 7. Acknowledgement

JS, KZ and RS are supported by the German Federal Ministry of Research and Education (BMBF grant 01KN1106). Peer Eysel conceived of the study, which forms the basis of this manuscript.

## 8. References

An, H. S.; Vaccaro, A. R.; Dolinskas, C. A.; Cotler, J. M.; Balderston, R. A. & Bauerle, W. B. (1991). Differentiation between spinal tumors and infections with magnetic resonance imaging. Spine, Vol. 16, No. 8 (August 1991), pp. 334-338, ISSN 0362-2436

Al-Sheikh, W.; Sfakianakis, G. N.; Mnaymneh, W.; Hourani, M.; Heal, A.; Duncan, R. C.; Burnett, A.; Ashkar, F. C. & Serafini, A. N. (1985). Subacute and chronic bone infections: diagnosis using In-111, Ga-67 and Tc-99m MDP bone scintigraphy, and radiography. Radiology, Vol. 155, No.2 (May 1985), pp. 501-506, ISSN 0033-8419

Borowski, A. M.; Crow, W. N.; Hdjipavlou, A. G.; Chaljub, G.; Mader, J.; Cesani, F. & vanSonnenberg, E. (1998). Interventional radiology case conference: the University of Texa Medical Branch. Percutaneous management fo pyogenic spondylodiscitis. American Journal of Radiology, Vol. 170, No. 6 (June 1998), pp. 1587-1592, ISSN 0361-803X

Buchelt, M.; Lack, W.; Kutschera, H. P.; Katterschafka, T.; Kiss, H.; Schneider, B. & Kotz, R. (1993). Comparision of tuberculous and pyogenic spondylitis. An analysis of 122 cases. Clinical Orthopaedics and related research, Vol. 296 (November 1993), pp. 192-199, ISSN 0009-921X

Busch, V. J.; Regez R. M.; Heere, B. & Willems, W. J. (2007) Osteoarticular infections in HIV-infected patients: 23 cases among 1,515 HIV-infected patients. Acta Orthopaedica, Vol. 78, No. 6, ( December 2007), pp786-790, ISSN 1745-3674.

Carragee, E. J.; Kim, D.; van der Vlugt, T. & Vittum, D. (1997a). The clinical use of erythrocyte sedimentation rate in pyogenic vertebral osteomyelitis. Spine, Vol. 22, No.18 (September 1997), pp. 2089-2093, ISSN 0362-2436

Carragee, E. J. (1997b). Pyogenic vertebral osteomyelitis. Journal of Bone and Joint Surgery, Vol. 79, No. 6, (June 1997), pp.874-880, ISSN 0021-9355

Chang, M. C.; Wu, H. T.; Lee, C. H.; Liu, C. L. & Chen, T. H. (2006). Tuberculous spondylitis and pyogenic spondylitis: comparatative magnetic resonance imaging features. Spine, Vol 31, No. 7 (April 2006), pp. 782-788, ISSN 0362-2436

Dunbar, J. A.; Sandoe, J. A., Rao, A. S.; Crimmins, D. W.; Baig, W. & Rankine, J. J. (2010). The MRI appearances of early vertebral osteomyelitis and discitis. Clinical Radiology, Vol. 65, No. 12 (December 2010), pp. 974-981, ISSN 0009-9260

Frangen, T. M; Kälicke, T.; Gottwald, M.; Andereya, S.; Andress, H. J.; Russe, O. J.; Müller, E. J.; Muhr, G. & Schinkel, C. (2006). Der Unfallchirurg, Vol. 109, No. 9 (September 2006), pp. 743-753. ISSN 0177-5537

Frazier, D. D.; Campbell, D. R.; Garvey, T. A.; Wiesel, S; Bohlmann, H. H. & Eismont, F. J.(2001). Journal of Bone and Joint Surgery, Vol. 83, No. A4 (April 2001), 560-565, ISSN 0021-9355

Friedman, J. A.; Maher, C. O.; Quast, L. M.; McClelland, R. L. & Ebersold, M. J. (2002). Spontaneous disc space infections in adults. Surgical Neurology, Vol. 57, No. 2 (February 2002), pp. 81-86, ISSN 0090-3019

Golimbu, C.; Firooznia, H. & Rafii M. (1984). CT of osteomyelitis of the spine. American Journal of Roentgenology, Vol. 142, No. 1 (January 1984), pp. 159-163. ISSN 0361-803X

Gouliouris, T.; Aliju S. H. & Brown, N. M. (2010). Spondylodiscitis: update on diagnosis and management. Journal of Antimicrobial Chemotherapy, Vol. 65, No. 3, (November 2010), pp. 11-24, ISSN 0305-7453

Govender, S.; Parbhoo, A. H.; Kumar, K. P. & Annamalai, K. (2001). Anterior spinal decompression in HIV-positive patients with tuberculosis. A prospective study. Journal of Bone & Joint Surgery, Vol. 83, No. 6 (August 2001), pp. 864-867), ISSN 0301-620X

Grados, F.; Lescure, F. X.; Senneville, E.; Flipo, R. M.; Schmit, J. L.; Fardellone, P. (2007). Suggestions for managing pyogenic (non-tuberculous) discitis in adults. Joint, Bone, Spine, Vol 74, No. 2 (March 2007), pp. 133-139, ISSN 1297-319X

Grammatico, L.; Baron, S.; Rusch, E.; Lepage, B.; Surer, N.; Desenclos, J. C. & Besnier, J. M. (2008). Epidemiology of vertebral osteomyelitis (VO) in France: analysis of hospital-discharge data 2002-2003. Epidemiology and Infection, Vol. 136, No. 5 (May 2008), pp. 653-660, ISSN 0950-2688

Hoekman, P.; van de Perre, P.; Nelissen, J.; Kwisanga, B.; Bogaerts, J. & Kanyangabo, F. (1991). Increased frequency of infection after open reduction of fractures in patients who are seropositive for human immunodeficiency virus. Journal of Bone and Joint Surgery, Vol. 73, No. 5 (June 1991), ISSN 0021-9355

Horberg, M. A.; Hurley, L. B.; Klein, D. B; Follansbee, S.E.; Quesenberry, C.; Flamm, J. A.; Green, G. M. & Luu, T. (2006). Surgical outcomes in human immunodeficiency virus-infected patients in the era of highly active antiretroviral therapy. Archives of Surgery, Vol. 141, No. 12 (December 2006), pp. 1238-1245, ISSN 0272-5533

Hsieh, P. C.; Wienecke, R. J.; O'Shaughnessy, B. A.; Koski, T. R. & Ondra, S. L. (2004). Surgical strategies for vertebral osteomyelitis and epidural abscess. Neurosurgical Focus, Vol. 17, No. 6 (December 2004), E4, ISSN 1092-0684

Jevtic, V. (2004). Vertebral infection. European Radiology, Vol. 14, No. 3 (March 2004), pp. 43-52, ISSN 0938-7994

Jimenez-Mejias, M. E.; De Dios Colmenero, J.; Sanchez-Lora, F. J.; Palomino-Nicas, J.; Requera, J. M.; Garcia de la Heras, J.; Garcia-Ordonez, M. E.; Pachon, J. Postoperative spondylodiscitis: etiology, clinical findings, prognosis, and comparison with nonoperative pyogenic spondylodiscitis. Clinical Infectious diseases, Vol. 29, No. 2 (August 1999), pp.339-345, ISSN 1058-4838

Kulowski, J. (1936). Pyogenic osteomyelitis of the spine: an analysis and discussion of 102 cases. Journal of Bone and Joint Surgery, Vol. 18, No. 2, (April 1936), pp. 343-364. ISSN 0021-9355

Leibert, E.; Schluger, N. W.; Bonk, S. & Rom, W. N. (1996). Spinal tuberculosis in patients with human immunodeficiency virus infection: clinical presentation, therapy and outcome. Tubercle and lung disease: The official journal of the International Union against Tuberculosis and Lung Disease, Vol. 77, No. 4 (August 1996), pp. 329-34, ISSN 0962-8479

Lew, D. P.; Waldvogel, F. A. (2004). Osteomyelitis. Lancet, Vol. 364, No. 9431 (July 2004), pp. 369-379, ISSN 0140-6736

Lillie, P.; Thaker, H.; Moss, P.; Baruah, J.; Cullen, L.; Taylor, D. & Barlow, G. (2008). Healthcare associated discitis in the era of antimicrobial resistance. Journal of Clinical Rheumtology, Vol. 14, No. 4 (August 2008), pp. 234-237 ISSN 1076-1608

Lucio, E.; Adesokan, A.; Hadjipavlou, A. G.; Crow, W. N. & Adegboyega, P. A. (2000). Pyogenic spondylodiscitis: a radiologic/pathologic and culture correlation study.

Archives of Pathology and Laboratory Medicine, Vol. 124, No. 5 (May 2000), pp. 712-716, ISSN 0003-9985

Maiuri, F.; Iaconetta, G.; Gallicchio, B.; Manto, A.; Briganti, F. (1997). Spondylodiscitis. Clinical and magnetic resonance diagnosis. Spine, Vol. 22, No. 15 (August 1997), pp. 1741-1746, ISSN 0362-2436

Modic, M. T.; Feiglin, D. H.; Piraino, D. W.; Boumphrey, F.; Weinstein, M. A.; Duchesneau, P. M. & Rehm, S. (1985). Vertebral osteomyelitis: assessment using MR. Radiology, Vol. 157, No. 1 (October 1985), pp. 157-166. ISSN 0033-8419

Mulleman, D.; Philippe, P.; Senneville, E.; Costes, C.; Fages, L.; Deprez, X.; Flipo, R. M. & Duquesnoy, B. (Streptococcal and enterococcal spondylodiscitis (vertebral osteomyelitis). High incidence of infective endocarditis in 50 cases. Journal of Rheumatology, Vol. 33, No. 1 (January 2006), pp.91-97, ISSN 0315-162X

Müller, E. J; Russe, O. J. & Muhr, G. (2004). Osteomyelitis of the spine. Der Orthopäde, Vol. 33, No. 3 (March 2004), pp. 305-315, ISSN 0085-4530

Nichols, L.; Balogh, K. & Silverman, M. (1989). Bacterial infections in the acquired immune deficiency syndrome. Clinicopathologic correlations in a series of autopsy cases. American Journal of Clinical Pathology, Vol. 92, No. 6, pp. 787-790, ISSN 0002-9173

Nolla, J. M.; Ariza, J.; Gomez-Vaquero, C.; Fiter, J.; Bermejo, J.; Valverde, J; Escofet, D. R. & Gudiol, F. (2002). Spontaneous pyogenic vertebral osteomyelitis in nondrug users. Seminars in Arthritis and Rheumatism, Vol. 31, No. 4 (February 2002), pp. 271-278, ISSN 0049-0172

Price, A. C.; Allen, J. H.; Eggers, F. M.; Shaff, M. I.; James, A. E. Jr. (1983). Intervertebral disc-space infection: CT-changes. Radiology, Vol.149, No. 3 (December 1983), pp. 725-9, ISSN 0033-8419

Quinones-Hinojosa, A.; Jun, P.; Jacobs, R., Rosenberg, W. S. & Weinstein, P. R. (2004). General principles in the medical and surgical management of spinal infections: a multidisciplinary approach. Neurosurgical focus, Vol. 17, No. 6 (December 2004), pp. E1, ISSN 1092-0684

Rankine, J. J. ; Barron, D. A.; Robinson, P.; Millner, P. A; Dickson, R. A. (2004). Therapeutic impact of percutaneous spinal biopsy in spinal infection. Postgraduate Medical Journal, Vol. 80, No. 948 (October 2004), pp. 607-609, ISSN 0032-5473

Sackett, D. L.; Rosenberg, W. M.; Gray, J. A.; Haynes, R. B. & Richardson, W. S. (1996). Evidence based medicine: what it is and what it isn't. British Medical Journal, Vol. 312, No. 7023 (January 1996), pp. 71-72.

Sammak, B.; Abd El Bagi M.; Al Shahed, M.; Hamilton, D.; Al Nabulsi, J., Youssef, B. & Al Thagafi, M. (1999). Osteomyelitis: a review of currently used imaging techniques. European Radiology, Vol. 9, No. 5 (August 1999), ISSN 0938-7994

Sapico, F. L. & Montgomerie, J. Z. (1979). Pyogenic vertebral osteomyelitis: report on nine cases and review of the literature. Reviews of infectious diseases, Vol. 1, No. 5 (September-October 1979), pp. 754-776, ISSN 0162-0886

Sapico, F. L. (1996). Microbiology and antimicrobial therapy of spinal infections. The Orthopedic Clinics of North America, Vol. 27, No. 1 (January 1996), pp. 9-13, ISSN 0030-5898

Schlaeffer, F.; Mikolich, D. J. & Mates, S. M. (1987). Technetium Tc 99m diphosphonate bone scan. False-normal findings in elderly patients with hematogenous vertebral osteomyelitis. Archives of Internal Medicine, Vol. 147, No. 11 (November 1987), pp. 2024-2026.

Schmitz, A.; Risse, J. H.; Grünwald, F.; Gassel, F. & Biersack, H. J.; Schmitt, O. (2001). Fluorine-18 fluorodeoxyglucose positron emission tomography findings in spondylodiscitis: preliminary results. European Spine Journal, Vol. 10, No. 6 (December 2001), pp. 534-539. ISSN 0940-6719

Shaltot, A.; Michell, P. A.; Betts, J. A.; Darby, A. J.; Gishen, P. (1982). Jamshidi needle biopsy of bone lesions. Clinical radiology, Vol. 33, No. 2 (March 1982), ISSN 0009-9260

Sharif, H. S.; Aideyan, O. A.; Clark, D. C.; Madkour, M. M.; Aabed, M. Y.; Mattsson, T. A.; al-Deeb, S. M. & Moutaery, K. R. (1989). Brucellar and tuberculous spondylitis: comparative imaging features. Radiology, Vol 171, No. 2 (May 1989), pp. 419-425, ISSN 0938-7994

Sir D'Arcy Power, K. B. E. (1923). Pott's disease fo the spine. British Journal of Surgery, Vol. 11, No. 41 (July 1923), pp. 1-6, ISSN 1365-2168

Sobottke, R.; Seifert, H.; Fätkenheuer, G.; Schmidt, M.; Gossmann, A. & Eysel, P. (2008). Current diagnosis and treatment of spondylodiscitis. Deutsches Ärzteblatt, Vol. 105, No. 10 (March 2008), pp. 181-187, ISSN 1866-0452

Sobottke, R.; Zarghooni, K.; Krengel, M.; Delank, S.; Seifert, H; Fätgenheuer, G.; Ernestus, I.; Källicke, T.; Frangen, T.; Arasteh, K.; Oette, M. & Eysel, P. (2009). Treatment of spondylodiscitis in human immunodefiency virus-infected patients: a comparison of conservative and operative therapy. Spine, Vol. 34, No. 13 (June 2009), pp. E452-458, ISSN 0362-2436

Stumpe, K. D.; Zanetti, M.; Weishaupt, D., Hodler, J.; Boos, N. & von Schulthess, G. K. (2002). FDG positron emission tomography for differentiation of degenerative and infectious endplate abnormalities in the lumbar spine detected on MR imaging. American Journal of Roentgenology, Vol. 179, No. 5 (November 2002), pp. 1151-1157, ISSN 0361-803X

Tali, E. T. (2004). Spinal infections. European Journal of Radiology, Vol. 50, No. 2, (May 2004), pp. 120-133, ISSN 0720-048X

Tayles, N. & Buckley, H. R. (2004). Leprosy and tuberculosis in iron age southeast asia? American Journal of Physical Anthropology, Vol. 125, No. 3 (November 2004), pp. 239-256, ISSN 0002-9483

Turunc, T.; Demiroglu, Y. Z.; Uncu, H.; Colakoglu, S. & Arslan, H. (2007). A comparative analysis of tuberculous, brucellar and pyogenic spontaneous spondylodiscitis patients. Journal of Infection, Vol. 158, No. 63 (August 2007), pp.158-163, ISSN 0163-4453

Van Ooij, A.; Beckers, J. M.; Herpers, M. J. & Walenkamp, G. H. (2000). Surgical treatment of aspergillus spondylodiscitis. European Spine Journal, Vol. 9, No. 1 (February 2000), ISSN 0940-6719

Vassilopoulos, D.; Chalasani, P., Jurado, R. L.; Workowski, K. & Agudelo, C. A. (1997). Medicine, Vol. 76, No. 4 (July 1997), pp. 284-294, ISSN 0025-7974

Weinstein, M. A. & Eismont, F. J. (2005). Infections of the spine in patients with human immunodeficiency virus. Journal of Bone and Joint Surgery, Vol. 87, No. 3 (March 2005), pp. 604-609, ISSN 0021-9355

Wiley, A. M. & Trueta, J. (1959). The vascular anatomy of the spine and its relationship to pyogenic vertebral osteomyelits. Journal of Bone and Joint Surgery, Vol: 41-B (Novemeber 1959), pp. 796-809, ISSN 0301-620X

World Health Organization (2009). Global tuberculosis control epidemiology, strategy and financing. WHO report 2009.World Health Organization Press, Geneva, Switzerland.

# 3

# Natural Killer Cells from HIV Infected Slow Progressors who Carry the Protective HLA-B*27 Allele and Inhibitory KIR3DL1 Receptors have Elevated Poly-Functional Potential Compared to Bw6 Homozygotes

Nicole F. Bernard[1,2,3,10] et al.*
*for the Canadian Cohort of HIV Infected Slow Progressors*
*[1]Research Institute of the McGill University Health Centre*
*[2]Division of Experimental Medicine, McGill University, Clinique du Quartier*
*[3]Division of Clinical Immunology and Allergy,*
*McGill University Health Centre, Toronto, Ontario*
*[10]Centre de Recherche du Centre Hospitalier de l'Université de Montréal*
*Montréal, Québec,*
*Canada*

## 1. Introduction

NK cells are a key component of the innate immune system, which can act early in defences against virally infected and tumor cells (Robertson and Ritz 1990; Bottino, Moretta, and Moretta 2006; Bancroft 1993). They have the capacity to secrete proinflammatory cytokines and lyse their targets without prior antigen sensitization (Cooper, Fehniger, and Caligiuri 2001). They are also involved in regulation of the adaptive immune response through their interaction with dendritic cells (DCs)(Sanabria et al. 2008; Smyth et al. 2005).

---

* Carlos Melendez-Pena[1,2], Philomena Kamya[1,2], Christos M. Tsoukas[1,2,3], Mohamed-Rachid Boulassel[4], Jean-Pierre Routy[1,4], Réjean Thomas[5], Pierre Côté[6], Colin Kovacs[7], Stephen A. Migueles[8], Mark Connors[8], Martin Potter[1], Marianne Harris[9] and Cecile L. Tremblay[10]
*[1]Research Institute of the McGill University Health Centre, Montréal, Québec, Canada*
*[2]Division of Experimental Medicine, McGill University, Montréal, Québec, Canada*
*[3]Division of Clinical Immunology and Allergy, McGill University Health Centre, Montréal, Québec, Canada*
*[4]Immunodeficiency Service and Division of Hematology, Royal Victoria Hospital, Canada*
*McGill University Health Center, Montreal, Quebec, Canada*
*[5]Clinique L'Actuel, Montréal, Québec, Canada*
*[6]Clinique Quartier Latin, Montréal, Québec, Canada*
*[7]Maple Leaf Medical Clinic, Toronto, Canada*
*[8]National Institutes of Allergy and Infectious Diseases, National Institutes of Health, Bethesda, Maryland, United States of America*
*[9]AIDS Research Program, St. Paul's Hospital, University of British Columbia, Vancouver, BC, Canada*
*[10]Centre de Recherche du Centre Hospitalier de l'Université de Montréal, Montréal, Québec, Canada*

Activation of NK cells is regulated through the integration of signals from a number of activating and inhibitory receptors(Lanier 2005). Many of the inhibitory receptors use major histocompatibility complex (MHC) class I or class I-like proteins as their ligands(Lanier 2005). The interaction between inhibitory NK receptors and their ligands during NK cell development is important in educating these cells for subsequent function and for avoiding reactivity to normal cells expressing self MHC class I (Kim et al. 1969; Anfossi et al. 2006). In humans one large family of NK receptors are encoded by the Killer Immunoglobulin-like Receptors (KIR) region that maps to chromosome 19q13.4 (Lanier 2005). The most polymorphic locus among the KIR region genes is *KIR3DL1*, which encodes both inhibitory KIR3DL1 (3DL1) and activating KIR3DS1 (3DS1) alleles (Norman et al. 2007). *3DL1* alleles can be further classified according to their expression levels on the cell surface into high (**h*), low/intermediate (**l*) and null (**004*) (not cell surface expressed) alleles (Yawata et al. 2006; Norman et al. 2007; Gardiner et al. 2001; Pando et al. 2003). Genotypes homozygous for *3DL1* can be divided into 2 groups: **h/*y*, where **y* can be either another **h* allele or **004* with no **l* alleles, and **l/*x*, where **x* can be an **l*, **x* or **004* allele (Martin et al. 2007). 3DL1 receptors recognize a subset of MHC class I HLA-B molecules known as Bw4. HLA-Bw4 differ from the remaining HLA-Bw6 antigens encoded at this locus, which do not interact with 3DL1, in the amino acids present between positions 77 and 83 of the HLA heavy chain (Wan et al. 1986). Bw4 allotypes with isoleucine at position 80 (Bw4*80I) have been reported to be better ligands for many of the 3DL1 alleles (Cella et al. 1994). However, there is evidence that Bw4 antigens with threonine at position 80 (Bw4*80T), particularly HLA-B*2705, interact strongly with certain 3DL1 receptors (Luque et al. 1996).

Epidemiological studies have reported that several *KIR/HLA* combinations are associated with slower progression to AIDS and suppression of viral load (VL) (Martin et al. 2007). Compared to *Bw6* homozygotes (hmz) the *3DL1/HLA-B* combination having the most potent influence on slowing time to AIDS and VL control is *3DL1*h/*y* with *HLA-B*57* (**h/*y+B*57*)(Martin et al. 2007). Previous work from our group showed that NK cells from individuals carrying this genotype combination demonstrated higher functional potential than those from carriers of either the NK receptor genotype or *HLA-B*57* alone or from *Bw6 hmz* (Boulet et al. 2010). In these studies functional potential was defined as the percent contribution of NK cells secreting interferon-γ (IFNγ) and tumor necrosis factor-α (TNF-α) and expressing CD107a, a marker of degranulation to the total response to stimulation with the HLA devoid K562 cell line. Furthermore, NK cells from carriers of **h/*y+B*57* had higher functional potential than carriers of *3DL1*h/*y* with other *Bw4* alleles(Boulet et al. 2010). HLA-B*57 is an HLA antigen considered to be protective in the context of HIV infection(Kaslow, Dorak, and Tang 2005; Altfeld et al. 2003; Leslie et al. 2004; Carrington, Martin, and van Bergen 2008). While the protective effect conferred by HLA-B*57 is mediated at least in part through $CD8^{+}$ T cell recognition of HIV epitopes restricted by this antigen, epidemiological studies and our results support the possibility that HLA-B*57's protective effect may also be mediated through its ability to educate NK cells for superior functional potential (Martin et al. 2002; Martin et al. 2007; Leslie et al. 2004; Miura et al. 2009; Leslie et al. 2005).

Murine models have shown using single MHC class I transgenic mice that MHC class I molecules can differ from each other in the potency of their NK education signals, which directly translates into activation potency upon encountering cells lacking that MHC ligand (Brodin, Karre, and Hoglund 2009). Since NK cells from **h/*y+B*57* carriers had higher functional potential than carriers of *3DL1*h/*y* with other *Bw4* alleles, HLA-B*57 may be an example in humans of an MHC class I antigen with an NK education potency that is superior to that of most other HLA-Bw4 molecules. HLA-B*27 is another allele considered to be protective in the context of HIV infection (Kaslow et al. 1996; Carrington and Bontrop 2002; Goulder, Edwards et al. 1997; Trachtenberg et al. 2003). Like HLA-B*57, its protective effect is mediated at least in part through immune pressure exerted by CD8+ T cells (Schneidewind et al. 2009; Goulder, Phillips et al. 1997; den Uyl, van der Horst-Bruinsma, and van Agtmael 2004; Goulder et al. 2001). In this report we questioned whether HLA-B*27, like HLA-B*57, could also act as a ligand for 3DL1 NK receptors that was superior to other HLA-Bw4 alleles in terms of its ability to educate NK cells for functional potential. *HLA-B*27* is found at a higher frequency among the approximately 5% of HIV infected individuals that we have classified as Slow Progressors (SP) compared with HIV infected individuals exhibiting a typical rate of disease progression or uninfected subjects (Carrington, Martin, and van Bergen 2008; Kaslow, Dorak, and Tang 2005). SP are defined by either exhibiting spontaneous control of viremia or maintaining CD4 counts >400 cells/mm3 for at least 7 years post-infection (Madec et al. 2005; Deeks and Walker 2007). In order to determine whether HLA-B*27, like HLA-B*57, could educate NK cells from *3DL1* hmz individuals for superior functional potential we compared the functional potential of NK cells from *3DL1 hmz+B*27* (*3DL1+B*27*) carriers with that from *3DL1 hmz* who were *Bw6 hmz* (*3DL1+Bw6*) or who expressed at least 1 *Bw4* alleles other than *B*57* or *B*27* (*3DL1+Bw4*). NK cells from *3DL1+B*27* carriers had a significantly higher functional potential than those from *3DL1+Bw6*. When the functional potential of NK cells from carriers of the 3DL1 NK receptor /HLA-B ligand pairs **h/*y+B*57*, *3DL1+B*27* and *3DL1+Bw4* were compared we observed decreasing levels in the functional potential where NK cells responded to missing self with a *h/*y+B*57* > *3DL1+B*27* > *3DL1+Bw4* hierarchy.

## 2. Materials and methods

### 2.1 Study population

A total of 51 HIV-infected SP were studied. Forty four were from the Canadian Cohort of HIV Infected Slow Progressors and 7 were from a cohort followed at the National Institutes of Allergy and Infectious Diseases (NIAID) (Migueles et al. 2008). The term SP was used here to define treatment naïve HIV infected subjects who maintained absolute CD4 counts above 400 cells/mm$^3$ for more than 7 years or who were followed for at least 1 year with VL <3000 copies/ml of plasma. Information on CD4, CD8 T cell counts, VL and duration of infection at time of testing, *3DL1* genotype and *HLA-B* allotype of the study population is provided in Table 1. All individuals in the study populations are *3DL1 hmz* to eliminate the possible confounding effect on NK function of expressing the activating 3DS1 receptor, which is an allele at this locus (Martin et al. 2007; Boulet et al. 2008; Yawata et al. 2006). The study population is classified into 4 groups: group 1 (n=12) carry the *3DL1+B*27* genotype, group 2 (n=13) are *3DL1+Bw4*, group 3 (n=14) are *3DL1+Bw6* and group 4 (n=12) are **h/*y+B*57*. Informed consent was obtained from all study subjects and research conformed to the ethical guidelines of the authors' institutions.

### 2.2 MHC and KIR typing

All subjects were typed for MHC class I alleles by sequence-based typing using kits from Atria Genetics (South San Francisco, CA) and Assign software to interpret sequence information for allele typing (Conexio Genetics, Perth, Australia) as previously described

(Boulet et al. 2010). *HLA-Bw6 hmz* subjects lacked any *HLA-Bw4* alleles at the *HLA-A* or *B* locus. *3DL1/S1* genotyping was performed using two sets of primers specific for the *3DL1* and *3DS1* alleles at the 3DL1 locus as previously described (Boulet et al. 2008). Subjects were subsequently *3DL1* allotyped by identifying single nucleotide polymorphisms (SNP) corresponding to high frequency *3DL1* alleles as previously described (Boulet et al. 2010). In our study we categorized *3DL1*005, *006, *007, *053, *054* as **l* alleles, *3DL1*001, *002, *008, *009, *015, *020* as **h* alleles and **004* as a null allele.

| Subjects ID | gender[1] | Age[2] | Time infected[2] | Group[3] | *HLA-B1* | *HLA-B2* | *KIR* genotype[4] | CD4[5] | CD8[5] | VL[6] |
|---|---|---|---|---|---|---|---|---|---|---|
| 1001 | M | 59 | 2.9 | 1 | B15:01 | B27:05 | *h/*y | 760 | 900 | 1.7 |
| 1002 | M | 59 | 14.6 | 1 | B15:01 | B27:05 | *h/*y | 788 | 2498 | 4.12 |
| 1003 | M | 61 | 23.5 | 1 | B27:02 | B67:01 | *h/*y | 670 | 1050 | 4.7 |
| 1004 | M | 49 | 20.2 | 1a | B27:05 | B57:01 | *h/*y | 830 | 1700 | 3.91 |
| 1005 | M | 37 | 2.5 | 1 | B27:05 | B40:02 | *h/*y | 1040 | 1090 | 1.7 |
| 1006 | M | 40 | 3.7 | 1 | B14:02 | B27:05 | *h/*y | 820 | 570 | 1.7 |
| 1007 | M | 71 | 5.2 | 1 | B27:03 | B51:01 | *l/*x | 590 | 114 | 1.7 |
| 1008 | F | 31 | 1.2 | 1a | B27:05 | B57:01 | *l/*x | 489 | 672 | 1.7 |
| 1009 | F | 59 | 13.2 | 1 | B27:03 | B49:01 | *l/*x | 692 | 627 | 1.7 |
| 1010 | M | 38 | 2.3 | 1 | B15:01 | B27:05 | *l/*x | 396 | 936 | 1.7 |
| 1011 | M | 63 | 25.0 | 1 | B27:05 | B51:01 | *h/*y | 340 | 748 | 1.7 |
| 1012 | M | 41 | 6.4 | 1 | B07:02 | B27:05 | *l/*x | 710 | 970 | 3.25 |
| 2001 | M | 35 | 6.5 | 2 | B15:02 | B51:02 | *l/*x | 500 | NA | 3.24 |
| 2002 | F | 39 | 15.9 | 2 | B49:01 | B58:02 | *h/*y | 400 | 510 | 3.54 |
| 2003 | M | 15 | 8.0 | 2 | B38:01 | B51:01 | *h/*y | 596 | 1614 | 2.08 |
| 2004 | M | 45 | 16.2 | 2 | B07:02 | B51:01 | *h/*y | 440 | 350 | 3.54 |
| 2005 | F | 46 | 14.7 | 2 | B07:02 | B38:01 | *l/*x | 720 | 720 | 1.7 |
| 2006 | M | 47 | 17.0 | 2 | B39:01 | B35:01 | *h/*y | 546 | 572 | 5.21 |
| 2007 | M | 46 | 1 | 2 | B53:01 | B58:01 | *l/*x | 870 | 550 | 1.7 |
| 2008 | M | 49 | 7.3 | 2 | B44:03 | B53:01 | *l/*x | 360 | 1610 | 2.8 |
| 2009 | F | 40 | 2.8 | 2 | B07:02 | B13:01 | *h/*y | 1487 | 712 | 3.76 |
| 2010 | F | 50 | 6.9 | 2 | B15:03 | B44:02 | *h/*y | 590 | 1650 | 3.73 |
| 2011 | F | 44 | 22.2 | 2 | B44:02 | B52:02 | *h/*y | 420 | 1180 | 3.15 |
| 2012 | F | 32 | 5.1 | 2 | B14:02 | B44:03 | *l/*x | 715 | 384 | 1.7 |
| 2013 | F | 36 | 6.3 | 2 | B49:01 | B53:01 | *h/*y | 535 | 793 | 2.43 |
| 3001 | M | 34 | 3.0 | 3 | B07:02 | B14:02 | *l/*x | 680 | 890 | 2.85 |
| 3002 | M | 40 | 14.4 | 3 | B14:02 | B15:01 | *h/*y | 343 | 804 | 1.7 |
| 3003 | M | 40 | 4.7 | 3 | B14:02 | B14:02 | *h/*y | 350 | 730 | 3.41 |
| 3004 | M | 40 | 3.4 | 3 | B07:02 | B07:02 | *h/*y | 985 | 605 | 3.3 |
| 3005 | M | 46 | 5.6 | 3 | B15:10 | B41:01 | *l/*x | 530 | 390 | 1.7 |
| 3006 | F | 42 | 4.0 | 3 | B07:05 | B35:01 | *l/*x | 919 | 1557 | 1.7 |
| 3007 | F | 57 | 3.1 | 3 | B07:02 | B42:01 | *l/*x | 636 | 663 | 1.7 |

| Subjects ID | gender[1] | Age[2] | Time infected[2] | Group[3] | *HLA-B1* | *HLA-B2* | *KIR* genotype[4] | CD4[5] | CD8[5] | VL[6] |
|---|---|---|---|---|---|---|---|---|---|---|
| 3008 | M | 53 | 4.1 | 3 | B07:02 | B14:02 | *h/*y | 447 | 455 | 3.3 |
| 3009 | M | 29 | 4.2 | 3 | B07:02 | B14:02 | 3DL1 hmz | 516 | 788 | 2.89 |
| 3010 | F | 61 | 14.3 | 3 | B07:02 | B18:01 | *l/*x | 810 | 1050 | 1.7 |
| 3011 | F | 39 | 6.6 | 3 | B42:01 | B45:01 | *h/*y | 620 | 408 | 2.69 |
| 3012 | M | 39 | 9.9 | 3 | B14:02 | B40:06 | *h/*y | 720 | 1820 | 2.59 |
| 3013 | M | 46 | 7.0 | 3 | B07:02 | B07:05 | *h/*y | 970 | 1210 | 1.94 |
| 3014 | M | 62 | 17.5 | 3 | B14:01 | B81:01 | *h/*y | 650 | 2110 | 4.46 |
| 4001 | F | 39 | 3.0 | 4 | B57 | B7 | *h/*y | 1443 | 895 | 1.7 |
| 4002 | F | 55 | 23.8 | 4 | B57 | B57 | *h/*y | 277 | 385 | 1.7 |
| 4003 | M | 58 | 20.5 | 4 | B57 | B15 | *h/*y | 883 | 590 | 1.7 |
| 4004 | M | 41 | 11.2 | 4 | B40:01 | B57:01 | *h/*y | 1200 | 860 | 1.7 |
| 4005 | M | 61 | 11.0 | 4 | B40:02 | B57:01 | *h/*y | 770 | 990 | 3.9 |
| 4006 | M | 45 | 14.9 | 4 | B07:02 | B57:01 | *h/*y | 650 | 1460 | 4.21 |
| 4007 | F | 39 | 2.6 | 4 | B35:01 | B57:01 | *h/*y | 530 | NA | 1.7 |
| 4008 | M | 24 | 2.0 | 4 | B07:02 | B57:01 | *h/*y | 680 | 880 | 3.1 |
| 4009 | M | 49 | 10.0 | 4 | B57 | B13 | *h/*y | 955 | 881 | 1.7 |
| 4010 | M | 58 | 18.0 | 4 | B57 | B44 | *h/*y | 1329 | 1243 | 1.7 |
| 4011 | M | 46 | 21.0 | 4 | B57 | B81 | *h/*y | 1362 | 1055 | 1.7 |
| 4012 | M | 36 | 7.0 | 4 | B57 | B52 | *h/*y | 780 | 739 | 1.7 |

Table 1. Study population characteristics. [1] M=male/ F=female, [2] in years, [3] 1= 3DL1+B*27; 2=3DL1+Bw4; 3=3DL1+Bw4; 4=*h/*y+B*57. The 2 subjects with the 1a designation carry both a B*27 and B*57 allele, [4] the individual classified as 3DL1 hmz has not been allotyped for KIR3DL1 alleles, [5] cells/mm$^3$, [6] VL= $\log_{10}$ viral load copies/ml plasma.

### 2.3 Cells

Peripheral blood mononuclear cells (PBMC) were isolated by density gradient centrifugation (Ficoll-Paque Pharmacia Upsala, Sweden) from whole blood obtained by venipuncture into tubes containing EDTA anti-coagulant or by leukaphersis as previously described (Boulassel et al. 2003). Cells were cryopreserved in 10% DMSO (Sigma-Aldrich, St. Louis, MO) with 90% fetal bovine serum (FBS, Wisent, St. Bruno, Quebec, Canada).

### 2.4 NK cell functional potential

Cryopreserved PBMC were thawed and resuspended at $10^6$ cells/ml in RPMI 1640 (Wisent) that contained 10% FBS (Wisent), 2mM L-glutamine and 50 IU penicillin and 50µg/ml streptomycin (Wisent). Brefeldin A (at 5µg/ml, Sigma-Aldrich), Monensin (at 6µg/ml, Golgi-Stop; BD Biosciences, Mississauga, Ontario, Canada) and anti-CD107a–FITC mAb (BD Biosciences) were added to the cells. One million PBMCs were stimulated with media alone or HLA devoid K562 cells (American Type Culture Collection Manassas, VA) at a PBMC to K562 cell ratio of 5:1 or with 1.25µg/ml phorbol 12-myristate 13-acetate (PMA); 0.25µg/ml ionomycin, (Sigma-Aldrich) as a positive control for 6 hours at 37°C in a humidified 5% $CO_2$

incubator. All stimulation data shown is from cells that generated a positive result in the PMA and ionomycin stimulation condition.

Cells were stained for viability using the Aqua LIVE/DEAD® fixable dead cell stain kit (Invitrogen, Burlington, Ontario, Canada) following manufacturer's instructions. Cells were then stained for cell surface markers with anti-CD56-APC, anti-CD16-Pacific Blue (BD Biosciences), anti-CD3-ECD and CD158e-PE (ie: Z27-PE, Beckman Coulter, Mississauga, Ontario, Canada) for 30 min. After washing with phosphate buffered saline (PBS) containing 1% FBS (Wisent), cells were fixed and permeabilized using the Fix and Perm Kit (Invitrogen) and stained for intracellular cytokines using anti-IFN-γ-Alexa 700 and anti-TNF-α-PE-Cy7 (BD Biosciences). Cells were washed and fixed with 1% paraformaldehyde solution (Fisher Scientific, Ottawa Ontario, Canada) and kept in the dark at 4°C until acquisition.

### 2.5 Flow cytometry analysis

Between 400,000 and 500,000 events were acquired per sample using an LSRII flow cytometer (BD Biosciences). Analysis for NK cell activation was performed using FlowJo software version 9.1 (Tree Star, San Carlos, CA). The functional profiles of stimulated NK cells were determined using a gating strategy where NK cells were defined as $CD3^-CD56^{+/-}$ $CD16^{+/-}$. Boolean gating was used to identify seven NK cell functional profiles, i.e. tri-functional NK cells ($CD107a^+$ $IFN\text{-}\gamma^+$ $TNF\text{-}\alpha^+$), bi-functional NK cells (any combination of two of these functions) and mono-functional NK cells (any single one of these functions). All results for the frequency of individual functional subsets were background corrected by subtracting the frequency of positive NK cells in the unstimulated subset. Corrected results were used to generate the percent contribution of each functional subset to the total NK cells response to K562. Results reported as subset frequency or percent contribution of a subset to the total K562 response showed a high level of correlation with each other (Boulet et al. 2010).

### 2.6 Statistical analysis

GraphPad Instat 3.05 and GraphPad Prism 5.04 were used for statistical analyses and graphical presentations. A Kruskal-Wallis test was used to assess the significance of between group differences in age, duration of infection at the time point tested, CD4 counts, CD8 counts and VL. Mann-Whitney *U* tests were used to test the significance of between group differences in the percent contribution of an NK cell functional subset to the total NK cell response. A Spearman correlation test was used to test the significance of the trend towards declining tri-functional potential with 3DL1/HLA-B genotype combinations. A *p* value of <0.05 was considered significant.

## 3. Results

### 3.1 Study population

Table 2 provides information on the average and standard deviation for age, duration of infection, CD4 count, CD8 count and $log_{10}$VL at the time point tested for NK functional potential for SP classified as *3DL1+B*27, 3DL1+Bw4, 3DL1+Bw6* and **h/*y+B*57* described in Table 1. No between-group differences were seen for any of these parameters (Krukal-Wallis test).

| | *3DL1+B*27* (n=12) | *3DL1+Bw4* (n=13) | *3DL1+Bw6* (n=14) | **h/*y+B*57* (n=12) |
|---|---|---|---|---|
| **Age[1]** | 50.7 ± 12.8[3] | 40.1 ± 9.5 | 44.9 ± 10.0 | 45.9 ± 11.0 |
| **Duration of infection[1]** | 10.1 ± 8.9 | 10.0 ± 6.5 | 7.2 ± 4.8 | 12.1 ± 7.6 |
| **CD4[2]** | 677 ± 198 | 619 ± 306 | 655 ± 211 | 904 ± 363 |
| **CD8[2]** | 989 ± 606 | 887 ± 494 | 963 ± 533 | 907 ± 292 |
| **$Log_{10}$ VL** | 2.53 ± 1.2 | 2.95 ± 1.0 | 2.57 ± 0.86 | 2.21 ± 0.95 |

Table 2. Summary of study population characteristics. [1] In years, [2] Cells/$mm^3$, [3] Means ± standard deviation.

### 3.2 NK cells from *3DL1+B*27* carriers have a higher functional potential than those from *3DL1+Bw6*

To investigate whether NK cells from HIV-infected SPs carrying the *3DL1+B*27* genotype for an NK receptor/HLA-B ligand pair differ in their NK cell functional potential compared to *Bw6 hmz* with no ligand for 3DL1 receptors, we measured the frequency of NK cells expressing CD107a and secreting IFN-γ and TNF-α from K562-stimulated NK cells using eight colour multi-parametric flow cytometry. In this analysis CD107a expressing NK cells were the sum of the mono-, bi- and tri-functional functional subsets expressing CD107a. This was also the case for IFN-γ and TNF-α secreting NK cells. As shown in Figure 1A the median (range) frequency of NK cells from *3DL1+B*27* versus *3DL1+Bw6* carriers expressing CD107a was 6.92% (3.01%, 17.15%) versus 4.27% (0.74%, 13.32%), secreting IFN-γ was 8.91% (4.25%, 21.52%) versus 5.17% (0.55%, 25.92%) and secreting TNF-α was 0.92% (0.11%, 3.67%) versus 0.23% (0.01%, 3.06) ($p<0.05$ for all comparisons; Mann-Whitney test). Therefore, the frequency of NK cells with any of these functions was significantly greater when NK cells were from *3DL1+B*27* individuals than from *3DL1+Bw6*.

Since we simultaneously measured these three functions following K562 stimulation we were able to assess the frequency of seven possible NK cell functional profiles and their percent contribution to the total K562 response. Figure 1B shows the percent contribution of each NK cell functional profile in PBMC from 12 *3DL1+B*27* and 14 *3DL1+Bw6* subjects. Of the seven possible NK cell functional profiles, only the percent contribution of tri-functional NK cells to the total K562 response was significantly higher in the *3DL1+B*27* group versus *3DL1+Bw6* SPs (2.99% [0.00%, 6.43%]) and (0.52% [0.00%, 7.36%]) for 3DL1+*B*27* and *3DL1+Bw6*, respectively, $p=0.019$; Mann-Whitney *U* test). Based on these results we concentrated on the tri-functional NK subset in subsequent analyses.

We next compared the K562 stimulated NK cells from *3DL1+B*27* individuals to that from carriers of *3DL1+Bw4*. NK cells from **h/*y+B*57* carriers have previously been shown to have superior tri-functional potential compared to *3DL1+Bw6* and *h/*y+*Bw4* subjects (Boulet et al. 2010; Kamya et al. 2011). Since *HLA-B*57* is a *Bw4* allele we excluded carriers of either *HLA-B*57* or *HLA-B*27* alleles from the *3DL1+Bw4* group. Although the tri-functional potential of NK cells from 13 *3DL1+Bw4* subjects was lower (1.78% [0.00%, 5.71%]) than that from *3DL1+B*27* individuals the difference did not achieve statistical significance ($p=0.2644$; Mann-Whitney *U* test) (**Figure 2A**).

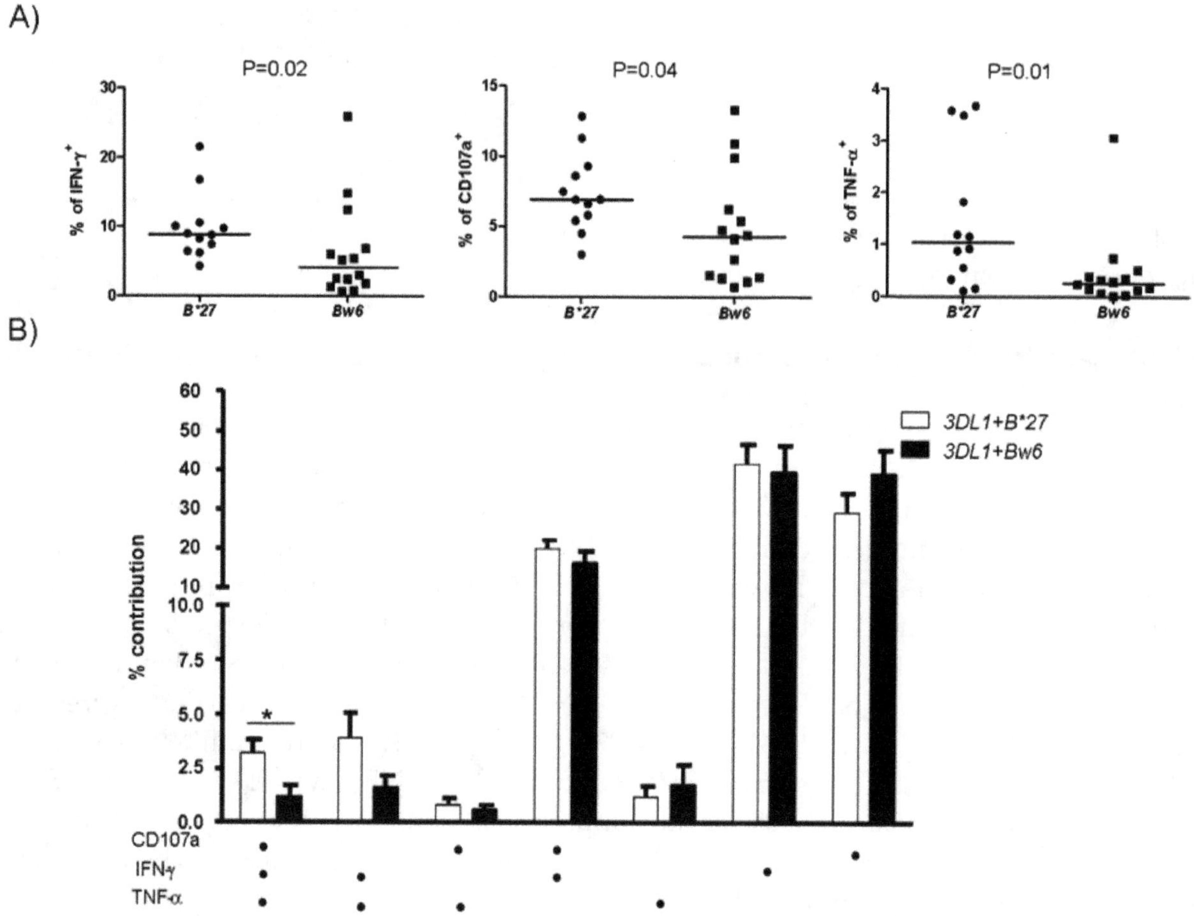


Fig. 1. NK cells from individuals carrying the 3DL1+HLA B*27 NK receptor-ligand pair have an increased functional potential. The frequency of NK cells that secrete IFN-γ (left), express CD107a (middle) or secrete TNF-α (right) in 3DL1 *hmz* individuals who carry *HLA-B*27* or *HLA-Bw6*. Each data point represents a separate individual. The bar through each scatter plot indicates the median frequency for the group. A Mann-Whitney U test was used to assess the significance of between-group comparisons (A). The percent contribution of seven different functional profiles to the total NK cell response to K562 *HLA*-devoid cells from individuals carrying *3DL1+B*27* (n=12) and *3DL1+Bw6* (n=14). Below the *x*-axis, dots refer to the presence of each functional marker (CD107a, IFN-γ and TNF-α) in that profile. The height of each bar represents the median for the group and the height of the error bar the interquartile range for that group. An asterisk (*) over the line linking two bars indicates that the contribution of that functional subset of the NK cell response was significantly different in the two study populations. A Mann-Whitney U test was used to assess the significance of between-group comparisons and $p<0.05$ was considered significant (B).

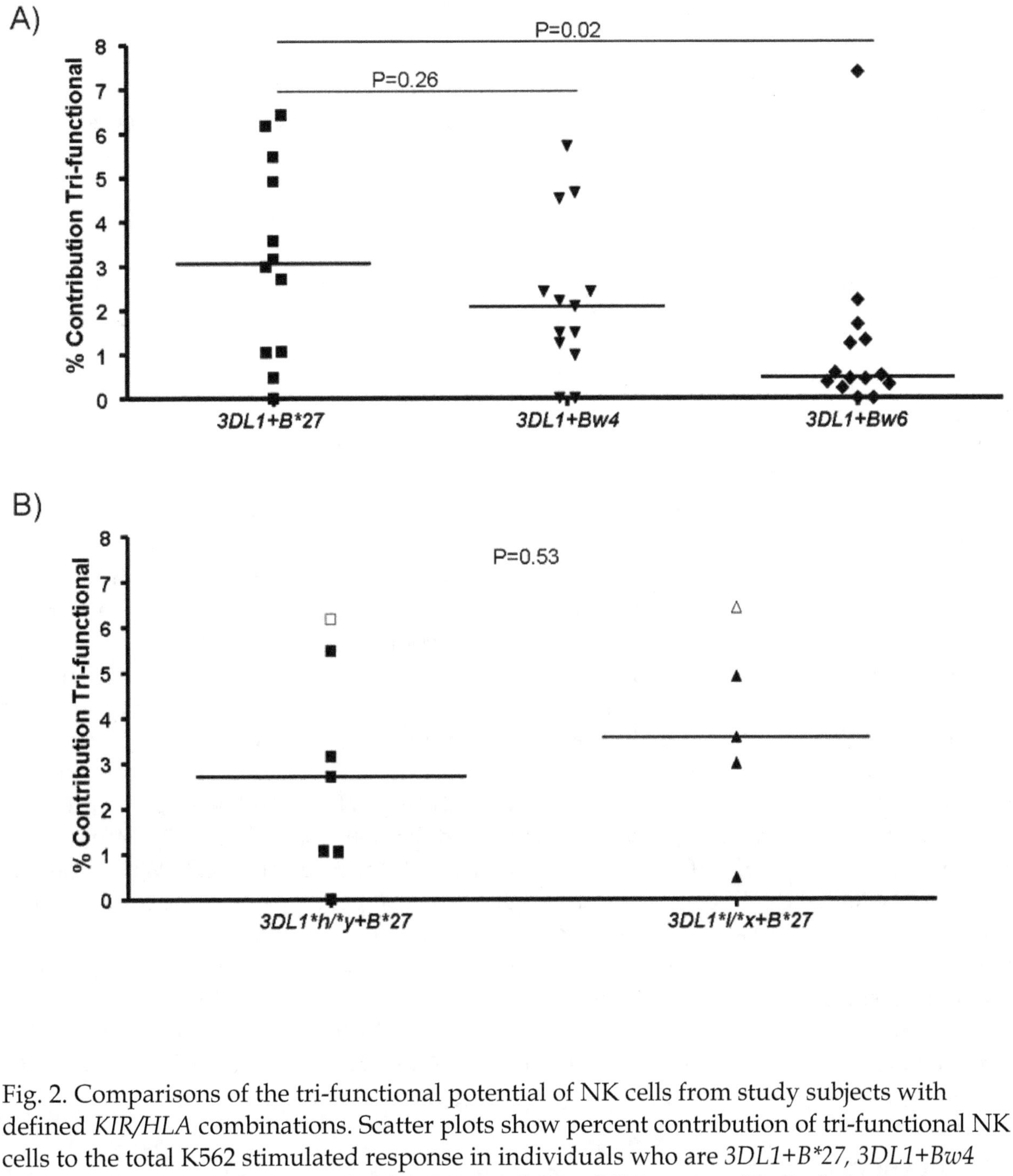


Fig. 2. Comparisons of the tri-functional potential of NK cells from study subjects with defined *KIR/HLA* combinations. Scatter plots show percent contribution of tri-functional NK cells to the total K562 stimulated response in individuals who are *3DL1+B*27, 3DL1+Bw4* and *3DL1+Bw6* carriers (A), and **h/*y+B*27* and **l/*x+B*27* carriers (B). Each data point represents results from a separate individual. The data point represented by an empty square and triangle refer to individuals that carry both *B*27* and *B*57*. The bar through each scatter plot indicates the median frequency for the group. A Mann-Whitney U test was used to assess the significance of between-group differences.

*3DL1 hmz* genotypes can be classified as either **h/*y* or **l/*x* depending on the 3DL1 alleles expressed. Previous work showed that NK cells from **h/*y+B*57* subjects had a significantly higher tri-functional potential than those from **l/*x+B*57* subjects. We therefore questioned whether NK cells from the 7 **h/*y+B*27* and 5 **l/*x+B27* individuals differed from each other in their tri-functional potential. The median (range) NK tri-functional potential was 2.56% (0.00%, 6.18%) and 3.57% (0.47%, 6.43%) for NK cells from carriers of the **h/*y+B*27* and **l/*x+B*27* genotypes, respectively (p=0.53; Mann-Whitney test), a difference that was not statistically significant (Figure 2B). Therefore, HLA-B*27 appears to be able to interact with NK receptor alleles in either the 3DL1 *h/*y and *l/*x genotype categories to educate NK cells for equivalent NK functional potential.

### 3.3 NK cells from *3DL1+B*27 and *h/*y+B*57* carriers have a similar tri-functional potential

Next we questioned whether the level of tri-functional potential of NK cells from *3DL1+B*27* carriers was of a similar magnitude to that seen in NK cells from **h/*y+B*57* carriers. For this analysis we excluded the 2 *3DL1+B*27* individuals who also expressed a *B*57* allele and compared NK tri-functional potential in this group to that in 12 **h/*y+B*57* carriers. As seen in Figure 3A, although the tri-functional potential of NK cells from **h/*y+B*57* carriers was higher than that from *3DL1+B*27* carriers this difference did not achieve statistical significance (p=0.09; Mann-Whitney test).

Pair-wise comparisons of the tri-functional potential of NK cells from carriers of **h/*y+B*57*, *3DL1+B*27* and *3DL1+Bw4* revealed that only the comparison of **h/*y+B*57* and *3DL1+Bw4* was statistically significant. NK cells from each of these groups had higher tri-functional potential than those from the *3DL1+Bw6* group (not shown). Small group sizes and large variability within groups likely contributed to the lack of statistical significance in the tri-functional potential between the **h/*y+B*57* and *3DL1+B*27* and the *3DL1+B*27* and *3DL1+Bw4* groups. We performed another analysis testing for the significance of a trend towards declining NK functional potential among subjects with these *3DL1/HLA-B* genotypes. The rationale for this came from epidemiological studies showing that the effect of *B*57* on time to AIDS and VL control was greater in the presence of **h/*y* than **l/*x 3DL1* genotypes and greater than that of *B*27* on these outcomes in the presence of either *3DL1* genotype (Martin et al. 2007). When the tri-functional potential of NK cells from these 3 *3DL1/HLA-B* genotypes were assessed. Using a test of trend we observed that this measure decreased as follows: **h/*y+B*57* > *3DL1+B*27* > *3DL1+Bw4* (r=-0.40, p=0.01; Spearman's correlation test). Together these results suggest that there is a hierarchy in the impact on NK cell education of HLA-B variants where B*57 is the most potent in the context of **h/*y* genotypes followed by B*27 in the context of *3DL1* genotypes. Furthermore the impact of these alleles is superior to that of other Bw4 alleles co-expressed with *3DL1* genotypes.

## 4. Discussion

We have presented results showing that NK cells from carriers of the *3DL1+B*27* KIR/HLA genotype combination have tri-functional responses to missing self that are 1) significantly higher than those from *3DL1+Bw6* and 2) have a tri-functional potential that falls between that of carriers of **h/*y+B*57* and *3DL1+Bw4*.

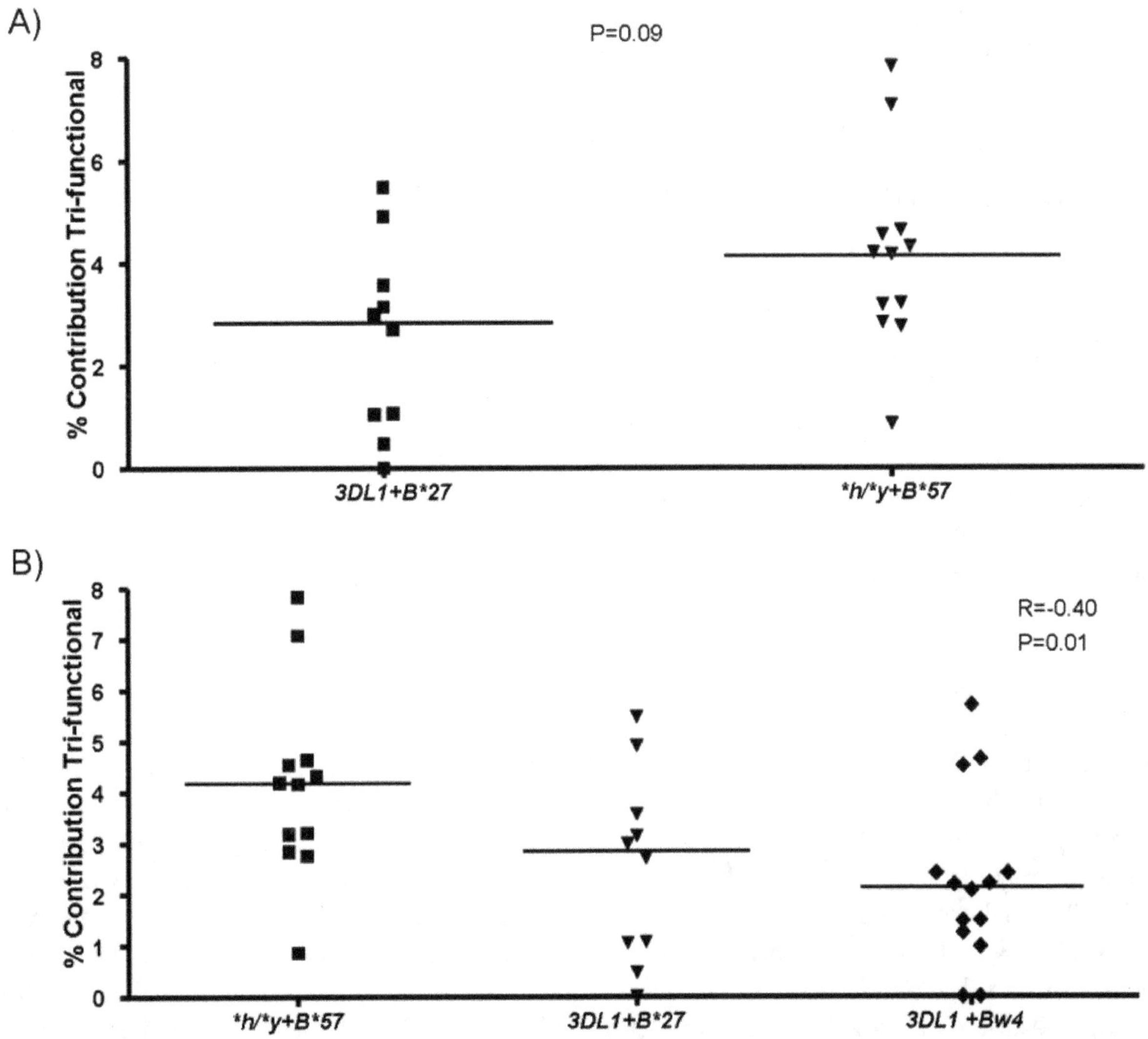


Fig. 3. Comparisons of the tri-functional potential of NK cells from individuals carrying *3DL1+B*27*, **h/*y+HLA-B*57* and *3DL1+Bw4*. Scatter plots show percent contribution of tri-functional NK cells to the total K562 stimulated response in individuals who are *3DL1+B*27* and **h/*y+B*57* carriers (A) or **h/*y+B*57*, *3DL1+B*27* and *3DL1+Bw4* carriers (B). Each data point represents results from a separate individual. The bar through each scatter plot indicates the median frequency for the group. A Mann-Whitney U test was used to assess the significance of between-group differences (A). A Spearman's correlation test was used to assess the significance of a trend towards decreasing functional potential in carriers of these genotype combinations (B).

We previously showed that B*57 is superior to most other Bw4 alleles in educating NK cells through its interaction with 3DL1 NK receptors for functional potential as measured by responses to missing self on K562 cells (Boulet et al 2010; Kamya et al. 2011). These results suggested that B*57, an allele associated with slow time to AIDS and VL control, may contribute to viral control not only through its interaction with HIV epitopes recognized by $CD8^+$ T cell but also through its interaction with 3DL1 inhibitory receptors on NK cells. B*27 is another allele associated with slow time to AIDS and VL control. We therefore sought to determine whether B*27 was also able to educate NK cells for potent responses to missing self. The rationale for investigating the role of B*27 in educating NK cells for NK functional potential in HIV infected SP is that this allele is over represented among SP compared to the uninfected or HIV susceptible subjects. Among 101 SPs enrolled in the Canadian Cohort of HIV Infected SP typed to date 18 (17.8%) were B*27 positive whereas in HIV susceptible subject enrolled in a Primary HIV Infection cohort 26 of 434 (6%) expressed this allele ($p<0.001$; Fisher's Exact test), an allele frequency similar to that seen in uninfected Caucasian (www.allelefrequencies.net). The frequency of individuals expressing both a *B*27* allele and a homozygous *3DL1* genotype would be expected to be even lower. This provided the rationale for investigating this phenomenon in SPs in whom the frequency of the *KIR/HLA* genotype under investigation was higher than in uninfected subjects. We also reasoned that SPs with either controlled viremia or long term non progression would constitute a population with limited NK dysfunction due to HIV infection.

Others have reported that HIV infection dysregulates NK cell subset distribution such that there is a reduction in the frequency of the $CD56^{+}CD16^{+}$ NK subset with cytolytic activity with an associated increase the frequency of an anergic $CD56^{-}/CD16^{+}$ subset (Mavilio et al. 2005; Tarazona et al. 2002). VL seems to play a key role in this redistribution of NK cell subsets. Even though a decrease of cytotoxic NK cells is observed in SPs compared to healthy controls it is not as pronounced as that observed in viremic HIV infected progressor subjects (O'Connor et al. 2007; Barker et al. 2007). NK function may be altered by direct contact with HIV. The gp120 Envelope glycoprotein has been shown to suppress the activity, proliferation and survival of NK cells (Kottilil et al. 2006). Perturbations in the NK cell receptor repertoire have been reported in HIV infection, affecting both inhibitory and activating receptors (Kottilil et al. 2004; Mavilio et al. 2003; De Maria et al. 2003; O'Connor et al. 2007). Furthermore, HIV can escape NK cell recognition by restricting upregulation of activating NK cell receptor ligands such as NKp44L (Fausther-Bovendo et al. 2009), MICA and ULBP1 and 2 (Cerboni et al. 2007) and by preventing downregulation of HLA-C/E (Bonaparte and Barker 2004). Results reported by Kamya et al. demonstrated a negative correlation between NK cell tri-functional potential and VL suggesting VL and HIV infection negatively impact NK function (Kamya et al. 2011). In summary, although NK function in SPs may be affected by HIV infection the effect would be expected to be limited in this population. Our results demonstrate that NK cells from *3DL1+B*27* SPs can produce IFN-γ and TNF-α and express CD107a following K562 stimulation to a greater extent than those from *3DL1+Bw6*. This finding is unlikely to be due to difference of VL as these 2 groups had a similar VL (Table 2).

We have previously shown that NK cells from SP who carry **h/*y+B*57* have a level of tri-functional potential that is significantly higher than those from individuals carrying either *3DL1*h/*y* or *3DL1*l/*x* genotypes with *Bw4* alleles other than *B*27* or *B*57*. The elevated tri-functional potential of NK cells from **h/*y+B*57* carriers depends on the presence of both the *3DL1*h/*y* receptor genotype and *HLA-B*57* since carriers of *3DL1*l/*x* with *HLA-B*57* also have significantly lower NK tri-functional potential (Kamya et al. 2011). In contrast, we observed no differences in tri-functional potential in NK cells from *HLA-B*27* positive SPs carrying either the *3DL1*h/*y* or **l/*x* receptor genotypes. It should be noted that a limitation in making this assertion is the small number of subject who were **h/*y+B*27* versus **l/*x+B*27* available to make this comparison. Epidemiological studies found that compared to *Bw6 hmz* the *B*57* effect on time to AIDS and VL control was enhanced in the presence of *3DL1*h/*y* compared to *3DL1*l/*x*. Overall, the effect of *B*27* on these outcomes was more moderate than that of *B*57* in the presence of *3DL1 *h/*y*. Compared to *Bw6 hmz* the *B*27-80T* allele *B*2705* was more protective in the presence of *3DL1*l/*x* than in the presence of *3DL1*h/*y* (Martin et al. 2007). All but one of the *3DL1+B*27* group of subjects in our study population expressed *B*27-80T* alleles (Carrington, Martin, and van Bergen 2008). Furthermore, there is also evidence that B*2705 has a greater affinity for one or more of the KIR3DL1*l allotypes (Luque et al. 1996). Our findings that NK cells from **h/*y+B*27* and **l/*x+B*27* carriers have similar levels of tri-functional potential that may be more modest than of **h/*y+B*57 carriers* is in line with B*27 being able to interact with receptors encoded by *3DL1*h/*y* and **l/*x* genotypes in *3DL1+B*27* carriers and this more effectively that B*57 interacting with receptors encoded by *3DL1*l/*x* genotypes (Kamya et al. 2011). There is also a trend towards NK cells from *3DL1+B*27* carriers having higher function that those from *3DL1+Bw4* individuals. These results argue in favour of HLA-B*27 and B*57 being unique among HLA-Bw4 antigens in their impact on educating NK cells for subsequent activity, although the effect of B*27 is more modest than that of B*57.

According to the rheostat model of NK education, the strength of the inhibitory input received by NK cells determines the threshold of activation that is set in each NK cell. The higher the inhibitory input, the more likely the NK cell will pass the threshold required to respond to stimuli with an increased frequency of effector cells and an increased number of effector functions (Brodin, Karre, and Hoglund 2009). During development, NK cells must acquire sufficient inhibitory signals to prevent autoreactivity through recognition of ligands for inhibitory NK receptors (Valiante et al. 1997; Hoglund et al. 1997). The larger the contribution of given receptor-ligand pairing to NK cell inhibition under homeostatic conditions the more potent a missing self response will be when the ligand is lost. This situation would be encountered in a setting of HIV infection where HIV encoded Nef downmodulates HLA-A and B molecules from the cells surface abrogating inhibitory signals mediated by 3DL1 receptors (Collins et al. 1998; Cohen et al. 1999).

In this report we have focused on comparisons of the tri-functional subset of NK cells. This was done because the percent contribution of this subset to the entire K562 stimulated response was the only functional subset that differed between carriers *3DL1+B*27* and a KIR/HLA receptor-ligand combination unable to signal through 3DL1 NK receptors. NK cells able elicit 3 functions are more potent in terms of the intensity of each of their functions than corresponding mono-functional NK cells (Kamya et al. 2011). This is similar to what has been reported for poly- versus mono-functional $CD8^+$ T cells (Darrah et al. 2007; Betts et al. 2006) Poly-functional HIV-specific $CD8^+$ T cells in SPs may play a role in superior anti-HIV activity (Betts et al. 2006; Makedonas and Betts 2011). This is still a controversial area as the low VL seen in SPs may preserve multi-functional HIV-specific immune response. Although the biological relevance of poly-functional antigen specific $CD8^+$ T cells in HIV infection is not yet clear, they do serve as an indicator of an effective response to HIV. Our experiments did not directly test the anti-viral activity of NK cells since we did not use HIV infected cells as stimuli. The role of tri-functional NK cells in inhibition of viral replication warrants further investigation.

If stimulation with HIV infected cells produces higher functionality in NK cells from *3DL1+B*27* versus *3DL1+Bw6* carriers and tri-functional NK cells are endowed with a superior capacity to suppress viral replication it would be interesting to study the ability of NK cells from *3DL1+Bw6* for other NK cells functions. Our results demonstrate that these individuals have a limited NK cell tri-functional potential upon missing self stimulation. Since these SPs are able to control viral replication and/or maintain CD4 counts above 400 for 7 or more years it is not unreasonable to assume that NK cells from these subjects possess other NK function. NK cells are known to mediated antibody-dependent cell-mediated cytotoxicity which has been shown to play a role in controlling viral replication (Forthal, Landucci, and Daar 2001) and may play a role in preventing infection (Rerks-Ngarm et al. 2009). In addition, NK cells are also able to regulate antiviral immunity by modulating DC function (Gerosa et al. 2002; O'Leary et al. 2006). In the presence of HIV replication the cross talk between NK cells and DC is impaired (Mavilio et al. 2006; Melki et al. 2010; Alter et al. 2010). It would be interesting to assess whether the interaction between NK cells and DC is maintained in SPs, particularly in *3DL1+Bw6* carriers.

## 5. Conclusion

We have demonstrated that NK cells from *3DL1+B*27* SPs have a higher tri-functional potential following K562 stimulation than those from *3DL1+Bw6*. A test of trend found that NK tri-functional potential declines significantly in NK isolated from carriers of the following genotypes: **h/*y+B*57* > *3DL1+B*27* > *3DL1+Bw4*. Our results suggest that although the protective effect on HIV infection conferred by HLA-B*27 is mediated in part by CD8$^+$ T cells recognizing HIV epitopes restricted by this allele, the protective effect of this alleles may also be mediated by its interaction with inhibitory 3DL1 receptors. HLA-B*27, like HLA-B*57, appears to have an impact on NK education that is superior to that of other Bw4 alleles. Although this remains to be demonstrated experimentally we hypothesize that in carriers of certain *3DL1* and *HLA-B*27* or *HLA-B*57* genotypes, virus-infected cells that have down modulated the HLA ligand for their inhibitory 3DL1 NK receptors may be able to recruit a larger number NK cells with multiple functions, which can play a role in viral control. Such information is relevant to vaccine design by providing a rationale for modulating NK activity at the time of vaccination to favor developing protective immunity.

## 6. Acknowledgements

The authors wish to thank the study participants of the Canadian Cohort of HIV Infected SPs and the NIAID Cohort. We are grateful to the following physicians, who recruited and followed study subjects enrolled in the Canadian Cohort for HIV Infected SPs: Drs. Bernard Lessard, Danielle Legault, Benoit Trottier, Michel Boissonault, Serge Dufresne, Jean-Guy Baril, Danièle Longpré, Benoit Trottier, Danielle Rouleau, Howard Turner, Julian Falutz, Joseph Cox, James Allan, John MacLoed, Marina B Klein and Roger LeBlanc. We are also grateful to Ms. Stephanie Matte for Cohort coordination. We thank Mr. Benjamin Tallon, Ms. Marie-Pierre Boisvert, Ms. Tsoarello Mabanga and Mr. Saied Sharafi for the expert technical assistance with HLA and KIR allotyping. This work was supported by grants #HOP-86862 and MOP-111155 from the Canadian Institutes for Health Research (CIHR), and a grant from the Fonds de Recherche en Santé du Québec (FRSQ) AIDS and Infectious Disease Network. CMP was supported by a Ph.D. scholarship from CIHR.

## 7. References

Alter, G., D. Kavanagh, S. Rihn, R. Luteijn, D. Brooks, M. Oldstone, J. van Lunzen, and M. Altfeld. 2010. IL-10 induces aberrant deletion of dendritic cells by natural killer cells in the context of HIV infection. *J Clin Invest* 120 (6):1905-13.

Altfeld, M., M. M. Addo, E. S. Rosenberg, F. M. Hecht, P. K. Lee, M. Vogel, X. G. Yu, R. Draenert, M. N. Johnston, D. Strick, T. M. Allen, M. E. Feeney, J. O. Kahn, R. P. Sekaly, J. A. Levy, J. K. Rockstroh, P. J. Goulder, and B. D. Walker. 2003. Influence of HLA-B57 on clinical presentation and viral control during acute HIV-1 infection. *AIDS* 17 (18):2581-91.

Anfossi, N., P. Andre, S. Guia, C. S. Falk, S. Roetynck, C. A. Stewart, V. Breso, C. Frassati, D. Reviron, D. Middleton, F. Romagne, S. Ugolini, and E. Vivier. 2006. Human NK cell education by inhibitory receptors for MHC class I. *Immunity* 25 (2):331-42.

Bancroft, G. J. 1993. The role of natural killer cells in innate resistance to infection. *Curr Opin Immunol* 5 (4):503-10.

Barker, E., J. Martinson, C. Brooks, A. Landay, and S. Deeks. 2007. Dysfunctional natural killer cells, in vivo, are governed by HIV viremia regardless of whether the infected individual is on antiretroviral therapy. *AIDS* 21 (17):2363-5.

Betts, M. R., M. C. Nason, S. M. West, S. C. De Rosa, S. A. Migueles, J. Abraham, M. M. Lederman, J. M. Benito, P. A. Goepfert, M. Connors, M. Roederer, and R. A. Koup. 2006. HIV nonprogressors preferentially maintain highly functional HIV-specific CD8+ T cells. *Blood* 107 (12):4781-9.

Bonaparte, M. I., and E. Barker. 2004. Killing of human immunodeficiency virus-infected primary T-cell blasts by autologous natural killer cells is dependent on the ability of the virus to alter the expression of major histocompatibility complex class I molecules. *Blood* 104 (7):2087-94.

Bottino, C., L. Moretta, and A. Moretta. 2006. NK cell activating receptors and tumor recognition in humans. *Curr Top Microbiol Immunol* 298:175-82.

Boulassel, M. R., G. Spurll, D. Rouleau, C. Tremblay, M. Edwardes, R. P. Sekaly, R. Lalonde, and J. P. Routy. 2003. Changes in immunological and virological parameters in HIV-1 infected subjects following leukapheresis. *J Clin Apher* 18 (2):55-60.

Boulet, S., S. Sharafi, N. Simic, J. Bruneau, J. P. Routy, C. M. Tsoukas, and N. F. Bernard. 2008. Increased proportion of KIR3DS1 homozygotes in HIV-exposed uninfected individuals. *AIDS* 22 (5):595-9.

Boulet, S., R. Song, P. Kamya, J. Bruneau, N. H. Shoukry, C. M. Tsoukas, and N. F. Bernard. 2010. HIV protective KIR3DL1 and HLA-B genotypes influence NK cell function following stimulation with HLA-devoid cells. *J Immunol* 184 (4):2057-64.

Brodin, P., K. Karre, and P. Hoglund. 2009. NK cell education: not an on-off switch but a tunable rheostat. *Trends Immunol* 30 (4):143-9.

Carrington, M., and R. E. Bontrop. 2002. Effects of MHC class I on HIV/SIV disease in primates. *AIDS* 16 Suppl 4:S105-14.

Carrington, M., M. P. Martin, and J. van Bergen. 2008. KIR-HLA intercourse in HIV disease. *Trends Microbiol* 16 (12):620-7.

Cella, M., A. Longo, G. B. Ferrara, J. L. Strominger, and M. Colonna. 1994. NK3-specific natural killer cells are selectively inhibited by Bw4-positive HLA alleles with isoleucine 80. *J Exp Med* 180 (4):1235-42.

Cerboni, C., F. Neri, N. Casartelli, A. Zingoni, D. Cosman, P. Rossi, A. Santoni, and M. Doria. 2007. Human immunodeficiency virus 1 Nef protein downmodulates the ligands of the activating receptor NKG2D and inhibits natural killer cell-mediated cytotoxicity. *J Gen Virol* 88 (Pt 1):242-50.

Cohen, G. B., R. T. Gandhi, D. M. Davis, O. Mandelboim, B. K. Chen, J. L. Strominger, and D. Baltimore. 1999. The selective downregulation of class I major histocompatibility complex proteins by HIV-1 protects HIV-infected cells from NK cells. *Immunity* 10 (6):661-71.

Collins, K. L., B. K. Chen, S. A. Kalams, B. D. Walker, and D. Baltimore. 1998. HIV-1 Nef protein protects infected primary cells against killing by cytotoxic T lymphocytes. *Nature* 391 (6665):397-401.

Cooper, M. A., T. A. Fehniger, and M. A. Caligiuri. 2001. The biology of human natural killer-cell subsets. *Trends Immunol* 22 (11):633-40.

Darrah, P. A., D. T. Patel, P. M. De Luca, R. W. Lindsay, D. F. Davey, B. J. Flynn, S. T. Hoff, P. Andersen, S. G. Reed, S. L. Morris, M. Roederer, and R. A. Seder. 2007. Multifunctional TH1 cells define a correlate of vaccine-mediated protection against Leishmania major. *Nat Med* 13 (7):843-50.

De Maria, A., M. Fogli, P. Costa, G. Murdaca, F. Puppo, D. Mavilio, A. Moretta, and L. Moretta. 2003. The impaired NK cell cytolytic function in viremic HIV-1 infection is associated with a reduced surface expression of natural cytotoxicity receptors (NKp46, NKp30 and NKp44). *Eur J Immunol* 33 (9):2410-8.

Deeks, S. G., and B. D. Walker. 2007. Human immunodeficiency virus controllers: mechanisms of durable virus control in the absence of antiretroviral therapy. *Immunity* 27 (3):406-16.

den Uyl, D., I. E. van der Horst-Bruinsma, and M. van Agtmael. 2004. Progression of HIV to AIDS: a protective role for HLA-B27? *AIDS Rev* 6 (2):89-96.

Fausther-Bovendo, H., N. Sol-Foulon, D. Candotti, H. Agut, O. Schwartz, P. Debre, and V. Vieillard. 2009. HIV escape from natural killer cytotoxicity: nef inhibits NKp44L expression on CD4+ T cells. *AIDS* 23 (9):1077-87.

Forthal, D. N., G. Landucci, and E. S. Daar. 2001. Antibody from patients with acute human immunodeficiency virus (HIV) infection inhibits primary strains of HIV type 1 in the presence of natural-killer effector cells. *J Virol* 75 (15):6953-61.

Gardiner, C. M., L. A. Guethlein, H. G. Shilling, M. Pando, W. H. Carr, R. Rajalingam, C. Vilches, and P. Parham. 2001. Different NK cell surface phenotypes defined by the DX9 antibody are due to KIR3DL1 gene polymorphism. *J Immunol* 166 (5):2992-3001.

Gerosa, F., B. Baldani-Guerra, C. Nisii, V. Marchesini, G. Carra, and G. Trinchieri. 2002. Reciprocal activating interaction between natural killer cells and dendritic cells. *J Exp Med* 195 (3):327-33.

Goulder, P. J., C. Brander, Y. Tang, C. Tremblay, R. A. Colbert, M. M. Addo, E. S. Rosenberg, T. Nguyen, R. Allen, A. Trocha, M. Altfeld, S. He, M. Bunce, R. Funkhouser, S. I. Pelton, S. K. Burchett, K. McIntosh, B. T. Korber, and B. D. Walker. 2001. Evolution and transmission of stable CTL escape mutations in HIV infection. *Nature* 412 (6844):334-8.

Goulder, P. J., A. Edwards, R. E. Phillips, and A. J. McMichael. 1997. Identification of a novel HLA-B*2705-restricted cytotoxic T-lymphocyte epitope within a conserved region of HIV-1 Nef. *AIDS* 11 (4):536-8.

Goulder, P. J., R. E. Phillips, R. A. Colbert, S. McAdam, G. Ogg, M. A. Nowak, P. Giangrande, G. Luzzi, B. Morgan, A. Edwards, A. J. McMichael, and S. Rowland-Jones. 1997. Late escape from an immunodominant cytotoxic T-lymphocyte response associated with progression to AIDS. *Nat Med* 3 (2):212-7.

Hoglund, P., J. Sundback, M. Y. Olsson-Alheim, M. Johansson, M. Salcedo, C. Ohlen, H. G. Ljunggren, C. L. Sentman, and K. Karre. 1997. Host MHC class I gene control of NK-cell specificity in the mouse. *Immunol Rev* 155:11-28.

Kamya, P., S. Boulet, C. M. Tsoukas, J. P. Routy, R. Thomas, P. Côté, M. R. Boulassel, J. G. Baril, C. Kovacs, S. A. Migueles, M. Connors, T. J. Suscovich, C. Brander, C. L. Tremblay, and N. Bernard for the Canadian Cohort of HIV Infected Slow Progressors. 2011. Receptor-ligand requirements for increased NK cell polyfunctional potential in slow progressors infected with HIV-1 coexpressing KIR3DL1*h/*y and HLA-B*57. *J Virol.* 85(12):5949-60.

Kaslow, R. A., M. Carrington, R. Apple, L. Park, A. Munoz, A. J. Saah, J. J. Goedert, C. Winkler, S. J. O'Brien, C. Rinaldo, R. Detels, W. Blattner, J. Phair, H. Erlich, and D. L. Mann. 1996. Influence of combinations of human major histocompatibility complex genes on the course of HIV-1 infection. *Nat Med* 2 (4):405-11.

Kaslow, R. A., T. Dorak, and J. J. Tang. 2005. Influence of host genetic variation on susceptibility to HIV type 1 infection. *J Infect Dis* 191 Suppl 1:S68-77.

Kim, H. W., J. A. Bellanti, J. O. Arrobio, J. Mills, C. D. Brandt, R. M. Chanock, and R. H. Parrott. 1969. Respiratory syncytial virus neutralizing activity in nasal secretions following natural infection. *Proc Soc Exp Biol Med* 131 (2):658-61.

Kottilil, S., K. Shin, J. O. Jackson, K. N. Reitano, M. A. O'Shea, J. Yang, C. W. Hallahan, R. Lempicki, J. Arthos, and A. S. Fauci. 2006. Innate immune dysfunction in HIV infection: effect of HIV envelope-NK cell interactions. *J Immunol* 176 (2):1107-14.

Kottilil, S., K. Shin, M. Planta, M. McLaughlin, C. W. Hallahan, M. Ghany, T. W. Chun, M. C. Sneller, and A. S. Fauci. 2004. Expression of chemokine and inhibitory receptors on natural killer cells: effect of immune activation and HIV viremia. *J Infect Dis* 189 (7):1193-8.

Lanier, L. L. 2005. NK cell recognition. *Annu Rev Immunol* 23:225-74.

Leslie, A. J., K. J. Pfafferott, P. Chetty, R. Draenert, M. M. Addo, M. Feeney, Y. Tang, E. C. Holmes, T. Allen, J. G. Prado, M. Altfeld, C. Brander, C. Dixon, D. Ramduth, P. Jeena, S. A. Thomas, A. St John, T. A. Roach, B. Kupfer, G. Luzzi, A. Edwards, G. Taylor, H. Lyall, G. Tudor-Williams, V. Novelli, J. Martinez-Picado, P. Kiepiela, B. D. Walker, and P. J. Goulder. 2004. HIV evolution: CTL escape mutation and reversion after transmission. *Nat Med* 10 (3):282-9.

Leslie, A., D. Kavanagh, I. Honeyborne, K. Pfafferott, C. Edwards, T. Pillay, L. Hilton, C. Thobakgale, D. Ramduth, R. Draenert, S. Le Gall, G. Luzzi, A. Edwards, C. Brander, A. K. Sewell, S. Moore, J. Mullins, C. Moore, S. Mallal, N. Bhardwaj, K. Yusim, R. Phillips, P. Klenerman, B. Korber, P. Kiepiela, B. Walker, and P. Goulder. 2005. Transmission and accumulation of CTL escape variants drive negative associations between HIV polymorphisms and HLA. *J Exp Med* 201 (6):891-902.

Luque, I., R. Solana, M. D. Galiani, R. Gonzalez, F. Garcia, J. A. Lopez de Castro, and J. Pena. 1996. Threonine 80 on HLA-B27 confers protection against lysis by a group of natural killer clones. *Eur J Immunol* 26 (8):1974-7.

Madec, Y., F. Boufassa, K. Porter, and L. Meyer. 2005. Spontaneous control of viral load and CD4 cell count progression among HIV-1 seroconverters. *AIDS* 19 (17):2001-7.

Makedonas, G., and M. R. Betts. 2011. Living in a house of cards: re-evaluating CD8+ T-cell immune correlates against HIV. *Immunological reviews* 239 (1):109-24.

Martin, M. P., X. Gao, J. H. Lee, G. W. Nelson, R. Detels, J. J. Goedert, S. Buchbinder, K. Hoots, D. Vlahov, J. Trowsdale, M. Wilson, S. J. O'Brien, and M. Carrington. 2002. Epistatic interaction between KIR3DS1 and HLA-B delays the progression to AIDS. *Nat Genet* 31 (4):429-34.

Martin, M. P., Y. Qi, X. Gao, E. Yamada, J. N. Martin, F. Pereyra, S. Colombo, E. E. Brown, W. L. Shupert, J. Phair, J. J. Goedert, S. Buchbinder, G. D. Kirk, A. Telenti, M. Connors, S. J. O'Brien, B. D. Walker, P. Parham, S. G. Deeks, D. W. McVicar, and M. Carrington. 2007. Innate partnership of HLA-B and KIR3DL1 subtypes against HIV-1. *Nat Genet* 39 (6):733-40.

Mavilio, D., J. Benjamin, M. Daucher, G. Lombardo, S. Kottilil, M. A. Planta, E. Marcenaro, C. Bottino, L. Moretta, A. Moretta, and A. S. Fauci. 2003. Natural killer cells in HIV-1 infection: dichotomous effects of viremia on inhibitory and activating receptors and their functional correlates. *Proc Natl Acad Sci U S A* 100 (25):15011-6.

Mavilio, D., G. Lombardo, J. Benjamin, D. Kim, D. Follman, E. Marcenaro, M. A. O'Shea, A. Kinter, C. Kovacs, A. Moretta, and A. S. Fauci. 2005. Characterization of CD56-/CD16+ natural killer (NK) cells: a highly dysfunctional NK subset expanded in HIV-infected viremic individuals. *Proc Natl Acad Sci U S A* 102 (8):2886-91.

Mavilio, D., G. Lombardo, A. Kinter, M. Fogli, A. La Sala, S. Ortolano, A. Farschi, D. Follmann, R. Gregg, C. Kovacs, E. Marcenaro, D. Pende, A. Moretta, and A. S. Fauci. 2006. Characterization of the defective interaction between a subset of natural killer cells and dendritic cells in HIV-1 infection. *J Exp Med* 203 (10):2339-50.

Melki, M. T., H. Saidi, A. Dufour, J. C. Olivo-Marin, and M. L. Gougeon. 2010. Escape of HIV-1-infected dendritic cells from TRAIL-mediated NK cell cytotoxicity during NK-DC cross-talk--a pivotal role of HMGB1. *PLoS Pathog* 6 (4):e1000862.

Migueles, S. A., C. M. Osborne, C. Royce, A. A. Compton, R. P. Joshi, K. A. Weeks, J. E. Rood, A. M. Berkley, J. B. Sacha, N. A. Cogliano-Shutta, M. Lloyd, G. Roby, R. Kwan, M. McLaughlin, S. Stallings, C. Rehm, M. A. O'Shea, J. Mican, B. Z. Packard, A. Komoriya, S. Palmer, A. P. Wiegand, F. Maldarelli, J. M. Coffin, J. W. Mellors, C. W. Hallahan, D. A. Follman, and M. Connors. 2008. Lytic granule loading of CD8+ T cells is required for HIV-infected cell elimination associated with immune control. *Immunity* 29 (6):1009-21.

Miura, T., M. A. Brockman, A. Schneidewind, M. Lobritz, F. Pereyra, A. Rathod, B. L. Block, Z. L. Brumme, C. J. Brumme, B. Baker, A. C. Rothchild, B. Li, A. Trocha, E. Cutrell, N. Frahm, C. Brander, I. Toth, E. J. Arts, T. M. Allen, and B. D. Walker. 2009. HLA-B57/B*5801 human immunodeficiency virus type 1 elite controllers select for rare gag variants associated with reduced viral replication capacity and strong cytotoxic T-lymphocyte [corrected] recognition. *J Virol* 83 (6):2743-55.

Norman, P. J., L. Abi-Rached, K. Gendzekhadze, D. Korbel, M. Gleimer, D. Rowley, D. Bruno, C. V. Carrington, D. Chandanayingyong, Y. H. Chang, C. Crespi, G. Saruhan-Direskeneli, P. A. Fraser, K. Hameed, G. Kamkamidze, K. A. Koram, Z. Layrisse, N. Matamoros, J. Mila, M. H. Park, R. M. Pitchappan, D. D. Ramdath, M. Y. Shiau, H. A. Stephens, S. Struik, D. H. Verity, R. W. Vaughan, D. Tyan, R. W. Davis, E. M. Riley, M. Ronaghi, and P. Parham. 2007. Unusual selection on the KIR3DL1/S1 natural killer cell receptor in Africans. *Nat Genet* 39 (9):1092-9.

O'Connor, G. M., A. Holmes, F. Mulcahy, and C. M. Gardiner. 2007. Natural Killer cells from long-term non-progressor HIV patients are characterized by altered phenotype and function. *Clin Immunol* 124 (3):277-83.

O'Leary, J. G., M. Goodarzi, D. L. Drayton, and U. H. von Andrian. 2006. T cell- and B cell-independent adaptive immunity mediated by natural killer cells. *Nat Immunol* 7 (5):507-16.

Pando, M. J., C. M. Gardiner, M. Gleimer, K. L. McQueen, and P. Parham. 2003. The protein made from a common allele of KIR3DL1 (3DL1*004) is poorly expressed at cell surfaces due to substitution at positions 86 in Ig domain 0 and 182 in Ig domain 1. *J Immunol* 171 (12):6640-9.

Rerks-Ngarm, S., P. Pitisuttithum, S. Nitayaphan, J. Kaewkungwal, J. Chiu, R. Paris, N. Premsri, C. Namwat, M. de Souza, E. Adams, M. Benenson, S. Gurunathan, J. Tartaglia, J. G. McNeil, D. P. Francis, D. Stablein, D. L. Birx, S. Chunsuttiwat, C. Khamboonruang, P. Thongcharoen, M. L. Robb, N. L. Michael, P. Kunasol, and J. H. Kim. 2009. Vaccination with ALVAC and AIDSVAX to prevent HIV-1 infection in Thailand. *N Engl J Med* 361 (23):2209-20.

Robertson, M. J., and J. Ritz. 1990. Biology and clinical relevance of human natural killer cells. *Blood* 76 (12):2421-38.

Sanabria, M. X., D. A. Vargas-Inchaustegui, L. Xin, and L. Soong. 2008. Role of natural killer cells in modulating dendritic cell responses to Leishmania amazonensis infection. *Infect Immun* 76 (11):5100-9.

Schneidewind, A., Z. L. Brumme, C. J. Brumme, K. A. Power, L. L. Reyor, K. O'Sullivan, A. Gladden, U. Hempel, T. Kuntzen, Y. E. Wang, C. Oniangue-Ndza, H. Jessen, M. Markowitz, E. S. Rosenberg, R. P. Sekaly, A. D. Kelleher, B. D. Walker, and T. M. Allen. 2009. Transmission and long-term stability of compensated CD8 escape mutations. *J Virol* 83 (8):3993-7.

Smyth, M. J., E. Cretney, J. M. Kelly, J. A. Westwood, S. E. Street, H. Yagita, K. Takeda, S. L. van Dommelen, M. A. Degli-Esposti, and Y. Hayakawa. 2005. Activation of NK cell cytotoxicity. *Mol Immunol* 42 (4):501-10.

Tarazona, R., J. G. Casado, O. Delarosa, J. Torre-Cisneros, J. L. Villanueva, B. Sanchez, M. D. Galiani, R. Gonzalez, R. Solana, and J. Pena. 2002. Selective depletion of CD56(dim) NK cell subsets and maintenance of CD56(bright) NK cells in treatment-naive HIV-1-seropositive individuals. *J Clin Immunol* 22 (3):176-83.

Trachtenberg, E., B. Korber, C. Sollars, T. B. Kepler, P. T. Hraber, E. Hayes, R. Funkhouser, M. Fugate, J. Theiler, Y. S. Hsu, K. Kunstman, S. Wu, J. Phair, H. Erlich, and S. Wolinsky. 2003. Advantage of rare HLA supertype in HIV disease progression. *Nat Med* 9 (7):928-35.

Valiante, N. M., M. Uhrberg, H. G. Shilling, K. Lienert-Weidenbach, K. L. Arnett, A. D'Andrea, J. H. Phillips, L. L. Lanier, and P. Parham. 1997. Functionally and structurally distinct NK cell receptor repertoires in the peripheral blood of two human donors. *Immunity* 7 (6):739-51.

Wan A. M., P. Ennis, P. Parham, and N. Holmes. 1986. The primary structure of HLA-A32 suggests a region involved in formation of the Bw4/Bw6 epitopes. *J Immunol* 137(11):3671-4.

Yawata, M., N. Yawata, M. Draghi, A. M. Little, F. Partheniou, and P. Parham. 2006. Roles for HLA and KIR polymorphisms in natural killer cell repertoire selection and modulation of effector function. *J Exp Med* 203 (3):633-45.

4

# HIV-Infection: The Role of Insulin Resistance and Alternative Treatments

Elaheh Aghdassi
*The University Health Network, Toronto, Canada*

## 1. Introduction

The impact of antiretroviral therapy (ART) on the natural history of HIV is indisputable, resulting in dramatic reductions in morbidity and mortality and improvements in quality of life. This recognition coincides with a change in view of HIV infection from a progressive fatal disease to a medically manageable chronic condition. However, the requirement for life-long therapy with ART has been associated with long-term metabolic toxicities (hyperlipidemia, insulin resistance, diabetes, and osteoporosis) and iatrogenic dysmorphias, termed lipodystrophy, that have increased the complexity of managing people living with HIV infection (PLWH), the manifestations of which include peripheral fat loss and central fat accumulation. Lipodystrophy has emerged as one of the most feared complications of ART for PLWH. The highly stigmatizing nature of this adverse event has been associated with feelings of low self-esteem, forced disclosure of HIV-status, and negative effect on antiretroviral adherence. Of more recent significant concern is the finding that the metabolic consequences of lipodystrophy and ART, as well as the inflammation caused by the virus, are strong mediators for the development of cardiovascular disease (CVD), diabetes, metabolic abnormalities, and fatty liver disease and will have important implications for the future health and survival of the PLWH. One of the possible mechanisms contributing to these metabolic abnormalities is insulin resistance (IR) that has been increasingly seen in PLWH. Interventions aimed at improving insulin sensitivity have been shown effective in alleviating some but not all of ART and/or HIV associated adverse outcomes. This chapter will review the evidence for IR as a potential mechanism involved in HIV-related complications and the role of alternative treatments in improving IR in people living with HIV infection.

## 2. Metabolic abnormalities associated with HIV infection

The successful introduction of highly active antiretroviral therapy (HAART), a combination of potent antiretroviral agents, including protease inhibitors (PIs), nucleoside reverse transcriptase inhibitors (NRTIs), and nonnucleoside reverse transcriptase inhibitors (NNRTIs), has impacted positively on morbidity and mortality among HIV-positive patients. However, over time, HAART has been associated with a number of metabolic and anthropometric abnormalities, including dyslipidemia [1-3], hypertension [4-8] and insulin resistance[9-11], as well as subcutaneous fat loss and abdominal obesity, all included in the definition of metabolic syndrome[12] and potentially contributing to CVD risk . In a cohort of HIV-infected adults (296 participants: 217 men and 79 women) of mixed ethnicity with a mean age of 45.3 years, an appreciable prevalence of metabolic syndrome (30.0%) has been reported with the frequency increasing to 42.5% in those over 50 years of age. More women had abdominal obesity (59.5%) than men (20.7%, $P<0.001$) and the frequency of elevated plasma glucose was also higher in females (37.2%) compared to males (16.9%, $P=0.004$). High frequencies of decreased high-density lipoprotein cholesterol (HDL-C) and elevated blood pressure were seen in both sexes. In those under 50 years of age, the 10-year Framingham coronary heart disease risk score for men was double that for women (6.2% vs. 2.7%, $P<0.001$). In older participants, the risk was similar between the sexes, with a third having scores over 10 %[(13)].

These metabolic disturbances are of complex origin, and their development may be affected by ART as well as the underlying HIV infection [(14)]. HIV infection itself has been reported to impair triglycerides (TG) metabolism and lipoprotein-lipase (LPL) activity, and reduced plasma HDL cholesterol, Apo-B and Apo-A1, with higher LDL TG, and higher total cholesterol/HDL ratio[(1-3-,15)]. Cytokines, such as interferon alpha, may play a role in the abnormal lipid homeostasis seen in PLWH (16,17). The use of PIs has been linked to further abnormalities in the serum lipid profile in PLWH (18, 19). Increased total cholesterol (TC), TG rich VLDL, and LDL-C are seen in PI-treated patients (19-21). Data from prospective cohort studies report new-onset hypercholesterolemia and hypertriglyceridemia after 5 years of HAART in 24 and 19% of subjects, respectively (22, 23). Individual PIs likely have substantially different affects on the lipid profile. Data from the Swiss Cohort study suggest that ritonavir, but not indinavir or nelfinavir, is associated with increased TG levels (22). Purnell(24) demonstrated significant effects of ritonavir on TG levels after 2 weeks in HIV-negative patients. Similarly, low dose ritonavir in combination with lopinavir over 4 weeks also increased TG levels in HIV-negative men (25). The newer PI atazanavir appears to have a significantly less pronounced effect on serum lipid levels (26, 27). The mechanism by which PIs influence serum TG is not clear. Animal studies (28, 29) suggest that PIs may prevent proteosomal degradation of nascent ApoB, a principle protein component of circulating TGs, leading to increased production of VLDL particles. Furthermore, as opposed to the "traditional" metabolic syndrome, which involves high free fatty acid (FFA) levels due to the inability for appropriate storage into fat cells in the presence of IR, patients receiving HAART develop a lipotoxicity due to mitochondrial dysfunction resulting in the excess release of FFA [(30)], resulting in increased production of VLDL and small, dense LDL as well as low plasma levels of HDL. This increase in lipolysis appears to cause the characteristic subcutaneous lipoatrophy in the face, legs, and buttocks with accumulation of fat in the visceral area and the back of the neck. PIs may also induce the lipoatrophy by inhibiting sterol regulatory enhancer-binding protein (SREBP-1) [(30,31)] and peroxisome proliferator-activated receptor-γ.(PPAR-γ)[(32)], which are both involved in lipogenesis.

Other antiretroviral medications may also affect serum lipids. Kumar(33) reported, in treatment-naïve HIV+ subjects, PI sparing regimens (zidovudine/lamivudine + abacavir) raised fasting TC and TG least in comparison with regimens containing a PI (zidovudine/lamivudine + nelfinavir) or stavudine and a PI. The DAD study ($n$ = 7483 patients)(34) reported that exposure to non-nucleoside reverse transcriptase inhibitors (NNRTIs) is also associated with modest yet significantly increased TG levels (odds ratio, 1.90; 95% confidence interval, 1.06–3.39), but not with low HDL-C or increased LDL-C.

Fat redistribution has also been reported frequently in PLWH. NRTIs used to treat HIV-1 infection are particularly associated with the lipoatrophy in subcutaneous fat [(35)], whereas PIs are considered more likely to cause systemic metabolic alterations such as insulin resistance [36]. Non-nucleoside-analog reverse transcriptase inhibitors are not thought to contribute to the development of lipodystrophy, although some data have led to a reconsideration of the effects of some of these drugs on peripheral fat accumulation [37]. There have been attempts to treat HIV-1-lipodystrophy using drugs of known effects against dyslipidemia (fibrates) or insulin resistance (thiazolidinediones), but results on the overall lipodystrophy syndrome have been poor [45,46].

There is a growing concern about an increased risk for cardiovascular disease (CVD) in PLWH especially those receiving ART. This risk could be related to hypertension or metabolic abnormalities such as dyslipidemia, diabetes mellitus and central fat deposition which are increasingly seen with long-term use of ART [19, 38-41]. This is also supported by epidemiological studies showing an increased risk for CVD in PLWH [42-44].

## 3. Insulin resistance (IR) as one of the possible mechanisms involved

Insulin resistance a risk factor for CVD is increasingly seen in PLWH and it is often accompanied by elevated blood pressure, dysfunctional glucose homeostasis, obesity, and dyslipidemia[47,48]. It has been shown [49] that the presence of dyslipidemia (i.e. hypertriglyceridemia and low plasma HDL concentration) is highly indicative of underlying IR in patients with HIV despite fasting normoglycemia. Patients with the HIV-metabolic syndrome were also found to have a redistribution of adipose tissue to the intraperitoneal compartment and have markedly elevated intrahepatic lipid content [50].

Insulin resistance is also a component of the lipodystrophy syndrome, and fasting insulin levels appear to correlate with waist to hip ratio. Multivariate modeling was used to estimate an approximate 1% increase in fasting insulin level for every 1% increase in visceral fat or every 1% increase in abdominal subcutaneous fat [51]. Insulin levels and IR are higher in patients with both peripheral lipoatrophy and visceral adiposity than in those who have either alone [52]. Intra-abdominal fat delivers excess free fatty acids directly into the portal blood system[53] and secrete cytokines and other factors that contribute to IR, impaired fibrinolysis[54,55], and endothelial dysfunction leading to increased risk for CVD[56].

It is unclear whether IR is a direct result of HIV infection alone or it is a complication of ART. Chronic infection with HIV may contribute to glucose abnormalities among HIV-infected patients. In the Multicenter AIDS Cohort Study, insulin resistance markers were higher in all groups of HIV-infected men compared with HIV-uninfected control subjects, even among those who were not receiving ART [57], suggesting an effect of HIV infection itself. A potential factor by which HIV could induce IR is TNF-α, which is chronically released by peripheral blood mononuclear cells in PLWH. Systemic inflammation has been associated with incident of diabetes in multiple cohorts in the general population [58-60]. Proinflammatory cytokines, such as tumor necrosis factor (TNF)-α, may induce insulin resistance by binding to insulin-responsive elements in skeletal muscle [61]. Among HIV-infected patients, markers of systemic inflammation decrease quickly with ART initiation [62] but do not normalize [63]. It is speculated that this residual inflammation with effective ART may contribute to the pathogenesis of co-morbidities in HIV-infected patients, including diabetes [64].

Insulin resistance could also be a consequence of drug treatments in HIV. Among PLWH on ART, an IR prevalence rate of about 20-85% has been reported [9, 10, 65,66]. There are differences in the pathways through which various PIs induce IR and in their propensity to do so. Certain PIs, such as indinavir (IDV), lopinavir, and ritonavir, have been shown to reversibly induce IR, probably by inhibition of glucose translocation through GLUT4 [67]. In contrast, atazanavir had no effect on IR.The NRTIs, zidovudine and stavudine, also have direct and indirect effects on glucose metabolism [68,69]. In a case-control study [70], comparing 55 previously ART-naive individuals who developed diabetes 48 weeks after ART initiation (case subjects) with 55 individuals who did not develop diabetes during a comparable follow-up (control subjects), subjects with higher levels of high-sensitivity C-reactive protein (hs-CRP), soluble TNFR1 (sTNFR1), and sTNFR2 at 48 weeks had an increased odds of subsequent diabetes, after adjustment for baseline marker level, age, BMI at week 48, CD4 count at week 48, and indinavir use. After further adjustment for week 48 glucose, effects were attenuated and only sTNFR1 remained significant (odds ratio, highest quartile vs. lowest 23.2 [95% CI 1.28–423], $P = 0.03$).

Insulin resistance, glucose and lipid metabolism were also found to be directly related to circulating adipokines suggesting that abnormalities in adipocytes may contribute to IR in patients with HIV. A known side effect of NRTIs is reduction in the production of adiponectin by lipoatrophy. Because adiponectin improves insulin sensitivity by increasing transportation/oxidation of FFAs and inhibition of hepatic glucose output, hypoadiponectinemia due to effects of NRTIs is thought to be a pathway for IR [7]. Serum adiponectin level has been shown to inversely correlate with fasting insulin concentration and with hepatic fat content [71]. Adiponectin also has anti-inflammatory properties. It suppresses inflammatory cell infiltration of the vascular intimal space (72-74), and deficiency of adiponectin up-regulates endothelial adhesion molecules [73]. In a study by Cade et al[74] who performed adipose tissue biopsies in a cohort of HIV-infected patients, he found that the use of PIs is associated with down-regulation of adiponectin mRNA in appendicular adipocytes. These findings suggest a mechanistic link between PI use and development of dyslipidemia and IR. They also found that patients with HIV-metabolic syndrome have blunted insulin-mediated suppression of protein breakdown, unlike patients with type 2 diabetes. These findings imply a shared signalling defect in patients with HIV-metabolic syndrome that affects lipid, glucose and protein metabolism.

## 4. Treatment challenge

Because HIV infection frequently occurs in young individuals, long-term HAART is necessary and, thus, risk-factor modification is increasingly important to prevent the development of CVD. There is no single pharmacologic agent available with effects on multiple targets. The efficacy and safety of combining anti-inflammatory, antihypertensives, hypoglycemic and lipid lowering agents and their interactions with ART must be considered and favourable effects on reversing these abnormalities have not been uniformly reported.

For example, dyslipidemia is common in HIV-infected patients, but treatment outcomes are often unsatisfactory. In one study [75] responses to lipid-lowering therapy were compared between 829 HIV-infected patients and 6941 uninfected controls, all with laboratory evidence of dyslipidemia. The HIV-infected patients had significantly smaller LDL declines in response to statins therapy than their HIV-negative counterparts (reduction, 25.6% vs. 28.3%); within the HIV population, pravastatin was less effective than other agents (simvastatin, lovastatin, or atorvastatin). This drug is cited in current guidelines as a preferred agent because it has fewer interactions with ART than do other statins. The various classes of ART respond to lipid-lowering therapy differently; for example, PIs blunted response to fibrate therapy, but NNRTIs did not [75].

There have also been attempts to treat HIV-1-lipodystrophy using drugs of known effects against dyslipidemia (fibrates) or insulin resistance (thiazolidinediones), but results on the overall lipodystrophy syndrome have been poor [(45,46)]. Therefore, drug treatment needs to be balanced against the potentially significant drug–drug interactions.
Until definitive data are available on the efficacy of these medications, the primary focus of treatment should be on lifestyle modification, including diet, exercise since they are shown to improve IR and CVD risk in the general population. As well, patients with HIV infection have been shown to have inadequate dietary intake and suboptimal levels of various micronutrients some of which play an important role in regulating insulin function and CVD risk [(76-78)].
Therefore, addressing nutritional deficiencies and modifiable risk factors such as smoking, obesity, and sedentary lifestyle can have a far greater impact on IR and CVD than changes in antiretroviral therapy.

## 5. Dietary factors, physical activity and insulin resistance

The identification of dietary factors that influence energy and lipid metabolism is an important research field of nutrition science and has become a growing requirement in the context of the HIV/AIDS epidemic in an attempt to attenuate the metabolic abnormalities and CVD risk associated with antiretroviral therapy.
Consumption of energy-dense / high fat diets is strongly and positively associated with the overweight state, that in turns induces IR, particularly when the excess body weight is located in the abdominal region [(79, 80)]. In patients with HIV infection, we collected 7-day food diary from 60 males who also had metabolic abnormalities [(77)]. We estimated their energy, macro- and micronutrient intakes and compared it to the Dietary Reference Intakes for Canadians. A large proportion (41.5% and 63.1%) of subjects had intakes of fat and saturated fat exceeding the recommended levels of intake. None of the subjects met the recommended level of intake for fiber and 90.8% did not meet the recommended levels of intake for vitamin E. These findings have also been confirmed in other studies [(79, 81)].
**Dietary fat quality**: IR is also independently affected by the type of dietary fat. In animal studies, saturated fat increases whereas omega-3 polyunsaturated fatty acids (PUFA) from fish and seafood reduce IR [(82, 83)]. Several human studies [(84-91)] have also shown that saturated fat is significantly associated with worsening of IR, independent of body fat, while monounsaturated and PUFA improves IR. Based on fatty acid composition in plasma and muscle, studies also consistently show that increased unsaturated fat intake is associated with improved insulin sensitivity [(91-94)]. Reports from systematic reviews [(95, 96)] also concluded that omega-3 PUFA reduce IR and serum triglycerides. Based on this, the American Diabetes Association [(97)] and American Heart Association [(98)] have recommended the consumption of 2-3 servings of fish/week. In one of our ongoing study (unpublished data) in males with HIV infection (n=27) who were found to have non-alcoholic fatty liver disease and several metabolic abnormalities, the omega-3 index (a combination of 2 long-chain omega-3 PUFA, Eicosapentaenoic acid and Docosahexaenoic acid) in the red blood cells was significantly lower when compared to HIV-negative male subjects (n=6) with minimal findings in their liver biopsies (3.44±0.35 vs. 6.20±1.15; P=0.022). This was accompanied with a significantly higher omega-6 to omega-3 PUFA ratio in HIV-infected group (5.58±0.57 vs. 3.40±0.31; P=0.028) in favor of inflammatory processes in the body.
The levels of the omega-3 PUFA in the blood and in the tissues are determined by diet and probably also by a genetic component. Changes in the levels of omega-3 PUFA are expected

in a given individual after a change in diet and during treatment with omega-3 PUFA. In a study [99] of 54 persons with HIV and elevated serum triglycerides (>150 mg/dL) and/or abnormal Quantitative Insulin Sensitivity Check Index values (<0.35 but >0.30) in which total fat, type of fat, fiber, and glycemic load were controlled along with supplementation with n-3 fatty acids to achieve an intake of 6 g/d, serum triglycerides in the intervention group decreased from a median of 180 mg/dL to 114 mg/dL from baseline to 3 weeks, whereas they remained stable in the control group (P = 0.003). Serum phospholipid fatty acids indicated a decrease in de novo lipogenesis and a decrease in arachidonic acid in the intervention group. At 3 weeks, the insulin area under the curve decreased but not significantly.

In another randomized placebo-controlled trial [100], 51 patients with HIV infection received either 2 capsules of Omacor (an omega-3 PUFA supplement) twice daily or 2 capsules of placebo. Plasma triglycerides were reduced in the n-3 PUFA group by 0.14 mmol/l after 12 weeks of treatment (n=26), while plasma triglycerides increased by 0.36 mmol/l in the control group (n=25). There was a significant increase in leukotriene B5 (LTB5) and LTB5/LTB4 ratio in the omega-3 PUFA group compared to the control group, inducing anti-inflammatory effects by increasing formation of anti-inflammatory LTB5.

**Calcium:** The importance of dietary calcium in the regulation of body weight and lipid metabolism has been the object of scientific investigations throughout the years. This relationship was first studied by Zamel et al [101-103], and today it continues to be an object of scientific interest [104, 105]. Some epidemiological studies show that, in the general population, a high calcium and dairy product intake were associated with less fat accumulation and higher insulin sensitivity. It also presents an inverse relationship with metabolic syndrome components, especially hypertension [106, 107]. On the other hand, the results of other investigations have indicated that calcium supplementation (1500 mg day$^{-1}$) did not induce changes in body weight or lipid metabolism [108]. It has been proposed that low calcium intake inhibits lipolysis and stimulates *de novo* synthesis, reducing fat oxidation, which results in an increased waist circumference. Through these mechanisms, a low dietary calcium intake leads to weight gain, whereas a high dietary calcium intake exerts the opposite effects [104]. Another hypothesis suggests that calcium may have a modulating effect on the foecal excretion of fats [109]. Reports from dietary assessments in the HIV infected patients have shown suboptimal intake of calcium [77, 79, 81]. In these studies, over 90% of the patients did not meet the recommended level of intake of 1000 g/day of calcium. In one study, patients who had dietary calcium intake below 700 mg day$^{-1}$ had greater waist circumference and body mass index (BMI) [81]. Dairy food consumers (>2 servings per day) showed lower BMI ($P < 0.01$), waist circumference ($P = 0.05$), systolic and diastolic blood pressure, all components of the metabolic syndrome [81].

**Chromium:** The metabolic abnormalities reported in PLWH are very similar to the abnormalities seen in patients with Type 2 diabetes and in those with chromium (Cr) deficiency. Chromium is a nutrient that potentiates insulin action and thus is an essential element for glucose and lipid metabolism [110-116]. Improvements in glucose tolerance [117-128], plasma TG, total and HDL-cholesterol [128-131] after Cr supplementation is well documented in humans and in animals. In Type 2 diabetic patients, Cr supplementation resulted in an improvement in insulin sensitivity [132-134] and other metabolic parameters [135,136]. Studies involving patients on total- parenteral- nutrition (TPN) led to conclusive documentation of the essential role of Cr in human nutrition [117, 123,124]. These patients developed diabetic symptoms including glucose intolerance, weight loss, impaired energy utilization, and nerve and brain disorders that were refractory to insulin. After adding Cr to TPN fluids, diabetic symptoms were alleviated, and exogenous insulin was no longer required. Furthermore, children, the elderly and people with type I and II diabetes mellitus have all been shown to display positive effects on blood glucose and lipids in response to supplemental Cr (128,129, 136, 137). Finally, in a meta-analysis of 41 randomized trials involving 1198 participants, Cr supplementation significantly improved glycemia and dyslipidemia among patients with diabetes but had no effect in those without diabetes (138).

The metabolic abnormalities including IR documented in PLWH may be related to suboptimal chromium status. We were the first to show (139) that the blood level of Cr was significantly lower and the urinary excretion was higher in antiretroviral-treated PLWH when compared with healthy control subjects. In a subsequent randomized, double blind, placebo-controlled trial (140), 50 HIV-positive subjects with evidence of body fat redistribution, elevated lipids or glucose and who were found to have IR based on the calculation of homeostatic model of assessment (HOMA= (fasting blood glucose x fasting insulin) / 22.5) were randomized to receive either 400 ug of Cr-nicotinate or placebo for a period of 16 weeks. For inclusion, the HOMA had to be> 2.5. Body weight and medication profile remained stable throughout the study period for both groups. Cr supplementation resulted in a significant decrease in blood insulin, blood triglycerides and HOMA. Blood glucose, C-peptide, total cholesterol, LDL and HDL cholesterol and Hb A1c remained unchanged. Biochemical parameters did not change in the placebo group except for LDL cholesterol that increased significantly post supplementation with placebo. In subjects supplemented with Cr, those who had body fat redistribution, had a more pronounced drop in blood triglycerides (-0.70±0.29 mmol/l) than those without (0.02 ±0.20 mmol/L) (P=0.056). The severity of IR at baseline determined the response to Cr supplementation as there was a strong correlation between baseline insulin level and the post-supplementation drop in blood: insulin (r= -0.852, p= 0.0001), triglycerides (r= -0.602, p=0.001) and c-peptide (r= -0.401, p=0.065).

Analysis by dual energy X-ray absorptiometry (DEXA) scan also showed a significant decrease in total body fat mass (kg) in the Cr- supplemented group. This was accompanied by a significant reduction in percent total body fat mass and a significant increase in percent total lean body mass. Further analysis of the regional fat distribution showed a significant decrease in percent trunk fat mass as well as percent fat mass in the arms and legs. In the Cr-supplemented group, the change in trunk fat mass was much more pronounced in subjects with body fat redistribution (-654.6 ±233.7 g) compare to those without this abnormality (-33.66 ±218.2 g) (P=0.068). As well, in subjects with body fat redistribution, Cr supplementation resulted in a decrease in trunk fat mass (-654.6 g ±233.7) whereas in the placebo group, trunk fat mass increased (1803±356 g). The difference between the two groups was statistically significant (P=0.05). Trunk fat mass correlated significantly with waist circumference (r=0.854, p=0.0001), and HOMA at baseline (r=0.275, p=0.036).

A detailed understanding of the molecular action of Cr is lacking; several lines of evidence point to enhancement of insulin action. Chromium increases insulin-stimulated glucose uptake in cultured muscle cells (141) and adipocytes (142). Chromium may increase insulin binding to cells, insulin receptor number, and insulin receptor tyrosine kinase activity (143). The enhancement of insulin action by Cr is associated with phosphorylation of insulin receptor substrate-1 (IRS-1) (141) and phosphatidylinositol 3-kinase (PI 3-kinase) (144) and is inhibited by wortmanin, an inhibitor of PI 3-kinase. Activation of these proteins in the insulin-signalling transduction pathway leads to translocation of glucose transporters from the cytosol to the plasma membrane. Indeed, Cr-picolinate supplementation was shown to significantly enhance the membrane-associated Glut-4 content of skeletal muscle and rate of glucose disappearance in obese rats after insulin stimulation [145]. In a follow-up study it was reported that improved glucose disposal rates in Cr-fed, obese, insulin-resistant animals were attributable to enhanced insulin-stimulated IRS-1 and PI 3-kinase activity in skeletal muscle [146].

The form or availability of Cr in specific foods is generally not known. A balanced diet will provide Cr with an average availability of 1-2% [147,148]. Processed meats; liver; whole-grains including some ready-to-eat bran cereals; some pulses, such as dried beans; some vegetables, including broccoli and mushrooms; and spices are some of the best sources of Cr. Dairy products, and most fruits and vegetables, contain low amounts of Cr. Rice and sugar are poor sources.

The suggested safe and adequate intake for Cr is established at 50-200 ug/day for adolescents and adults, and 10-120 ug/day for infants and children [149]. It is reported that Cr intake by even healthy subjects consuming average Westernized diets is suboptimal [150] and is below the recommended level of 50 ug. One third of the diets, designed by a nutritionist to be well-balanced and to contain the recommended daily intake of vitamins and minerals (except chromium) contained less than the minimal safe and adequate intake of 50 ug of Cr [151]. Anderson and Kozolvsky [150] measured the daily Cr intake of 22 female and 10 male subjects for 7 days. Not a single subject had a mean daily Cr intake of 50 ug or more. On the other hand, consuming less than 50 ug/d of Cr does not mean that one would eventually become Cr deficient. For example, in one study [152], 11 elderly women had an average intake of 20.1 ug/day and 11 elderly men had an average intake of 29.8 ug per day; the range of intakes was 13.6-47.7 ug among the 22 subjects. Of these, 16 maintained equilibrium, 4 exhibited positive balances, and 2 exhibited slight and one exhibited severe negative balance. The intake at which Cr is low enough to induce changes responsive to Cr supplementation is not well established. Moreover, because other substances in the diet influence absorption and metabolism of Cr, the point at which Cr intake becomes inadequate depends in part on the other foods consumed, medical conditions and medication profile.

Chromium chloride, chromium nicotinate, and chromium picolinate are commonly used formulations of trivalent chromium in the supplements. The studies that reported positive effects of supplemental chromium on people with diabetes usually involve 400 ug or more of Cr.

Chromium supplements are inexpensive [153], and the limited safety data suggest that Cr is safe even at high doses [154]. Therefore, Cr supplementation would be an attractive option for management of diabetes and for control of insulin and lipid concentration of PLWH. The role of Cr supplementation in conjunction with the initiation of HAART should be studied prospectively as a cost-effective approach to reducing CVD.

**Physical activity:** At the present time, overweight and obese individuals constitute a much larger segment of the HIV-infected population than patients with wasting syndrome [155]. As with individuals in the general population, an obese patient with HIV should be advised about the benefits of weight loss and regular physical activity; this is applicable not only to patients with high risk of diabetes but also to individuals who have already developed glucose intolerance or frank diabetes. There is considerable evidence that lifestyle changes, including changes in diet (eg, calorie restriction and reduction in intake of carbohydrates, saturated fats, and cholesterol) and increased physical activity can help reverse the progression to type II diabetes and improve glycemic control in individuals already diagnosed with the condition (156-159). In a randomized study, aggressive lifestyle modification was more effective than metformin in preventing the development of diabetes in individuals with elevated fasting glucose (160); however, adherence to lifestyle changes is difficult to maintain over time. The expected improvement in Hb A1C levels in individuals who are able to follow lifestyle modification recommendations is 1%-2%, similar to goals that are attainable with some drug regimens.

Clear evidence has established that adults who engage in regular physical activity and/or exhibit high cardiorespiratory fitness have a reduced risk of developing type II diabetes (161). Furthermore, the beneficial effects of a physically active lifestyle seem to hold true for normal-weight, overweight, and obese individuals alike. It is hypothesized that the mechanisms underlying this protective effect may be due, at least in part, to the insulin-sensitizing properties of physical activity on skeletal muscle.

From controlled studies, exercise training is associated directly with improved insulin sensitivity (162-165). Hughes et al (166) showed that exercise training of between 50% and 75% of maximal capacity can improve insulin sensitivity in individuals with impaired glucose tolerance. From community studies, increased levels of overall habitual physical activity have been positively associated with surrogate measures of insulin sensitivity among individuals without diabetes (167-168) and among those with impaired glucose tolerance (169), independent of obesity. In another study (170), including 1467 men and women of African American, Hispanic, and non-Hispanic white ethnicity, aged 40 to 69 years, with glucose tolerance ranging from normal to mild non–insulin-dependent diabetes mellitus, increased participation in non-vigorous as well as overall and vigorous physical activity was associated with significantly higher insulin sensitivity.

However, questions remain regarding the nature and amount of physical activity required to have a sustained, beneficial impact on glucose and insulin metabolism at the individual and the community levels. The Centers for Disease Control and Prevention (CDC), and the American College of Sports Medicine (ACSM), have recently recommended that every US adult should accumulate at least 30 minutes of moderate-intensity physical activity (3 to 6 metabolic equivalents [METs]) on most, preferably all, days of the week (171). The same recommendation was put forth by a 1996 National Institute of Health Consensus Statement (172).

## 6. References

[1] Grunfeld C, Kotler DP, Hamadeh R, et al. Hypertriglyceridemia in the acquired immunodeficiency syndrome. Am J Med 1989; 86:27–31.

[2] Grunfeld C, Pang M, Doerrler W, et al. Lipids, lipoproteins, triglyceride clearance and cytokines in human immunodeficiency virus infection and the acquired immunodeficiency syndrome. J Clin Endocrinol Metab 1992; 74:1045–1052.

[3] Aznar R, Egido M, Puzo J, et al. Lipid profiles in untreated HIV infected asymptomatic patients. 13th International AIDS Conference, Durban, South Africa 2000, p B758 (Abstract).

[4] Sutinen J, Korsheninnikova E, Funahashi T, et al. Circulating concentration of adiponectin and its expression in subcutaneous adipose tissue in patients with highly active antiretroviral therapy-associated lipodystrophy. J Clin Endocrinol Metab 2003; 88:1907–1910.

[5] Lihn AS, Richelsen B, Pedersen SB, et al. Increased expression of TNF-{alpha}, IL-6, and IL-8 in HIV-associated lipodystrophy. Implications for the reduced expression and plasma levels of adiponectin. Am J Physiol Endocrinol Metab 2003; 285(5):E1072-80.

[6] Vigouroux C, Maachi M, Nguyen TH, et al. Serum adipocytokines are related to lipodystrophy and metabolic disorders in HIV-infected men under antiretroviral therapy. AIDS 2003; 17:1503–1511.

[7] Addy CL, Gavrila A, Tsiodras S, et al. Hypoadiponectinemia is associated with insulin resistance, hypertriglyceridemia, and fat redistribution in human immunodeficiency virus-infected patients treated with highly active antiretroviral therapy. J Clin Endocrinol Metab 2003;88:627-636.

[8] Tong Q, Sankale JL, Hadigan CM, et al. Regulation of adiponectin in human immunodeficiency virus-infected patients: relationship to body composition and metabolic indices. J Clin Endocrinol Metab 2003; 88:1559–1564.

[9] Hadigan C, Miller K, Corcoran C, et al. Fasting hyperinsulinemia and changes in regional body composition in human immunodeficiency virus-infected women. J Clin Endocrinol Metab. 1999;84:1932-1937.

[10] Limone P, Biglino A, Valle M, et al. Insulin resistance in HIV-infected patients: relationship with pro-inflammatory cytokines released by peripheral leukocytes. J Infect 2003;47:52-58.

[11] Virkamaki A, Puhakainen I, Koivisto VA, et al. Mechanisms of hepatic and peripheral insulin resis tance during acute infections in humans. J Clin Endocrinol Metab 1992;74:673-679.

[12] World Health Organization. Definition, Diagnosis and Classification of Diabetes Mellitus and its Complications. Report of a WHO Consultation. Geneva: World Health Organization, 1999.

[13] Adeyemi O, Rezai K, Bahk M, et al. Metabolic Syndrome in Older HIV-Infected Patients: Data from the CORE50 Cohort. *AIDS Patient Care and STDs 2008;* 22(12): 941-945.

[14] Villarroya F, Domingo P, Giralt M. Lipodystrophy in HIV 1-infected patients: lessons for obesity research. Int J Obes (Lond) 2007; 31:1763–1776.

[15] Hellerstein MK, Grunfeld C, Wu K, et al. Increased de novo hepatic lipogenesis in human immunodeficiency virus infection. J Clin Endocrinol Metab 1993; 76:559–565.

[16] Christeff N, De Truchis P, Melchior JC, et al. Longitudinal evolution of HIV-1-associated lipodystrophy is correlated to serum cortisol:DHEA ratio and IFN-alpha. Eur J Clin Invest 2002; 32:775–784.

[17] Grunfeld C, Pang M, Doerrler W. Circulating interferon alpha levels and hypertriglyceridemia in the acquired immunodeficiency syndrome. Am J Med 1991; 90:154–162.

[18] Depairon M, Chessex S, Sudre P, et al. Premature atherosclerosis in HIV-infected individuals–focus on protease inhibitor therapy. AIDS 2001; 15:329–334.

[19] Behrens G, Dejam A, Schmidt H. Impaired glucose tolerance, ß cell function and lipid metabolism in HIV patients under treatment with protease inhibitors. AIDS 1999; 13:F63–F70.

[20] Penzak SR, Chuck SK, Stajich GV. Safety and efficacy of HMG-CoA reductase inhibitors for treatment of hyperlipidemia in patients with HIV infection. Pharmacotherapy 2000; 20:1066–1071.

[21] Mooser V, Carr A. Antiretroviral therapy-associated hyperlipidaemia in HIV disease. Curr Opin Lipidol 2001; 12:313–319.

[22] Periard D, Telenti A, Sudre P, et al. Atherogenic dyslipidemia in HIV-infected individuals treated with protease inhibitors. The Swiss HIV Cohort Study. Circulation 1999; 100:700–705.

[23] Tsiodras S, Mantzoros C, Hammer S, Samore M. Effects of protease inhibitors on hyperglycemia, hyperlipidemia, and lipodystrophy: a 5-year cohort study. Arch Intern Med 2000; 160:2050–2056.

[24] Purnell JQ, Zambon A, Knopp RH, et al. Effect of ritonavir on lipids and post-heparin lipase activities in normal subjects. AIDS 2000; 14:51–57.

[25] Lee GA, Seneviratne T, Noor MA, et al. The metabolic effects of lopinavir/ritonavir in HIV-negative men. AIDS 2004; 18:641–649.

[26] Sanne I, Piliero P, Squires K, et al. Results of a phase 2 clinical trial at 48 weeks (AI424-007): a dose-ranging, safety, and efficacy comparative trial of atazanavir at three doses in combination with didanosine and stavudine in antiretroviral-naive subjects. J Acquir Immune Defic Syndr 2003; 32:18–29.

[27] Parker RA, Wang S, Mulvey R, et al. Differential effects of HIV protease inhibitor on proteosome, gene expression, and lipogenesis provide a mechanism for PI-associated dyslipidemia and Atazanavir's favorable lipid profile. Eleventh Conference on Retroviruses and Opportunistic Infections 2004, [abstract 706].

[28] Liang JS, Distler O, Cooper DA, et al. HIV protease inhibitors protect apolipoprotein B from degradation by the proteasome: a potential mechanism for protease inhibitor-induced hyperlipidemia. Nat Med 2001; 7:1327–1331.

[29] Riddle TM, Schildmeyer NM, Phan C, et al. The HIV protease inhibitor ritonavir increases lipoprotein production and has no effect on lipoprotein clearance in mice. J Lipid Res 2002; 43:1458–1463.

[30] Caron M, Auclair M, Vigouroux C, et al. The HIV protease inhibitor indinavir impairs sterol regulatory element-binding protein-1 intranuclear localization, inhibits preadipocyte differentiation, and induces insulin resistance. Diabetes 2001; 50:1378–1388.

[31] Riddle TM, Kuhel DG, Woollett LA, et al. HIV protease inhibitor induces fatty acid and sterol biosynthesis in liver and adipose tissues due to the accumulation of activated sterol regulatory element-binding proteins in the nucleus. J Biol Chem 2001; 276:37514–37519.

[32] Kannisto K, Sutinen J, Korsheninnikova E, et al. Expression of adipogenic transcription factors, peroxisome proliferator-activated receptor gamma co-activator 1, IL-6 and CD45 in subcutaneous adipose tissue in lipodystrophy associated with highly active antiretroviral therapy. AIDS 2003; 17:1753–1762.

[33] Kumar P, Rodriguez-French A, Thompson M. Prospective study of hyperlipidemia in ART-naive subjects taking combivir/abacavir, combivir/nelfinavir, or stavudine / lamivudine / nelfinavir. Ninth Conference on Retroviruses and Opportunistic Infections, Seattle, WA, 2002 [abstract 33].

[34] Fontas E, van Leth F, Sabin CA, et al. Lipid profiles in HIV-infected patients receiving combination antiretroviral therapy: are different antiretroviral drugs associated with different lipid profiles? J Infect Dis 2004; 189:1056–1074.

[35] Boyd MA, Carr A, Ruxrungtham K, et al. Changes in body composition and mitochondrial nucleic acid content in patients switched from failed nucleoside analogue therapy to ritonavir-boosted indinavir and efavirenz. J Infect Dis 2006; 194:642–650.

[36] Flint OP, Noor MA, Hruz PW, et al. The role of protease inhibitors in the pathogenesis of HIV-associated lipodystrophy: cellular mechanisms and clinical implications. Toxicol Pathol 2009; 37:65–77.

[37] Haubrich RH, Riddler SA, DiRienzo AG, et al. Metabolic outcomes in a randomized trial of nucleoside, nonnucleoside and protease inhibitor-sparing regimens for initial HIV treatment. AIDS 2009; 23:1109–1118.

[38] Carr A, Samaras K, Burton S, et al. A syndrome of peripheral lipodystrophy, hyperlipidaemia and insulin resistance in patients receiving HIV protease inhibitors. AIDS 1998; 12:F51–F58.

[39] Carr A, Samaras K, Thorisdottir A, et al. Diagnosis and prediction and natural course of HIV protease inhibitor (PI)-associated lipodystrophy, hyperlipidaemia and diabetes mellitus: a cohort study. Lancet 1999; 353:2093–2099.

[40] Saint-Marc T, Partisani M, Poizot-Martin I, et al. Fat distribution evaluated by computed tomography and metabolic abnormalities in patients undergoing antiretroviral therapy: preliminary results of the LIPOCO study. AIDS 2000; 14:37–49.

[41] Vigouroux C, Gharakhanian S, Salhi Y, et al. Diabetes, insulin resistance and dyslipidaemia in lipodystrophic HIV-infected patients on highly active antiretroviral therapy (HAART). Diabetes Metab 1999; 25:225–232.

[42] Grinspoon S, Carr A. Cardiovascular risk and body-fat abnormalities in HIV-infected adults, N Engl J Med 2005; 352:48–62.

[43] Hsue PY, Lo JC, Franklin A, et al. Progression of atherosclerosis as assessed by carotid intima-media thickness in patients with HIV infection, Circulation 2004; 109: 1603–1608.

[44] The Data Collection on Adverse Events of Anti-HIV Drugs (DAD) Study Group, Combination antiretroviral therapy and the risk of myocardial infarction, N Engl J Med 2003; 349:1993–2003.

[45] Raboud JM, Diong C, Carr A, et al. A meta-analysis of six placebo-controlled trials of thiazolidinedione therapy for HIV lipoatrophy. HIV Clinical Trials 2010; 11(1):39-50.

[46] Martínez E, Domingo P, Ribera E, et al. Effects of metformin or gemfibrozil on the lipodystrophy of HIV-infected patients receiving protease inhibitors. Antivir Ther 2003; 8:403–410.

[47] Brown TT, Cole SR, Li X, et al. Antiretroviral therapy and the prevalence and incidence of diabetes mellitus in the multicenter AIDS cohort study. Arch Intern Med 2005;165:1179–1184.

[48] Bastard JP, Bouteloup V, Leport C, et al. High incidence and risk factors for diabetes over 9-year follow-up after first generation protease inhibitor initiation in the ARNS CO8 APROCO-COPILOTE cohort. Antivir Ther 2009;14(Suppl. 2):A5.

[49] Reeds, D.N. Metabolic Syndrome risks of cardiovascular disease: differences between HIV-positive and HIV-negative? J. Cardiometab. Syndr 2008; 3:79–82.

[50] Reeds DN, Yarasheski KE, Fontana L, et al. Alterations in liver, muscle, and adipose tissue insulin sensitivity in men with HIV infection and dyslipidemia. Am J Physiol Endocrinol Metab 2006; 290: E47–E53.

[51] Meininger G, Hadigan C, Rietschel P, Grinspoon S. Body-composition measurements as predictors of glucose and insulin abnormalities in HIV-positive men. Am J Clin Nutr 2002;76:460-465.

[52] Hadigan C, Meigs JB, Corcoran C, et al. Metabolic abnormalities and cardiovascular disease risk factors in adults with human immunodeficiency virus infection and lipodystrophy. Clin Infect Dis 2001; 32:130-139.

[53] Bjorntorp P. "Portal" adipose tissue as a generator of risk factors for cardiovascular disease and diabetes. Arteriosclerosis 1990; 10:493–496.

[54] Alessi MC, Peiretti F, Morange P, et al. Production of plasminogen activator inhibitor-1 by human adipose tissue: possible link between visceral fat accumulation and vascular disease. Diabetes 1997; 46:860–867.

[55] Mertens I, Van der Planken M, Corthouts B, et al. Visceral fat is a determinant of PAI-1 activity in diabetic and non-diabetic overweight and obese women. Horm Metab Res 2001; 33:602–607.

[56] Hashimoto M, Akishita M, Eto M, et al. The impairment of flow-mediated vasodilatation in obese men with visceral fat accumulation. International Journal of Obesity & Related Metabolic Disorders: Journal of the International Association for the Study of Obesity 1998; 22(5):477-84.

[57] Pradhan AD, Manson JE, Rifai N, et al. C-reactive protein, interleukin 6, and risk of developing type 2 diabetes mellitus. JAMA 2001; 286:327–334.

[58] Hu FB, Meigs JB, Li TY, et al. Inflammatory markers and risk of developing type 2 diabetes in women. Diabetes 2004; 53:693–700.

[59] Spranger J, Kroke A, Möhlig M, et al. Inflammatory cytokines and the risk to develop type 2 diabetes: results of the prospective population-based European Prospective Investigation into Cancer and Nutrition (EPIC)-Potsdam Study. Diabetes 2003; 52:812–817.

[60] Hotamisligil GS, Peraldi P, Budavari A, et al. IRS-1-mediated inhibition of insulin receptor tyrosine kinase activity in TNF-α- and obesity-induced insulin resistance. Science 1996; 271:665–668.

[61] Brown TT, McComsey GA, King MS, et al. Loss of bone mineral density after antiretroviral therapy initiation, independent of antiretroviral regimen. J Acquir Immune Defic Syndr 2009; 51:554–561.

[62] Brown TT, Patil SP, Jacobson LP, et al. Association between systemic inflammation and obstructive sleep apnea in men with or at risk for HIV-infection from the Multicenter AIDS Cohort Study. Antivir Ther 2009;14(2):A19.

[63] Deeks SG. Immune dysfunction, inflammation, and accelerated aging in patients on antiretroviral therapy. Top HIV Med 2009; 17:118–123.

[64] Grunfeld C. Insulin resistance in HIV infection: drugs, host responses, or restoration to health? Top HIV Med 2008;16:89–93.

[65] Hotamisligil GS, Shargill NS, Spiegelman BM. Adipose expression of tumor necrosis factor-alpha: direct role in obesity-linked insulin resistance. Science 1993; 259:87-91.

[66] Brown TT, Li X, Cole SR, et al. Cumulative exposure to nucleoside analogue reverse transcriptase inhibitors is associated with insulin resistance markers in the Multicenter AIDS Cohort Study. AIDS 2005;19:1375–1383.

[67] Blümer RM, van Vonderen MG, Sutinen J, et al. Zidovudine/lamivudine contributes to insulin resistance within 3 months of starting combination antiretroviral therapy. AIDS 2008; 22:227–236.

[68] Fleischman A, Johnsen S, Systrom DM, et al. Effects of a nucleoside reverse transcriptase inhibitor, stavudine, on glucose disposal and mitochondrial function in muscle of healthy adults. Am J Physiol Endocrinol Metab 2007; 292:E1666–E1673.

[69] Brown TT, Tissiopoulos K, Bosch RJ, et al. Association Between Systemic Inflammation and Incident Diabetes in HIV-Infected Patients After Initiation of Antiretroviral Therapy. Diabetes Care 2010; 33(10):2244-2249.

[70] Bajaj M, Suraamornkul S, Piper P, et al. Decreased plasma adiponectin concentrations are closely related to hepatic fat content and hepatic insulin resis tance in pioglitazone-treated type 2 diabetic patients. J Clin Endocrinol Metab 2004; 89:200-206.

[71] Ouchi N, Kihara S, Arita Y, et al. Adipocyte-derived plasma protein, adiponectin, suppresses lipid accumulation and class A scavenger receptor expression in human monocyte-derived macrophages. Circulation 2001; 103:1057–1063.

[72] Ouchi N, Kihara S, Arita Y, et al. Novel modulator for endothelial adhesion molecules: adipocyte-derived plasma protein adiponectin. Circulation 1999; 100:2473–2476.

[73] Okamoto Y, Arita Y, Nishida M, et al. An adipocyte-derived plasma protein, adiponectin, adheres to injured vascular walls. Horm Metab Res 2000; 32:47–50.

[74] Cade WT. Reeds DN. Mittendorfer B. Patterson BW. Powderly WG. Klein S. Yarasheski KE. Blunted lipolysis and fatty acid oxidation during moderate exercise in HIV-infected subjects taking HAART. American Journal of Physiology - Endocrinology & Metabolism 2007; 292(3):E812-9.

[75] Silverberg MJ, Leyden W, Hurley L, et al. Response to newly prescribed lipid-lowering therapy in patients with and without HIV infection. Ann Intern Med 2009; 150:301-313.

[76] Hendricks KM, Dong KR, Tang AM, et al. High-fiber diet in HIV-positive men is associated with lower risk of developing fat deposition. Am J Clin Nutr 2003; 78:790–795.

[77] Arendt BM, Aghdassi E, Mohammed SS, et al. Dietary intake and physical activity in Canadian populations sample of male with HIV infection and metabolic abnormalities. Curr. HIV Res 2008; 6:82–90.

[78] Hendricks KM, Tang AM, Ding B, et al. Dietary intake in human immunodeficiency virus-infected adults: a comparison of dietary assessment methods. J. Am. Diet. Assoc 2005; 105:532–540.

[79] Joy T, Keogh HM, Hadigan C, et al. Dietary fat intake and relationship to serum lipid levels in HIV-infected patients with metabolic abnormalities in the HAART era. AIDS 2007; 21:1591–1600.

[80] Riccardi G, Giacco R, Rivellese AA. Dietary fat, insulin sensitivity and the metabolic syndrome. Clinical Nutrition 2004;23:447-456.

[81] Leite LHM, Sampaio ABMM. Dietary calcium, dairy food intake and metabolic abnormalities in HIV-infected individuals. Journal of Human Nutrition and Dietetics 2010; 23 (10): 535–543.
[82] Jang IS, Hwang DY, Chae KR, et al. Role of dietary fat type in the development of adiposity from dietary obesity-susceptible Sprague-Dawley rats. Br J Nutr. 2003;89(3):429-38.
[83] Nakatani T, Kim HJ, Kaburagi Y, et al. A low fish oil inhibits SREBP-1 proteolytic cascade, while a high-fish-oil feeding decreases SREBP-1 mRNA in mice liver: relationship to anti-obesity. J Lipid Res 2003;44(2):369-79.
[84] Maron DJ, Fair JM, Haskell WL. Saturated fat intake and insulin resistance in men with coronary artery disease. The Stanford Coronary Risk Intervention Project Investigators and Staff. Circulation 1991;84:2020-2027.
[85] Parker DR, Weiss ST, Troisi R, et al. Relationship of dietary saturated fatty acids and body habitus to serum insulin concentrations - the normative aging study. Am J Clin Nutr 1993;58:129-136.
[86] Mayer EJ, Newman B, Quesenberry CP Jr, et al. Usual dietary fat intake and insulin concentrations in healthy women twins. Diabetes Care 1993;16:1459-1469.
[87] Feskens EJ, Loeber JG, Kromhout D. Diet and physical activity as determinants of hyperinsulinemia - the Zutphen elderly study. Am J Epidemiol 1994;140:350-360.
[88] Marshall JA, Bessesen DH, Hamman RF. High saturated fat and low starch and fibre are associated with hyperinsulinemia in non diabetic population - the San Luis Valley diabetes study. Diabetologia 1997;40:430-438.
[89] Mooy JM, Grootenhuis PA, de Vries H, et al. Determinants of specific serum insulin concentrations in a general Caucasian population aged 50 to 74 years (the Hoorn Study). Diabet Med 1998;15:45-52.
[90] Mayer-Davis EJ, Monaco JH, Hoen HM, et al. Dietary fat and insulin sensitivity in a triethnic population - the role of obesity. The insulin resistance atherosclerosis study (IRAS). Am J Clin Nutr 1997; 65:79-89.
[91] Pelikanova T, Kohout M, Valek J, et al. Insulin secretion and insulin action related to the serum phospholipid fatty acid pattern in healthy men. Metabolism 1989;38:188-192.
[92] Borkman M., Storlien L.H., Pan D.A., et al.The relation between insulin sensitivity and fatty- acid composition of skeletal-muscle phospholipids. N Engl J Med 1993;328:238-244.
[93] Vessby B, Tengblad S, Lithell H. Insulin sensitivity is related to the fatty acid composition of serum lipids and skeletal muscle phospholipids in 70-year-old men. Diabetologia 1994;37:1044-1050.
[94] Pan D.A., Lillioja S., Milner M.R., et al. Skeletal muscle membrane lipid composition is related to adiposity and insulin action. J Clin Invest 1995; 96:2802-2808.
[95] Harris WS. N-3 fatty acids and human lipoprotein metabolism: an update. Lipids 1999; 34S:S257–8.
[96] Balk E, Chung M, Lichtenstein A, et al. Effects of omega-3 fatty acids on cardiovascular risk factors and intermediate markers of cardiovascular disease. Evidence report/technology assessment no. 93. AHRQ publication no. 04-E010-2. Rockville (MD): Agency for Healthcare Research and Quality; 2004.

[97] American Diabetes Association. Evidence-based nutrition principles and recommendations for the treatment and prevention of diabetes and related complications. Diabetes Care 2002;25:S50-S60.

[98] Kris-Etherton PM, Harris WS, Appel LJ. AHA scientific statement: fish consumption, fish oil, omega-3 fatty acids, and cardiovascular disease. Circulation 2002;106:2747-57.

[99] Woods MN, Wanke CA, Ling PR, et al. Effect of a dietary intervention and n-3 fatty acid supplementation on measures of serum lipid and insulin sensitivity in persons with HIV. American Journal of Clinical Nutrition 2009; 90(6):1566-78.

[100] Thusgaard M, Christensen JH, Morn B, et al. Effect of fish oil (n-3 polyunsaturated fatty acids) on plasma lipids, lipoproteins and inflammatory markers in HIV-infected patients treated with antiretroviral therapy: a randomized, double-blind, placebo-controlled study. Scandinavian Journal of Infectious Diseases 2009; 41(10):760-6.

[101] Zemel MB. Role of dietary calcium and dairy products in modulating adiposity. Lipids 2003; 38, 139–146.

[102] Zemel MB. The role of dairy foods in weight management. J Am Coll Nutr 2005; 24:537S–546S.

[103] Zemel MB, Richards J, Milstead A, Campbell P. Effects of calcium and dairy on body composition and weight loss in African-American adults. Obes Res 2005; 13:218–225.

[104] Astrup A. The role of calcium in energy balance and obesity: the research for mechanisms. Am J Clin Nutr 2008; 88:873–874.

[105] Major GC, Chaput JP, Ledoux M, et al. Recent developments in calcium-related obesity research. Obes Rev 2008; 9:428–445.

[106] Beydoun MA, Gary TL, Caballero BH, et al. Ethnic differences in dairy and related nutrient consumption among US adults and their association with obesity, central obesity and metabolic syndrome. Am J Clin Nutr 2008; 87:1914–1925.

[107] Marques-Vidal P, Gonçalves A, Dias CM. Milk intake is inversely related to obesity in men and in young women: data from the Portuguese Health Interview Survey 1998–1999. Int. J. Obes. (Lond) 2006; 30:88–93.

[108] Sampath V, Havel PJ, King JC. Calcium supplementation does not alter lipid oxidation or lipolysis in overweight / obese women. Obesity 2008; 16:2400–2404.

[109] Parikh S, Yanovski JA. Calcium intake and adiposity. Am J Clin Nutr 2003; 77:281–287.

[110] Anderson RA, Polansky MM, Bryden NA, et al. Effect of supplemental chromium on patients with symptoms of reactive hypoglycemia. Metabolism 1987; 36:351-355.

[111] Saad MJA. Molecular mechanisms of insulin resistance. Brazilian J Med Biol Res 1994; 27:941-957.

[112] Kahn CR. Current concepts of the molecular mechanism of insulin action. Ann Rev Med 1985; 36:429-451.

[113] Roth RA, Lui F, Chin JE. Biochemical mechanisms of insulin resistance. Hormone Res 1994; 41:51-55.

[114] Davis CM, Vincent JB. Chromium oligopeptide activates insulin receptor kinase activity. Biochemistry 1997; 36:4382-4385.

[115] Imparl-Radosevich J, Deas S, Polansky MM, et al. Regulation of phosphotyrosine phosphatase (PTP-1) and insulin receptor kinase by fractions from cinnamon:

implications for cinnamon regulation of insulin signaling. Hormone Research 1998; 50(3):177-82.
[116] Davis CM, Sumall KH, Vincent JB. A biologically active form of chromium may activate a membrane phosphotyrosine phosphatase (PTP). Biochemistry 1996; 35:12963-12969.
[117] Jeejeebhoy KN, Chu RC, Marliss EB, et al. Chromium deficiency, glucose intolerance, and neuropathy reversed by chromium supplementation in a patient receiving long-term total parenteral nutrition. Am J Clin Nutr 1977; 30:531.
[118] Anderson RA. Recent advances in the clinical and biochemical effects of chromium deficiency. In: Essential and Toxic Trace Elements in Human Health and Disease. Prasad AS (editor). New York: Wiley Liss; 1993. pp 221-234.
[119] Anderson RA. Chromium, glucose tolerance, diabetes and lipid metabolism. J Adv Med 1995; 8:37-49.
[120] Mertz W. Chromium in human nutrition: a review. J Nutr 1993; 123:626-633.
[121] Riales R, Albrink MJ. Effect of chromium chloride supplementation on glucose tolerance and serum lipids including high density lipoprotein of adult men. Am J Clin Nutr 1981; 34:2670-2678.
[122] Anderson RA, Bryden NA, Polansky MM, Reiser S. Urinary chromium excretion and insulinogenic properties of carbohydrates. Am J Clin Nutr 1990; 51:864-868.
[123] Freund H, Atamian S, and Fischer JE. Chromium deficiency during total parenteral nutrition. JAMA 1979; 241:496.
[124] Brown RO, Forloines-Lynn S, Cross RE, Heizer WD. Chromium deficiency after long-term total parenteral nutrition. Dig Dis Sci 1986; 31:661.
[125] Schwarz K, Mertz W. Chromium(III) and the glucose tolerance factor. Arch Biochem Biophys 1959; 85:292-295.
[126] Anderson RA, Polansky MM. Bryden NA. Roginski E. Mertz E, Glinsmann W. Chromium supplementation of human subjects: effects on glucose, insulin and lipid variables. Metabolism: Clinical & experimental 1983; 32:894-899.
[127] Glinsmann WH, Mertz W. Effect of trivalent chromium on glucose tolerance. Metabolism 1966; 15:510-520.
[128] Levine RA, Streeten DHP, Doisy RJ. Effects of oral chromium supplementation on the glucose tolerance of elderly human subjects. Metabolism 1968; Clinical & Experimental 17:114-125.
[129] Mahdi GS, Naismith DJ. Role of chromium in barley in modulating the symptoms of diabetes. Ann Nutr Metab 1991; 35:65-70.
[130] Abraham AS, Brooks BA, Eylath U. The effects of chromium supplementation on serum glucose and lipids in patients with and without non-insulin dependent diabetes. Metabolism 1992; 41:768-771.
[131] Uyanik F. The effects of dietary chromium supplementation on some blood parameters in sheep. Biological trace Element Research 2001; 84: 93-99.
[132] Morris BW, Kouta S, Robinsont R, et al. Chromium supplementation improves insulin resistance in patients with type 2 diabetes. Diabetic Medicine 2000; 17:684-686.
[133] Morris BW, MacNeil S, Hardisty CA, et al. Chromium homeostasis in patients with type II (NIDDM) diabetes. Journal of Trace Elements in Medicine & Biology 1999;13(1-2):57-61.

[134] Evans GW. The effect of chromium picolinate on insulin controlled parameters in humans. Int J Biosoc Med Res 1989; 11:163-180.

[135] Anderson RA, Cheng N, Bryden NA, et al. Elevated intakes of supplemental chromium improve glucose and insulin variables in individuals with type 2 diabetes. Diabetes 1997; 46:1786-1791.

[136] Gurson CT, Saner G. Effect of chromium on glucose utilization in marasmic protein-calorie malnutrition. Am J Clin Nutr 1971; 24: 1313.

[137] Hopkins LL, Ransome-Kati O, Majaj AS. Improvement of impaired carbohydrate metabolism by chromium 3 in malnourished infants. Am J Clin Nutr 1968; 21:203-211.

[138] Balk EM, Tatsioni AT, Lichtenstein AH, et al. Effect of chromium supplementation on glucose metabolism and lipids. Diabetes care 2007; 30:2154-2163.

[139] Aghdassi E, Salit IE, Fung L, et al. Is chromium an important element in HIV-positive patients with metabolic abnormalities? An hypothesis generating pilot study. Journal of the American Collegue of Nutrition 2006; 25(1): 56-63.

[140] Aghdassi E, Arendt BE, Salit IE, et al. In patients with HIV-infection, chromium supplementation improves insulin resistance and other metabolic abnormalities: a randomized, double-blind, placebo controlled trial. Current HIV Research 2010; 8(2):113-20.

[141] Miranda ER, Dey CS. Effect of chromium and zinc on insulin signaling in skeletal muscle cells. Biol Trace Elem Res 2004; 101:19-36.

[142] Yoshimoto S, Sakamoto K, Wakabayashi I, Masui H. Effect of chromium administration on glucose tolerance in stroke-prone spontaneously hypertensive rats with streptozotocin-induced diabetes. Metabolism 1992; 41:636-642.

[143] Davis CM, Vincent JB. Isolation and characterization of a biologically active chromium oligopeptide from bovine liver. Arch Biochem Biophys 1997; 339:335-343.

[144] Wang ZQ, Zhang XH, Cefalu WT. Chromium picolinate increases phosphoinostide 3-kinase activity, glucose uptake, and glycogen content in cultured human skeletal muscle cells. Diabetes 2002; 51(Suppl 2)-abstract.

[145] Cefalu WT, Wang ZQ, Zhang XH, et al. Oral chromium picolinate improves carbohydrate and lipid metabolism and enhances skeletal muscle Glut-4 translocation in obese, hyperinsulinemic (JCR-LA corpulent) rats. J Nutr 2002; 132:110711-110714.

[146] Wang ZQ, Zhang XH, Russell JC, et al. Chromium picolinate enhances skeletal muscle cellular insulin signaling in vivo in obese, insulin-resistant JCR:LA-cp rats. J Nutr 2006; 136:415-420.

[147] Anderson RA, Bryden NA, Polansky MM. Chromium content of selected breakfast cereals. J Food Comp Anal 1988; 1:303-8.

[148] Anderson RA, Bryden NA, Polansky MM. Dietary chromium intake: Freely chosen diets, institution diets, and individual foods. Biol Trace Elem Res 1992; 32:117-21.

[149] National Research Council:' Recommended Dietary Allowance,' 10 ed. Washington DC: National Academy Press, 1989.

[150] Anderson RA, Kizlovsky AS. Chromium intake, absorption and excretion of subjects consuming self-selected diets. Am J Clin Nutr 1985; 41:1177.

[151] Anderson RA, Bryden NA, Polansky MM. Dietary chromium intake: Freely chosen diets, institution diets, and individual foods. Biol Trace Elem Res 1992; 32:117-21.

[152] Offenbacher EG. Chromium in the elderly. Biol Trace Elem Res 1992; 32:123-31.

[153] Nielson F. controversial chromium:does the superstar mineral of the mountbanks receive appropriate attention from clinicians and nutritionists? Nutr Today 1996; 31:226-33.

[154] Anderson R, Cheng N, Bryden N, et al. Elevated intakes of supplemental chromium improve glucose and insulin variables in individuals with type 2 diabetes. Diabetes 1997; 46:1786-91.

[155] Amorosa V, Synnestvedt M, Gross R, et al. A tale of 2 epidemics: the intersection between obesity and HIV infection in Philadelphia. J Acquir Immune Defic Syndr. 2005;39:557-561.

[156] American Diabetes Association. Standards of medical care in diabetes- 2008. Diabetes Care. 2008;31(Suppl 1):S12-S54.

[157] Jansson S, Engfeldt P. Changed life style can prevent type 2 diabetes. Intervention studies show good results in "pre-diabetics" [in Swedish]. Lakartidningen 2007;104:3771-3774.

[158] Ilanne-Parikka P, Eriksson JG, Lindström J, et al. Effect of lifestyle intervention on the occurrence of metabolic syndrome and its components in the Finnish Diabetes Prevention Study. Diabetes Care 2008;31:805-807.

[159] Riccardi G, Rivellese AA, Giacco R. Role of glycemic index and glycemic load in the healthy state, in prediabetes, and in diabetes. Am J Clin Nutr 2008; 87:269S-274S.

[160] Knowler WC, Barrett-Connor E, Fowler SE, et al. Reduction in the incidence of type 2 diabetes with lifestyle intervention or metformin. N Engl J Med 2002; 346:393-403.

[161] LaMonte MJ, Blair SN, Church TS. Physical activity and diabetes prevention. J Appl Physiol 2005; 205-1213.

[162] Holloszy JO, Schultz J, Kusnierkiewicz J, et al. Effects of exercise on glucose tolerance and insulin resistance. Acta Med Scand 1986;711:55-65.

[163] LeBlanc J, Nadeau A, Richard R, Tremblay A. Studies on the sparing effect of exercise on insulin requirements in human subjects. Metabolism1981; 30:1119-1124.

[164] Burstein R, Epstein Y, Shapiro Y, et al. Effect of an acute bout of exercise on glucose disposal in human obesity. J Appl Physiol 1990; 69:299-304.

[165] King DS, Dalsky GP, Staten MA, et al. Insulin action and secretion in endurance-trained and untrained humans. J Appl Physiol 1987;63:2247-2252.

[166] Hughes VA, Fiatarone MA, Fielding RA, et al. Exercise increases muscle GLUT-4 levels and insulin action in subjects with impaired glucose tolerance. Am J Physiol 1993; 264:E855-E862.

[167] Regensteiner JG, Mayer EJ, Shetterly SM, et al. Relationship between habitual physical activity and insulin levels among nondiabetic men and women: the San Luis Valley Diabetes Study. Diabetes Care 1991;14:1066-1074.

[168] Folsom AR, Jacobs DR, Wagenknecht LE, et al. Increase in fasting insulin and glucose over seven years with increasing weight and inactivity of young adults. Am J Epidemiol 1996;144:235-246.

[169] Regensteiner JG, Shetterly SM, Mayer EJ, et al. Relationship between habitual physical activity and insulin area among persons with impaired glucose tolerance: the San Luis Valley Diabetes Study. Diabetes Care 1995;18:490-497.

[170] Mayer-Davis EJ, D'Agostino R, Karter AJ, et al. Intensity and Amount of Physical Activity in Relation to Insulin Sensitivity. The Insulin Resistance Atherosclerosis Study. JAMA. 1998;279(9):669-674.

[171] Pate RR, Pratt M, Blair SN, et al. Physical activity and public health: a recommendation from the Centers for Disease Control and Prevention and the American College of Sports Medicine. JAMA 1995; 273:402-407.

[172] NIH Consensus Development Panel on Physical Activity and Cardiovascular Health. Physical activity and cardiovascular health. JAMA1996; 276:241-246.

5

# Nosocomial Infections in Patients with Human Immunodeficiency Virus (HIV)

Olga Perovic[1,2] and Ashika Singh[1]
[1]*National Institute for Communicable Diseases,*
*a Division of the National Health Laboratory Service*
[2]*University of Witwatersrand*
*South Africa*

## 1. Introduction

Human immunodeficiency virus (HIV) results in acquired immune deficiency syndrome (AIDS) and is characterized by a serious disorder of the immune system in which the protective defenses against infection cannot function leaving the individual vulnerable to severe infections and conditions. This results in opportunistic infections causing an unfavourable outcome. Since its discovery in 1981 when the first cases were described, HIV/AIDS continues to affect people globally. According to the UNAIDS (Joint United Nations Programme on HIV/AIDS) and WHO (World Health Organization) 2009 AIDS epidemic update report, the estimated number of people living with HIV worldwide in 2008 was 33.4 million (UNAIDS 2009). Ultimately there is a high prevalence of HIV infection among patients admitted to hospitals as well as a high prevalence of AIDS patients as a result of opportunistic infections related to their HIV status or advanced AIDS (Mbanya, Ateudjieu et al. 2010).

## 2. Bacterial colonization

A major risk factor for bacterial colonization is immunosuppression subsequently making HIV-infected individuals ideal candidates (Craven, Steger et al. 1996). Bacterial colonization refers to the presence of bacteria in a host but does not cause a specific immune response or infection. However, if the relationship between the host and bacterial agent is changed - such as immunosuppression of the host, this episode can result in infections (Mandell, Bennett et al. 2005). Colonization therefore seems to contribute significantly to the development of nosocomial infections in HIV-positive patients (Petrosillo, Pagani et al. 2003).
Colonization is the first step of microbial infection. It is the establishment of the pathogen at the suitable portal of entry for example, host tissues that are in contact with the external environment. Sites of entry include the conjunctiva, the digestive tract, the respiratory tract and the urogenital tract. Organisms such as *Staphylococcus aureus* have been found to have high rates of nasal colonization in HIV-infected patients (Raviglione, Mariuz et al. 1990; Weinke, Schiller et al. 1992). Additionally other body cavities may also provide productive environments for bacterial colonization. The oral cavity is proximal and contiguous with the trachea and is therefore a portal for respiratory pathogen colonization. The teeth and other

oral mucosal surfaces particularly in ICU patients operate as reservoirs for respiratory pathogen colonization (Raghavendran, Mylotte et al. 2007).

## 3. HIV and nosocomial infections

A nosocomial (hospital-acquired) infection is one in which there is no evidence that the infection was present or in an incubation period at the time of hospital admission except 48 hours after admission. The condition is classified as an infection when it is manifested as a clinical disease and not a colonization where microorganisms are present but have no harmful effects on the patient's health. However, asymptomatic patients are considered infected if the body fluid or body site that is normally sterile (e.g. blood or cerebrospinal fluid) contains pathogenic microorganisms (Emori and Gaynes 1993). Nosocomial infections constitute a significant public health concern. They contribute to long hospital-stays and additional health care costs and are a significant cause of morbidity and mortality in hospital environments (Petrosillo, Pagani et al. 2003; Singh, Goering et al. 2006). Nosocomial infections are common and not always avoidable because of the large turnover of patients with underlying conditions. Furthermore their immune systems are often in a weakened state. Horizontal transmission from one patient to another creates an opportunity for the spread of hospital pathogens. Various invasive surgical procedures such as indwelling catheters and medical devices bypass the natural body-protective barriers. Prior antimicrobial therapy and inappropriate use of antimicrobial agents resulting in the emergence of resistant strains are traditional risk factors for acquiring infections in the hospitals. Nosocomial infections are therefore a major challenge to the patients' safety in the hospital setting and HIV as an additional factor has lead to an increase in morbidity and mortality. This can be explained by the ability of opportunistic pathogens and microorganisms that are normally non-pathogenic to cause disease in immunocompromised individuals (Emori and Gaynes 1993; Craven, Steger et al. 1996; Vandenesch, Naimi et al. 2003; Singh, Goering et al. 2006; Panis, Matsuo et al. 2009). There are several pathogenic processes that are involved in the progression to AIDS in HIV-infected individuals such as: depletion in CD4 lymphocytes, defects in B lymphocytes, neutrophil dysfunction and the breakdown of the integument as a result of AIDS-related dermatological conditions for example bacterial and fungal dermatoses and Kaposi's sarcoma. These individual factors have significant implications regarding host susceptibility to nosocomial infections (Duse 1999). Noscomial infections appear to be more common in HIV-positive individuals with AIDS as opposed to HIV-negative individuals (Angus and Wax 2001). Studies have suggested that HIV-infected or AIDS patients are at high risk of acquiring nosocomial infections particularly sepsis and bacteraemia due to the implantation of invasive intravascular medical devices (Gobbi, Maggi et al. 1998; Tumbarello, Tacconelli et al. 1998; Laing 1999; Petrosillo, Pagani et al. 2003; Japiassú, Amâncio et al. 2010). Nosocomial urinary tract and respiratory tract infections are also common in HIV-infected AIDS patients following bacterial colonization (Petrosillo, Nicastri et al. 2005).

### 3.1 Bacteraemia

Bacteraemia or bloodstream infections are among the most severe of hospital-acquired infections and have been shown to cause significant mortality and prolonged hospital-stays in patients with HIV (Tumbarello, Tacconelli et al. 1998). Previous studies have shown that an increase in these bloodstream infections is associated with HIV infections (Beuheza, Beckelman et al. 1989; Fife, Crane et al. 1990).

### 3.1.1 Etiological agents

Coagulase-negative staphylococci have been implicated as important causes of nosocomial bloodstream infections particularly in patients that are immunocompromised (Tumbarello, Tacconelli et al. 1995; Pagano, Tacconelli et al. 1997) and in those infected with HIV (Weinke, Schiller et al. 1992; Tumbarello, Tacconelli et al. 1996; Tumbarello, Tacconelli et al. 1998). Globally, *Staphylococcus aureus* is the second most common pathogen that is responsible for causing bloodstream infections (Fluit, Jones et al. 2000; Luzzaro, Vigano et al. 2002) and in European countries it is the leading cause of nosocomial bloodstream infections (Luzzaro, Vigano et al. 2002). *S. aureus* is also the most common pathogen isolated from all bloodstream infections in the US (Shorr, Tabak et al. 2006). Bloodstream infections caused by these organisms are associated with a high frequency of life-threatening complications such as metastatic infections and infective endocarditis (del Rio, Cervera et al. 2009). *S. aureus* has also shown to be responsible for a significant number of in-hospital deaths in patients with long-term catheters, cardiovascular, orthopaedic and other medical devices (Chu, Crosslin et al. 2005). Methicillin-resistant strains of *S. aureus* also pose a major problem in nosocomial bloodstream infections (del Rio, Cervera et al. 2009).

Other studies have suggested an increased risk of nosocomial bloodstream infections due to aerobic gram-negative bacilli such as *Pseudomonas aeruginosa, Klebsiella pneumoniae* and *Escherichia coli* in patients that were HIV-infected particularly in those having invasive devices (Hickey and Shanson 1993; Sanford 1995; Zurlo and Lane 1997; Tumbarello, Tacconelli et al. 1998). Nontyphoidal *Salmonella* species is an infrequent cause of hospital infections (Jaspan 2008).

### 3.1.2 Clinical manifestations

Bloodstream infections may be defined as the presence of viable bacteria in the blood (bacteraemia) with a documented positive blood culture result and the presence of clinical symptoms of systemic infection (Garner, Jarvis et al. 1988). Primary bloodstream infection is a bloodstream infection without a documented primary source of infection (portal of entry or site of infection) and can be distinguished from a secondary bloodstream infection which is a bloodstream infection secondary to a localised site of infection - wound infection, skin and soft-tissue infection, biliary tract infection and pneumonia (Seifert 2009). Infections usually associated with secondary bloodstream infections include deep-seated abscesses, osteomyelitis and endocarditis (Fowler, Olsen et al. 2003). It has been reported that approximately one third of patients with *S. aureus* bloodstream infections develop local complications or distant septic metastases and affect the epidural space and intervertebral discs, bone and joints particularly when prosthetic material and native and prosthetic cardiac valves are being used (Ringberg, Thoren et al. 2000; Fowler, Olsen et al. 2003). Visceral abscesses in the spleen and kidney may also develop (del Rio, Cervera et al. 2009). Risk factors associated with complicated *S. aureus* bloodstream infections include the presence of persistent bacteraemia which is defined as the presence of positive blood cultures after 72-96 hours of appropriate treatment, the presence of skin lesions suggesting distant metastases, persistent fever and community acquisition (Fowler, Olsen et al. 2003).

Bloodstream infections are a major cause of illness in patients infected with HIV. A high percentage of bloodstream infections, ranging from 10% to 63% were observed in hospitalised HIV-infected individuals presenting with fever in a number of studies conducted in Sub-Saharan Africa (Archibald, den Dulk et al. 1998; Ssali, Kamya et al. 1998;

McDonald, Archibald et al. 1999; Peters, Zijlstra et al. 2004). Another study showed that bloodstream infection was associated with recent HIV diagnosis. Almost half the patients with bloodstream infections presented with a temperature of greater than 38°C. Lower T CD4$^{+}$ counts were also strongly associated with those patients having bloodstream infections. Symptoms of abdominal illness such as nausea, vomiting and loss of appetite were also associated with bloodstream infections caused by pathogens (Varma, McCarthy et al. 2010). HIV-infected patients may be predisposed to bloodstream infections due to several conditions such as defective cell-mediated immunity, altered B-cell function with a consequent lack of serum opsonins against some encapsulated bacteria and qualitative and quantitative deficits of neutrophils leading to an increase in the susceptibility of the patient to bacterial and fungal infections (Mertins, Ortona et al. 1990; Zurlo and Lane 1997).

### 3.1.3 Management

The clinical microbiology laboratory plays an important part in the management of patients with bloodstream infections. A highly specific indicator of bloodstream infections is the culturing of pathogenic microorganisms from blood. In addition antimicrobial susceptibility testing (AST) may assist in the choice of antimicrobial therapy to be administered (Bohte, van Furth et al. 1995; Chalasani, Valdecanas et al. 1995; Fine, Smith et al. 1996). The early and rapid administration of antimicrobial treatment to infected patients has initially shown to decrease mortality (Leibovici, Konisberger et al. 1992). However, due to the emergence of antibiotic resistance there is a need to develop new antimicrobial agents (Ibrahim, Sherman et al. 2000).

It is recommended that for those patients that are infected with coagulase-negative staphylococci due to the presence of catheters, the catheter should be removed and a short course (5-7 days) of antibiotics administered. If the patient has endovascular hardware present, persistent fever or bacteraemia may be experienced after the catheter has been removed, then a long course of antibiotics may be required (O'Grady and Chertow 2011).

The choice of antibiotics for enterococcal bloodstream infections depends on the susceptibility of the infecting isolate due to antibiotic resistance. Ampicillin is the preferred choice of drug for the treatment of ampicillin-susceptible enterococci. If the pathogen is resistant to ampiciliin, vancomycin should be used if the isolate is vancomycin-susceptible. Enterococci resistant to both ampicillin and vancomycin can be treated with new oxazolidinones, linezolid or lipopeptides, daptomycin. However, this depends on susceptibility testing (O'Grady and Chertow 2011). Some studies have shown that combination therapy may be more effective than monotherapy. This was seen in a number of patients with enterococcal bloodstream infections in which the catheter was not removed and a combination of ampicillin and gentamicin was used (Sandoe, Witherden et al. 2002).

For gram-negative bacilli removal of short-term catheters followed by 5-7 days of systemic antibiotic therapy is suggested based on antimicrobial susceptibility test results. Usually fourth generation cephalosporins, carbapenems or a combination of β-lactam and β-lactamase inhibitor may be used (O'Grady and Chertow 2011). However, extended-spectrum beta-lactamase-producing *Escherichia coli* and *Klebsiella pneumoniae* should not be treated with cephalosporins or piperacilin-tazobactam even if they may be susceptible as treatment with these drugs has been associated with poor clinical outcome (Paterson, Ko et al. 2001; Jacoby and Munoz-Price 2005).

Fluconazole may be used to treat individuals with bloodstream infections as a result of *Candida* species. Alternative therapy includes echinocandins as first-line therapy and lipid formulations of amphotericin B (Mora-Duarte, Betts et al. 2002; Reboli, Roststein et al. 2007).

A confirmed catheter-related bloodstream infection for gram-positive organisms requires at least two positive results drawn from different sites. These infections are difficult to treat unless the infected catheter is removed (Cotton, Gill et al. 1987; Peces, Gago et al. 1997).

### 3.2 Urinary tract infections

Other common nosocomial infections are associated with the urinary tract. Nosocomial urinary tract infection is a major infection acquired in both hospitals and nursing homes. In most cases these infections are commonly related to catheterization. Bacteriuria is a term referring to bacteria in the urine (Mandell, Bennett et al. 2005). Insertion of a catheter may predispose the bladder to the introduction of organisms that may colonize the site of insertion. Any disconnection of the catheter from the collection tube or breakage of the closed system may result in bacteriuria. The collection bag is drained regularly and if the lumen of the drainage tube is contaminated with bacteria, this provides a portal of entry for bacteria to the drainage bag, collection tube and catheter. A biofilm which secures the bacteria against the catheter or mucosal surface protects the bacteria from the mechanical flow of urine, host defences and antibiotics (Warren 2001). The rate of urinary tract infections particularly related to the use of urinary catheters plays a significant role in nosocomial infection in HIV patients (Gobbi, Maggi et al. 1998).

#### 3.2.1 Etiological agents

Common organisms isolated from urinary tract infections include *Escherichia coli, Pseudomonas aeruginosa, Klebsiella pneumoniae, Proteus mirabilis, Staphylococcus epidermis,* enterococci and *Candida* species (Warren 2001). Uropathic *E. coli* are responsible for most urinary tract infections. The *E. coli* serogroups most often implicated as the cause of high proportion of infection are O1, O2, O4, O6, O7, O8, O75, O150 and O18ab (Roberts and Phillips 1979; Rosen, Hooton et al. 2007). Hospital environments are a significant determinant of the type of organisms causing urinary tract infections. Staphylococci, enterococci, *Proteus, Klebsiella, Enterobacter* and *Pseudomonas* species are most often isolated from inpatients whereas *E. coli* infection predominate in the outpatient population (Bronsema, Adams et al. 1993). *Corynebacterium urealyticum* (*Corynebacterium* group D2) has been identified as an important nosocomial pathogen (Soriano, Aguado et al. 1990).

#### 3.2.2 Pathogenesis

Urinary tract infections are as a result of the interaction between bacterial virulence and the biologic and behavioural factors in the host. Bacteria may invade and spread within the urinary tract via three possible routes. These are the ascending, haematogenous and lymphatic pathways. The ascending pathway involves colonization of the urethra with bacteria. Microorganisms in the urine can enter the bladder. Once in the bladder, bacteria can multiply and pass up the ureters to the renal pelvis and parenchyma. The haematogenous pathway involves infection of the renal parenchyma by blood-borne organisms. The organisms most often implicated here are *S. aureus* and *Candida* species. In humans, infection of the kidney via the haematogenous route rarely involves gram-negative bacilli. Lymphatic pathway infection occurs when increased pressure in the bladder can cause lymphatic flow to be directed to the kidneys taking with it microorganisms (Mandell, Bennett et al. 2005).

### 3.2.3 Clinical manifestations

Urinary tract infection may involve the lower urinary tract or both the upper and lower urinary tracts. Lower urinary tract symptoms as a result from bacteria-producing irritation of the urethral and vesicle mucosa. This may cause frequent and painful urination of small amounts of urine that is turbid, suprapubic heaviness or pain and in some cases blood in the urine. Upper urinary tract infection includes fever, flank pain as well as symptoms such as increased frequency of urine, dysuria and the urgency to urinate. However these symptoms may vary greatly (Mandell, Bennett et al. 2005). Urinary tract infections in HIV-infected individuals include HIV-associated nephropathy, as well as skin and soft tissue infections (Eulalia Valencia, Enriquez et al. 1997).

### 3.2.4 Management

All symptomatic urinary tract infections should be treated whereas asymptomatic infection should be treated if at least two cultures of clean-voided, midstream urine grow the same organism in significant cell counts.

A high fluid intake is recommended resulting in a dilution of the bacteria in the urine. Rapid hydration may reduce bacterial counts but this usually returns to normal once hydration is stopped. Decreasing the urinary pH results in antibacterial activity e.g. ingesting large volumes of cranberry juice contributes to low pH as high concentrations of hippuric acid (derived from the precursors in the berry) penetrates into the bacterial cell preventing optimal functioning. Hippuric acid is a weakly ionisable organic acid and is therefore able to better penetrate bacterial cells. Analgesics may be administered to patients exhibiting pain.

Antimicrobial therapy is effective and guidelines are based on local antibiotic susceptibility patterns. However, antimicrobial drugs may either cure the infection or may cause bacterial persistence, relapse or re-infection. Bacterial cell counts should be reduced within 48 hours after the initiation of treatment with the antimicrobial drug that the microorganism is sensitive to *in vitro*. Bacteriologic cure is expected when the urine cultures are negative after 48 hours of initial treatment and during the follow-up period of 1-2 weeks. Bacteriologic persistence occurs when bacterial counts are not reduced after 48 hours of treatment initiation or if the infecting organism persists in low numbers in the urine after 48 hours. Bacteriologic relapse occurs within 1-2 weeks after treatment has ended. Re-infection occurs during the administration of the drug or anytime thereafter. This is referred to as superinfection and may be identified by a change in bacterial species.

Individuals that are severely ill with pyelonephritis should be hospitalised and parenteral therapy is required.

For hospitalised immunocompromised patients with infections caused by gram-negative bacteria, third generation cephalosporins, aminopenicillin inhibitor combinations and carbapenems may be used with or without aminoglycosides and fluoroquinolones are recommended.

## 3.3 Respiratory tract infections

Nosocomial pulmonary infections are more common in patients with AIDS and are related to the extent of immunosuppression, prior use of antibiotics, and the exposure to invasive procedures. Nosocomial *Mycobacterium tuberculosis* and bacterial pneumonia are common in HIV-positive individuals and are associated with significant morbidity and mortality (Petrosillo, Nicastri et al. 2005). The majority of tuberculosis cases and deaths occur in low resource areas; however nosocomial transmission to the patients with HIV occurs in both developed and developing countries mainly including multiple-drug resistant tuberculosis.

### 3.3.1 Pneumonia

Nosocomial pneumonia is the second leading cause of nosocomial infection and the leading cause of infection-related deaths in hospitalised patients (Mandell, Bennett et al. 2005). The morbidity associated with nosocomial pneumonia includes longer hospitalised stays and higher costs for health care (Wenzel 1989). Risk factors associated with nosocomial pneumonia are related to the patient's immune status, infection-control practices and introduction of invasive procedures or other intervention (American Thoracic Society 1996). Patient-related risk factors are: age greater than 70 years, malnutrition, coma, metabolic acidosis, severe underlying disease and the presence of any of a number of co-morbid illnesses such as alcoholism, central nervous system dysfunction, and azotemia. Infection-control-related risk factors are a lack of hand hygiene, a lack of glove-use practices and the use of contaminated respiratory equipment. Intervention-related risk factors include procedures and treatment that may challenge normal host defenses or allow exposure of the host to large inocula of bacteria. Sedatives and narcotics may be aspirated, cytotoxic agents and corticosteroids may inhibit the hosts normal responses to infection and prolonged use of antimicrobials may lead to the development of drug resistance. Surgical procedures associated with the chest and abdomen may predispose the patient to pneumonia as these are associated with changes in host defense. Ventilation is also a major risk factor for the development of pneumonia in intensive care units (Craven and Steger 1995; George 1995). Pneumonia often affects individuals with impaired host defense systems such as defects in antibody production, phagocytosis, ciliary function or decreased CD4+ T-lymphocyte counts as seen in AIDS (Braunwald, Fauci et al. 2004).

#### 3.3.1.1 Etiological agents

Reports of an increased risk of nosocomial respiratory tract infections due to aerobic gram-positive and negative bacteria such as *Staphylococcus aureus, Streptococcus pneumoniae, Pseudomonas aeruginosa, Haemophilus influenzae* and members of the enterobacteriaceae such as *Klebsiella pneumoniae, Escherichia coli, Serratia marcescens, Enterobacter* species in patients with HIV have been observed most frequently. Mortality rates are especially high in patients that have pneumonia caused by *Pseudomonas aeruginosa* or *Acinetobacter* species (Kollef, Bock et al. 1995; Tumbarello, Tacconelli et al. 1998; Mandell, Bennett et al. 2005). Anaerobic bacteria have been isolated from a number of patients with nosocomial pneumonia but only a small percentage of these cases are thought to be caused by these organisms (A'Court and Garrard 1992). *Legionella* species have also occasionally found to be the cause of nosocomial pneumonia and majority of these cases have been in immunocompromised individuals (Mandell, Bennett et al. 2005).

#### 3.3.1.2 Clinical manifestations

Symptoms may vary and may be non-specific. Initial symptoms include fever, chills and malaise. Progressive anorexia and weight loss is usually indicative of chronic illness. Pulmonary symptoms may initially occur but as the illness progresses, this may become more frequent. Patients presenting with prolonged illness and nonspecific complaints together with pulmonary symptoms including shortness of breath, increased respiratory rate, sputum production, new or persistent cough, hemoptysis, chest pain or dyspnea should be evaluated. Extrapulmonary symptoms may also occur. Chronic pneumonia may present with skin and mucous membrane lesions suggesting histoplasmosis, coccidioidomycosis, blastomycosis and in some epidemiologic settings paracoccidioidomycosis and may be differential in nosocomial settings. Cryptococcosis, nocardiosis and Karposi's sarcoma are important considerations in AIDS patients (Mandell, Bennett et al. 2005; Raghavendran, Mylotte et al. 2007).

### 3.3.1.3 Management

Important considerations for the treatment of nosocomial pneumonia include early administration of the appropriate antibiotic (Iregui, Ward et al. 2002). Delay or inappropriate antibiotic treatment results in increased morbidity and mortality. Timely, accurate and appropriate therapy is therefore of vital importance as overuse or the unnecessary use of broad-spectrum antibiotics may result in drug resistance, superinfection and increased drug toxicity rates resulting in an increase in morbidity and mortality (Raghavendran, Mylotte et al. 2007). Ventilator-associated pneumonia is common. The antibiotic therapy that is employed depends on the use of prior antibiotic treatment at the time of onset of ventilator-associated pneumonia. If there is no prior history of antibiotic usage for early onset ventilator-associated pneumonia, third and fourth generation cephalosporins such as ceftriaxone or cefotaxime are the preferred choices or alternatively fluoroquinolones and or macrolides as part of combination treatment. An antipseudomonad cephalosporin such as ceftazadime or cefipime, an antipseudomonad penicillin such as piperacillin, carbepenem such as imipenem or meropenem or aztreonam combined with an aminoglycoside either in the presence or absence of methicillin-resistant *S. aureus* coverage with vancomycin or linezolid particularly if gram-positive cocci have been identified in the sputum Gram-stain, may be an effective combined regimen for the treatment of late-onset ventiliator-associated pneumonia (Ost, Hall et al. 2003).

## 4. Intensive Care Unit (ICU) – Nosocomial infections in HIV-infected patients

Nosocomial infection rates are highest in patients from intensive care units (ICU) and infection rates in adult and paediatric ICUs are about three fold higher than elsewhere in the hospital. The sites of infection and pathogens involved vary depending on the type of ICU treatment (Fridkin, Welbel et al. 1997; Weinstein 1998). Since the beginning of the AIDS epidemic, admissions in the ICU of hospitals have markedly increased with HIV-infected patients being admitted with concomitant infections such as pneumocystis pneumonia, bacterial pneumonia and tuberculosis - all of which are important infectious causes of respiratory failure resulting in pulmonary disease.

*Pseudomonas aeruginosa* and *Staphylococcus aureus* as noted previously, are particularly significant causes of nosocomial bacterial pneumonias in ICU in both HIV-infected and HIV-uninfected patients. Therefore the management of hospital-acquired and ventilator-associated pneumonia is similar for both group of patients (American Thoracic Society 2005). However, the presence of methicillin-resistant *S. aureus* is an independent risk factor for death in HIV-infected patients and this should be considered in the initial treatment regimens (Franzetti, Grassini et al. 2006). Urinary tract infections in the ICU are as a result of fungal infections. *Candida* species including *Candida albicans* are the main cause of urinary tract infections in the ICU (Fridkin, Welbel et al. 1997). Another major cause of ICU admissions in HIV-infected patients is sepsis (Huang, Quartin et al. 2006; Japiassu, Amancio et al. 2010). Patients with invasive catheters and monitoring devices are predisposed to bloodstream infections caused by coagulase-negative staphylococci. Reports from one study demonstrated a 50% mortality rate in HIV-infected sepsis patients in ICU. The lung was the most common site of infection in this study followed by primary bloodstream infections, venous catheter-related bacteraemia and urinary tract infections. Nosocomial infections were source of the sepsis and accounted for 90% of cases in this cohort and were composed mostly of gram-negative rods such as *Pseudomonas aeruginosa, Klebsiella pneumoniae, Enterobacter* species, *Escherichia coli, Acinetobacter* species, *Serratia marcescens, Staphylococcus* species, *Stenotrophomonas maltophilia, Clostridium difficile, Citrobacter freundii, Burkholderia cepacia* and *Candida* species. *Mycobaterium tuberculosis* was the etiologic agent in some cases. The CD4 count of the patients in this cohort was very low. This could be associated with greater use of antibiotics for opportunistic infections or bacterial infections resulting in antibiotic resistance and consequently contributing to the development of nosocomial infections (Japiassú, Amâncio et al. 2010). It is challenging for clinicians practicing in the ICU setting to balance the need for providing adequate antimicrobial treatment to potentially infected individuals with the risks of overuse or unnecessary use of antibiotics. Most intensive care units have adopted the following strategy - to initiate broad-spectrum antibiotics followed by the appropriate antibiotic for the specific organism once identified and antimicrobial susceptibility testing is released (Ibrahim, Sherman et al. 2000). Comparison in characteristics of nososcomial infections between HIV positive verses. HIV negative patients is presented in Table 1.

| **Nosocomial Infections** | **HIV positive patients** | | **HIV negative patients** | |
|---|---|---|---|---|
| | **Rate** | **Common organisms** | **Rate** | **Common organisms** |
| **Bacteraemia** | Increased in patients with central venous catheter and a high proportion of resistant *K. pneumoniae* | Coagulase-negative staphylococci *Staphylococcus aureus, Klebsiella pneumoniae, Candida* species, *Salmonella* species | Lower mortality in HIV negative patients | *Staphylococcus aureus, Escherichia coli, Klebsiella pneumoniae* |
| **Urinary tract infections** | Higher in catheterized patients and associated with nephropathy | Staphylococci, enterococci, *Proteus, Klebsiella, Enterobacter, Pseudomonas* species and *Candida* species | High in catheterized patients | Staphylococci, enterococci, *Proteus, Klebsiella, Enterobacter* and *Pseudomonas* species |
| **Pneumonia** | The highest rate among all nosocomial infections and mostly increased in patients with CD4 lymphocyte T count < 200 cell/$m^3$ | *Mycobacterium tuberculosis, Pneumocystis jiroveci, Staphylococcus aureus, Streptococcus pneumoniae, Pseudomonas aeruginosa, Haemophilus influenzae* and members of the enterobacteriaceae such as *Klebsiella pneumoniae, Escherichia coli, Serratia marcescens, Enterobacter* species | Higher in the patients with risk factors such as: age >65, malnutrition, severe underlying diseases and patients with alcohol abuse | *Staphylococcus aureus, Streptococcus pneumoniae, Pseudomonas aeruginosa, Haemophilus influenzae* and members of the enterobacteriaceae such as *Klebsiella pneumoniae, Escherichia coli, Serratia marcescens, Enterobacter* species |
| **Intensive Care Units (ICUs)** | More severe and increased in HIV/AIDS patients | As above | Higher in patients with risk factors and prolonged duration of stay | As above |

Table 1. Characteristics of nosocomial infections between HIV positive and negative patients.

## 5. Hospital infection control

In any society, health is a priority and infections particularly infections acquired in the hospital setting are a significant cause of disease worldwide. It is therefore imperative that the correct measures to control such infections are structured accordingly. These include an individual commitment by healthcare workers ensuring careful hand washing, appropriate isolation and use of gloves and the proper and sterile use of medical devices. System issues also need to be addressed - soap and water need to be available and placed at convenient locations easily accessible to healthcare workers. Surgical patients need to be administered pre-operative antibiotics 1-2 hours prior to incision and patients with communicable diseases need to be isolated. In addition, a good starting point for an infection control programme is basic surveillance thereby allowing for the calculation of the rates of infections. The role of such a programme is to provide local data and can be very effective in tracking the spread of nosocomial infections (Wenzel, Bearman et al. 2008). This would allow infection control personnel to rationally identify potential sources of pathogens and aid infectious disease physicians in the development of treatment regimens to manage patients affected by the related organisms (Singh, Goering et al. 2006).

## 6. Conclusion

Nosocomial infections are a serious problem that are continually increasing and expanding creating a severe public health threat and exhaust the health budget. In immunocompromised HIV-infected patients this threat is further amplified. However there are publications readily available indicating increased rates of nosocomial infections in HIV-infected patients. There is a enormous array of factors that need to be taken into consideration when confronted with such infections. The importance of knowing the risk factors, etiological agents and antimicrobial susceptibility are essential and should not be underestimated. The lifesaving role of antiretroviral therapy has improved and prolonged the survival outcome but some dilemmas around chronic HIV infections persist. It may be related to the lack of case control studies that directly indicate relationship amongst nosocomial infections and HIV/AIDS. Importantly, in nosocomial settings ongoing infection control measures warrant prompt attention.

## 7. References

A'Court, C. and C. S. Garrard (1992). "Nosocomial pneumonia in the intensive care unit: mechanism and significance" Thorax 47: 465-473.

Angus, D. C. and R. S. Wax (2001). "Epidemiology of sepsis: an update." Crit Care Med 29(7 Suppl): S109-116.

Archibald, L. K., M. O. den Dulk, et al. (1998). "Fatal Mycobacterium tuberculosis bloodstream infections in febrile hospitalized adults in Dar es Salaam, Tanzania." Clin Infect Dis 26(2): 290-296.

Beuheza, J., R. Beckelman, et al. (1989). Impact of HIV epidemic on mortality trends in men 25-44 years of age in the United States International Conference on AIDS, Montreal, Quebec, Canada.

Bohte, R., R. van Furth, et al. (1995). "Aetiology of community-acquired pneumonia: a prospective study among adults requiring admission to hospital." Thorax 50: 543-547.

Braunwald, E., A. Fauci, et al. (2004). Harrison's Principles of Internal Medicine. 16. New York, NY: McGraw-Hill.

Bronsema, D. A., J. R. Adams, et al. (1993). "Secular trends and rates of etiology of nosocomial urinary tract infection at a university hospital." J Urol 150: 414-416.

Chalasani, N. P., M. A. L. Valdecanas, et al. (1995). "Clinical utility of blood cultures in adult patients with community-acquired pneumonia without defined underlying risks." Chest 108: 932-936.

Chu, V. H., D. R. Crosslin, et al. (2005). "Staphylococcus aureus bacteremia in patients with prosthetic devices: costs and outcomes." Am J Med 118(12): 1416.

Cotton, D. J., V. J. Gill, et al. (1987). "Clinical features and therapeutic interventions in 17 cases of Bacillus bacteremia in an immunosuppressed patient population." J Clin Microbiol 25: 672-674.

Craven, D. E. and K. A. Steger (1995). "Epidemiology of nosocomial pneumonia. New perspectives on an old disease." Chest 108(2 Suppl): 1S-16S.

Craven, D. E., K. A. Steger, et al. (1996). "Nosocomial colonization and infection in persons infected with human immunodeficiency virus." Infect Control Hosp Epidemiol 17(5): 304-318.

del Rio, A., C. Cervera, et al. (2009). "Patients at Risk of Complications of Staphylococcus aureus Bloodstream Infection." Clin Infect Dis 48: S246–253.

Duse, A. G. (1999). "Nosocomial infections in HIV-infected/AIDS patients." J Hosp Infect 43 Suppl: S191-201.

Emori, G. T. and R. P. Gaynes (1993). "An Overview of Nosocomial Infections, Including the Role of the Microbiology Laboratory." Clin Microbiol Rev 6(4): 428-442.

Eulalia Valencia, M., A. Enriquez, et al. (1997). "Nosocomial infection with methicillin resistant Staphylococcus aureus in 14 human immunodeficiency virus infected patients." Med Clin (Barc) 109(7): 261-263.

Fife, D., G. L. Crane, et al. (1990). "Cumulative AIDS incidence and altered mortality from bacterial infections." AIDS Res Hum Retroviruses 6(10): 1203-1208.

Fine, M. J., M. A. Smith, et al. (1996). "Prognosis and outcomes of patients with community-acquired pneumonia. A meta-analysis." JAMA 275(2): 134-141.

Fluit, A. C., M. E. Jones, et al. (2000). "Antimicrobial susceptibility and frequency of occurrance of clinical blood isolates in Europe from the SENTRY Antimicrobial Surveillance Programme, 1997 and 1998." Clin Infect Dis 30: 354-360.

Fowler, V. G., Jr., M. K. Olsen, et al. (2003). "Clinical identifiers of complicated Staphylococcus aureus bacteremia." Arch Intern Med 163(17): 2066-2072.

Franzetti, F., A. Grassini, et al. (2006). "Nosocomial bacterial pneumonia in HIV-infected patients: risk factors for adverse outcome and implications for rational empiric antibiotic therapy." Infection 34(1): 9-16.

Fridkin, S. K., S. F. Welbel, et al. (1997). "Magnitude and prevention of nosocomial infection in the intensive care unit." Infect Dis Clin North Am 11: 479-496.

Garner, J. S., W. R. Jarvis, et al. (1988). "CDC definitons for nosocomial infections." Am J Infect Control 16: 128-140.

George, D. L. (1995). "Epidemiology of nosocomial pneumonia in intensive care unit patients." Clin Chest Med 16(1): 29-44.

Gobbi, M., P. Maggi, et al. (1998). Incidence of nosocomial infections in HIV infected/AIDS patients. Int. Conf AIDS. Roma, Italy. 12:1080 (abstract no. 60438).

Hickey, M. M. and D. C. Shanson (1993). "Septicemia in patients with and without AIDS at Westminster Hospital, London." J Infect 27: 243-250.

Huang, L., A. Quartin, et al. (2006). "Intensive care of patients with HIV infection." N Engl J Med 355(2): 173-181.

Ibrahim, E. H., G. Sherman, et al. (2000). "The influence of inadequate antimicrobial treatment of bloodstream infections on patient outcomes in the ICU setting." Chest 118(1): 146-155.

Iregui, M., S. Ward, et al. (2002). "Clinical importance of delays in the initiation of appropriate antibiotic treatment for ventilator-associated pneumonia." Chest 122(1): 262-268.

Jacoby, G. A. and L. S. Munoz-Price (2005). "The new beta-lactamases." N Engl J Med 352(4): 380-391.

Japiassú, A. M., R. T. Amâncio, et al. (2010). "Sepsis is a major determinant of outcome in critically ill HIV/AIDS patients." Critical Care 14(R152).

Jaspan, B. H. (2008). "Bacterial Disease and Antimicrobial Susceptibility
Patterns in HIV-Infected, Hospitalized Children: A
Retrospective Cohort Study." PloS ONE 3(9): e3260.

Kollef, M. H., K. R. Bock, et al. (1995). "The safety and diagnostic accuracy of minibronchoalveolar lavage in patients with suspected ventilator-associated pneumonia." Ann Intern Med 122(10): 743-748.

Laing, R. B. S. (1999). "Nosocomial infections in patients with HIV diease." Journal of Hospital Infection 43(3): 179-185.

Leibovici, L., H. Konisberger, et al. (1992). "Bacteremia and fungemia of unknown origin in adults." Clin Infect Dis 14(2): 436-443.

Luzzaro, F., E. F. Vigano, et al. (2002). "Prevalence and drug susceptibility of pathogens causing bloodstream infections in northern Italy: a two-year study in 16 hospitals." Eur J Clin Microbiol Infect Dis 21(12): 849-855.

Mandell, G. L., J. E. Bennett, et al. (2005). Principles and practices of Infectious Diseases Sixth edition.

Mbanya, D., J. Ateudjieu, et al. (2010). "Risk Factors for Transmission of HIV in a Hospital Environment of Yaoundé, Cameroon." Int. J. Environ. Res. Public Health 7: 2085-2100.

McDonald, L. C., L. K. Archibald, et al. (1999). "Unrecognized Mycobacterium tuberculosis bacteremia among hospital inpatients in less developed countries." Lancet 354: 1159-1163.

Mertins, S. D., L. Ortona, et al. (1990). "Role of polymorphonuclear leukocytes in infection by retroviruses with emphasis on the human immunodeficiency virus." Viral Immunol 3(3): 173-194.

Mora-Duarte, J., R. Betts, et al. (2002). "Comparison of caspofungin and amphotericin B for invasive candidiasis." N Engl J Med 347(25): 2020-2029.

O'Grady, N. P. and D. S. Chertow (2011). "Managing bloodstream infections in patients who have short-term central venous catheters." Cleveland Clinic Journal of Medicine 78: 10-17.

Ost, D. E., C. S. Hall, et al. (2003). "Decision analysis of antibiotic and diagnostic strategies in ventilator-associated pneumonia." Am J Respir Crit Care Med 168(9): 1060-1067.

Pagano, L., E. Tacconelli, et al. (1997). "Bacteraemia in patients with haematological malignancies. Analysis of risk factors, etiological agents and prognostic indicators." Haematologica 82: 415-419.

Panis, C., T. Matsuo, et al. (2009). "Nosocomial infections in human immunodeficiency type 1 (HIV-1) infected and AIDS patients: major microorgansims and immunological profile." Brazilian Journal of Microbiology 40: 155-162.

Paterson, D. L., W. C. Ko, et al. (2001). "Outcome of cephalosporin treatment for serious infections due to apparently susceptible organisms producing extended-spectrum beta-lactamases: implications for the clinical microbiology laboratory." J Clin Microbiol 29: 2206-2212.

Peces, R., E. Gago, et al. (1997). "Relapsing bacteraemia due to Micrococcus luteus in a haemodialysis patient with a Perm-Cath catheter. ." Nephrol Dial Transplant 12: 2428-2429.

Peters, R. P., E. E. Zijlstra, et al. (2004). "A prospective study of bloodstream infections as cause of fever in Malawi: clinical predictors and implications for management." Trop Med Int Health 9: 928-934.

Petrosillo, N., E. Nicastri, et al. (2005). "Nosocomial pulmonary infections in HIV-positive patients." Curr Opin Pulm Med 11(3): 231-235.

Petrosillo, N., L. Pagani, et al. (2003). "Nosocomial infections in HIV-positive patients: an overview." Infection 31 Suppl 2: 28-34.

Raghavendran, K., J. M. Mylotte, et al. (2007). "Nursing home-associated pneumonia, hospital-acquired pneumonia and ventilator-associated pneumonia: the contribution of dental biofilms and periodontal inflammation." Periodontol 2000 44: 164-177.

Raviglione, M. C., P. Mariuz, et al. (1990). "High Staphylococcus aureus nasal carriage rate in patients with acquired immunodeficiency syndrome or AIDS-related complex." Am J Infect Control 18(2): 64-69.

Reboli, A. C., C. Roststein, et al. (2007). "Anidulafungin verses fluconzaole for invasive candidiasis." N Engl J Med 356: 2472-2482.

Ringberg, H., A. Thoren, et al. (2000). "Metastatic complications of Staphylococcus aureus septicemia: to seek is to find." Infection 28: 132-136.

Roberts, A. P. and R. Phillips (1979). "Bacteria causing symptomatic urinary tract infection or asymptomatic bacteriuria." J Clin Pathol 32(5): 492-496.

Rosen, D. A., T. M. Hooton, et al. (2007). "Detection of Intracellular Bacterial Communities in Human Urinary Tract Infection." PloS Med 4(12): 1949-1958.

Sandoe, J. A., I. R. Witherden, et al. (2002). "Enterococcal intravascular catheter-related bloodstram infection: management and outcome of 61 consecutive cases." J Antimicrob Chemother 50: 577-582.

Sanford, J. P. (1995). Principles and practices of infectious diseases : Pseudomonas species (including melioidosis and glanders). New York, Churchill Livingstone.

Seifert, F. (2009). "The Clinical Importance of Microbiological Findings in the Diagnosis and Management of Bloodstream Infections." Clin Infect Dis 48: S238–245.

Shorr, A. F., Y. P. Tabak, et al. (2006). "Healthcare associated bloodstream infection: a distinct entity? Insights from a large US database." Crit Care Med 34: 2588-2595.

Singh, A., R. V. Goering, et al. (2006). "Application of molecular techniques to the study of hospital infection." Clin Microbiol Rev 19(3): 512-530.

American Thoracic Society (1996). "Hospital-acquired pneumonia in adults: diagnosis, assessment of severity, initial antimicrobial therapy and prevention strategies." Am J Respir Crit Care Med 153: 1711-1725.

American Thoracic Society (2005). "Guidelines for the management of adults with hospital-acquired, ventilator-associated, and healthcare-associated pneumonia." Am J Respir Crit Care Med 171(4): 388-416.

Soriano, F., J. M. Aguado, et al. (1990). "Urinary tract infection caused by Corynebacterium group D2: Report of 82 cases and reviews." Rev Infect Dis 12: 1019-1034.

Ssali, F. N., M. R. Kamya, et al. (1998). "A prospective study of community-acquired bloodstream infections among febrile adults admitted to Mulago Hospital in Kampala, Uganda." Acquir Immune Defi c Syndr Hum Retrovirol 19: 484-489.

Tumbarello, M., E. Tacconelli, et al. (1995). "The impact of bacteraemia on HIV infection. Nine years experience in a large Italian univeristy hospital." J Infect 31: 123-131.

Tumbarello, M., E. Tacconelli, et al. (1998). "Nosocomial bloodstream infections in HIV-infected patients: attributable mortality and extension of hospital stay." J Acquir Immune Defic Syndr Hum Retrovirol 19(5): 490-497.

Tumbarello, M., E. Tacconelli, et al. (1996). "Predictors of Staphylococcus aures pneumonia associated with human immunodeficiency virus infection." Respir Med 90: 531-537.

UNAIDS (2009). "AIDS Epidemic Update."

Vandenesch, F., T. Naimi, et al. (2003). "Community-acquired methicillin-resistant Staphylococcus aureus carrying Panton-Valentine leukocidin genes: worldwide emergence." Emerg Infect Dis 9(8): 978-984.

Varma, J. K., K. D. McCarthy, et al. (2010). "Bloodstream Infections among HIV-Infected Outpatients, Southeast Asia." Emerg Infect Dis 16(10): 1569-1575.

Warren, J. W. (2001). "Catheter-associated urinary tract infections." Int J Antimicrob Agents 17(4): 299-303.

Weinke, T., R. Schiller, et al. (1992). "Association between Staphylococcus aureus nasopharyngeal colonization and septicemia in patients infected with human immunodeficiency virus." Eur J Clin Microbiol Infect Dis 11: 985-989.

Weinstein, R. A. (1998). "Nosocomial infection update." Emerg Infect Dis 4(3): 416-420.

Wenzel, R., G. Bearman, et al. (2008). A Guide to Infection Control in the Hospital Fourth Edition. Boston, MA, International Society for Infectious Diseases.

Wenzel, R. P. (1989). "Hospital-acquired pneumonia: overview of the current state of the art for prevention and control." Eur J Clin Microbiol Infect Dis 8(1): 56-60.

Zurlo, J. J. and H. C. Lane (1997). AIDS etiology, diagnosis, treatment and prevention : Other bacterial infections. Philadelphia, Lippincott-Raven.

6

# Pulmonary Manifestations of HIV Disease

Muhwa J. Chakaya
*Chief Research Officer, Centre for Respiratory Diseases Research,*
*Kenya Medical Research Institute,*
*Kenya*

## 1. Introduction

After the first cases of AIDS were described in 1981, the HIV pandemic rapidly expanded to become a major global public health problem with broad health, social, economic and developmental consequences that have not been seen with any other disease. In the 30 years that this disease has been known to mankind it has killed an estimated 25 million people and continues to affect not less than 33 million people many of whom could die if life saving therapies are not made available to them [1]. The African continent has borne the largest impact of this disease. Of the 33.3 million people that UNAIDS estimated were living with HIV in 2009, nearly 67% were living in Africa[1].

Pulmonary disease is a major contributor to the morbidity and mortality suffered by persons infected with HIV. It was the appearance of previously rare Pneumocytis pneumonia often accompanied by Kaposis sarcoma in previously healthy young gay men, intravenous drugs addicts and their sexual contacts that alerted the world to the new syndrome of the Acquired Immune Deficiency Syndrome (AIDS) caused by HIV [2,3,4,5,6]. Before combination anti retroviral treatment (cART) became available a high proportion of HIV infected individuals would experience respiratory symptoms, and serious life threatening lung disease. Lung disease was often the index diagnosis that would point to the presence of HIV infection[7,8]. In general the incidence of serious pulmonary disease has declined following the wide availability of cART. For example in the USA rates of opportunistic infections decreased from 89.0 per 1000 person years in 1994-1997 to 25 per 1000 person years in 1998-2002, and 13 per 1000 person years in 2003-2007[9]. However, the incidence of many infectious diseases remain relatively high even in the cART era [10,11] and worryingly as HIV infected persons live longer, they appear to face an increased risk of non infectious lung diseases such as lung cancer, chronic obstructive lung disease and pulmonary arterial hypertension[12,13].

The range of pulmonary diseases that occur in HIV infected individuals is wide and includes infections, neoplasms, vascular lesions, interstitial pneumonias and obstructive airways disease. This chapter will summarize the current knowledge base on HIV associated lung disease including the burden and spectrum of the common diseases, diagnostic evaluation and approaches to treatment and prevention.

## 2. Burden of pulmonary disease in HIV

Prospective cohort studies carried out in the pre cART era out in North America and Western Europe documented a high incidence of both Pneumocytis and bacterial

| **Pneumonia** | **Bacterial** | Streptococcus pneumoniae<br>Haempholius influenza<br>Staphylococus aureus<br>Pseudomonas aeruginosa<br>Mycobacterium tuberculosis<br>Others |
|---|---|---|
| | **Fungal** | Pneumocystic jirovecii<br>Aspergilus spp<br>Cryptococcus neoformans<br>Candida spp<br>Mycoses Endemic to specific geographic areas (Histoplasma spp, Coccidiodes spp, Paracoccidiodes, Pencillium marneffei) |
| | **Viral** | Cytomegalovirus<br>Herpes Simplex<br>Influenza<br>Others |
| | **Parastic** | Toxoplasma gondii<br>Strongyloides stercoralis |
| **Malignacies** | | Kaposis sarcoma<br>Lymphoma<br>Lung cancer |
| **Other non infectious diseases** | | Non specific Interstitial pneumonitis<br>Lymphoid Intersititial Pneumonitis<br>Pulmonary arterial hypertension<br>Chronic Obstructive Airway disease<br>Others |

Table 1. Common pulmonary complications of HIV/AIDS.

pneumonia[14,15]. The advent of cART markedly reduced the burden of both Pneumocytis and bacterial pneumonia but more so for Pneumocytis pneumonia[16,17,18,].
In contra distinction with situation in the developed world where Pneumocytis pneumonia was the hallmark of HIV lung disease, tuberculsosis (TB) has been the predominant disease in HIV infected persons in Sub - Saharan Africa. Tuberculosis case notification rates rapidly escalated as the HIV epidemic spread[19, 20, 21,]. In 2009 the World Health Organization estimated that HIV associated TB occurred in about 1.2 million people and was responsible for the deaths of about 200,000 people with nearly 85% of this burden occurring in Sub - Saharan Africa[22].

## 3. Clinical evaluation of HIV infected persons with respiratory symptoms

### 3.1 History

Even though advances have been made in medical technologies for the diagnosis of lung disease, a good clinical history remains essential in the clinical evaluation of HIV infected persons with lung disease. A thorough understanding of the patient's illness may assist to narrow down the specific diagnosis behind the patient symptoms. It is important to establish if the patient presenting with respiratory symptoms already knows his or her HIV status and

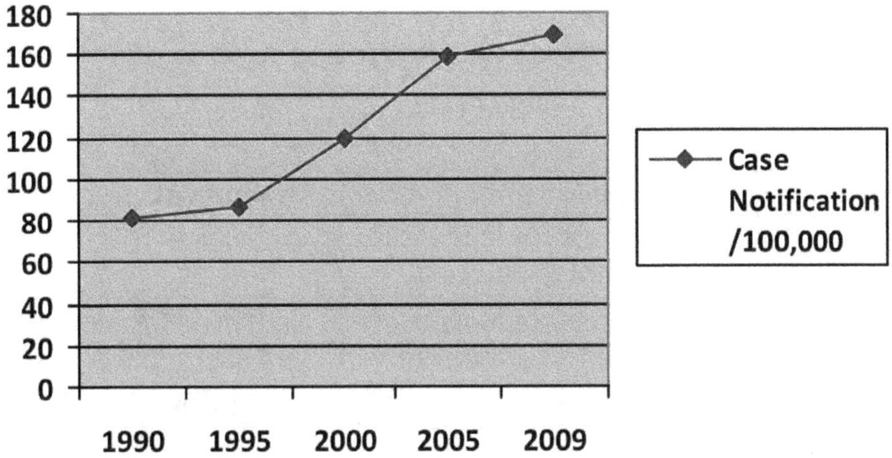


Source WHO, Global Tuberculosis Report, 2010

Fig. 1. TB Case Notification in Sub -Saharan Africa - 1990-2009.

if so how long that status has been known. It is also important to know if that person has suffered opportunistic infections in the past, and if the patient is taking cART and preventive therapy for opportunistic infections. If the patient has been taking cART current and previous regimens must be elucidated and enquiries on adherence to current and previous cART made. The appearance of a lung opportunistic infection in a patient who has been on cART may point to a failing regimen. Since certain infections occur only in specific geographic areas a travel history should be obtained. Other risk factors for disease occurrence or for poor outcomes must as far as feasible be sought. These risk factors include intravenous drug use, alcohol abuse and tobacco smoking. The pre morbid health status must also be known.

### 3.2 Clinical examination

The clinical examination is intended to establish if serious lung disease is present and thus if urgent interventions are required. A common sense approach will help identify most patients with serious lung disease. Assessment of the patients' mental status together with measurement of the respiratory rate, pulse, temperature, blood pressure and transcutaneous arterial oxygen saturation should rapidly reveal the presence or absence of serious life threatening lung disease.

### 3.3 Laboratory tests

The choice of laboratory and other tests to be carried out will depend on the clinical condition of the patient, the setting in which the patient is seen and the laboratory infrastructure available. Ideally most patients should have a plain chest radiograph to confirm the presence of lung disease and the extent of pulmonary involvement which will influence the placement of patients into specific risk groups for various outcomes and guide further management. Further medical tests may be carried out to identify co-morbid states or other organ involvement to assist with prognostication while others may be carried to diagnose the specific disease and thus assist in provision of targeted treatment. Tests designed to identify specific diseases include examination of body fluids such as sputum, blood, urine, bronchoalvelaor lavage fluid, pleural fluid and others for pathogens using various stains, cultures, antigen and nucleic acid detection tests. Fiberoptic bronchoscopy (FOB), where available, with lavage, brushing and biopsy has found a special place in the evaluation of HIV infected persons with respiratory symptoms. However FOB should not be used routinely in all HIV infected persons. This procedure may not provide treatment changing results in some settings.

**Evaluation of the patient with HIV Lung Disease**

| Test /procedure | Purpose | Comment |
|---|---|---|
| Chest x-ray | Detection of lung disease/ severity assessment | Universally done |
| CT scan | Detection of lung disease /severity assessment | Offers better detection and radiographic chacterization of lung disease/May be abnormal in the presence of a normal chest x-ray |
| Pulse oximetry | Severity assessment/ monitoring | Shoulde be used in all patients with severe disease |
| Arterial blood gases | Severity assessment/montoring | Shoulde be used in all patients with severe disease |
| Blood count (WBC, HB, Platelets)/ coagulation tests | Severity assessment/monitoring | Shoulde be used in all patients with severe disease |
| Renal and liver function tests | Severity assessment/monitoring | Shoulde be used in all patients with severe disease |
| Induced Sputum gram stain and culture | Microbiological aetiology | Shoulde be used in all patients with severe disease |
| Blood culture | Microbiological aetiology | Shoulde be used in all patients with severe disease |
| Antigen detection (Bllod/urine/sputum) | Microbiological aetiolgy | Especially for S. Pneumoniae and L. pneumophila sero group 1 |
| Serological tests | Microbiological aetiology | Most for the detection of "atypical pathogens". Provide retrospective diagnosis |
| Fiberoptic bronchoscopy witrh lavage, brushing and or biopsy | Microbiological aetiology/diagnosis of non infectious disease | Probably best reserved for patients with non diagnostic results with non invasive tests |
| Open Lung Biopsy | Histological diagnosis/Microbiological diagnosis | Used mostly if bronchoscopy with TBB fails to provide a diagnosis |
| Radio isotope studies | Diagnosis of infectious /non infectious disease | Gallium 67 citrate and $^{99m}$ TCDTPA: expensive, time consuming and require complex infrastructure |
| Other tests (lung function tests) | Diagnosis of non infectious disease (COPD) | TLCO, KCO, FEV1, FVC: Sensitive but not specific for any lung disease |

Table 2. Common tests and procedures for evaluating HIV associated lung disease.

## 4. Specific lung diseases

### 4.1 Fungal pneumonia in HIV infected persons

### 4.1.1 Pneumocytis pneumonia (PcP)

The causative organism of Pneumocystis pneumonia, *Pneumocystis jirovecii,* has had an interesting history in terms of its taxonomy. Initially the pathogen was thought to be protozoan in nature. Later it was placed on the fungal group based on its nucleic acid profile and the name of the human pathogen was changed from *Pneumocystis* carinii to Pneumocystis jirovecii based on the understanding that the species that affects humans is distinctly different from that which affects other animals including cats[23].

#### 4.1.1.1 Epidemiology

Pneumocystis pneumonia was the dominant opportunistic infection in the pre cART era in the North America and Europe[1, 2, 3,4,5,14,15]. In contrast to the dominance of PcP in North America and Western Europe, other regions of the world and especially Sub Saharan Africa, the current epicentre of the HIV/AIDS epidemic, did not experience this surge of PcP with rates of PcP ranging from 0- 21% in the earlier case series and cohort studies [24,25,26,27,]. In fact for a while this infection was thought to be absent from Africa[28]. As the HIV epidemic matured in Sub- Saharan Africa the prevalence of PcP in HIV infected patients appeared to have increased[29,30,31], but the rates of this infection did not reach the levels that were observed in Western Europe and North America during the early years of the HIV epidemic. Currently PcP remains relatively rare in Sub - Saharan Africa, with prevalence as low as 1% being reported[32, 33, 34,]. The reasons for the low prevalence of PcP in Sub - Saharan Africa are not fully known but racial factors influencing susceptibility to the development of disease following infection or colonization may partly play a role. It is also worth noting that African populations have been documented to have a high prevalence of exposure to this pathogen and therefore the low rates of PcP in Sub -Saharan Africa is not the result of the absence of the pathogen from the African environment[35].

#### 4.1.1.2 Risk factors

Several studies have examined the risk factors for PcP in HIV infected individuals. These studies indicate that the risk of PcP is highest in those with declining CD 4 T cell count especially when the count falls below 200, unexplained fever, history of AIDs defining illness, presence of oral thrush and not being on prophylaxis or when prophylaxis fails[36,37]. HIV infected persons of the negroid race may have a lower risk of of PcP compared to Caucasians[38].

#### 4.1.1.3 Clinical manifestations

**Symptoms**

Pneumocystis pneumonia usually presents with a sub acute onset of cough and shortness of breath. The cough is usually non productive or may be productive of scanty mucoid sputum while shortness of breath is slowly progressive and gradually limits activity. Many patients do not experience chest pain and do not have other constitutional disturbances, the symptom complex being largely dominated by shortness of breath.

**Signs**

The majority of patients will appear anxious when they are first examined. The breathing frequency is usually rapid and shallow. The pulse is also rapid but most often at the first evaluation the blood pressure is normal. Patients with PcP may have no fever at presentation. Lung signs including crackles may be absent and even when present are non specific. There may be evidence of other opportunistic infections such ano genital herpetic ulcers and oral thrush.

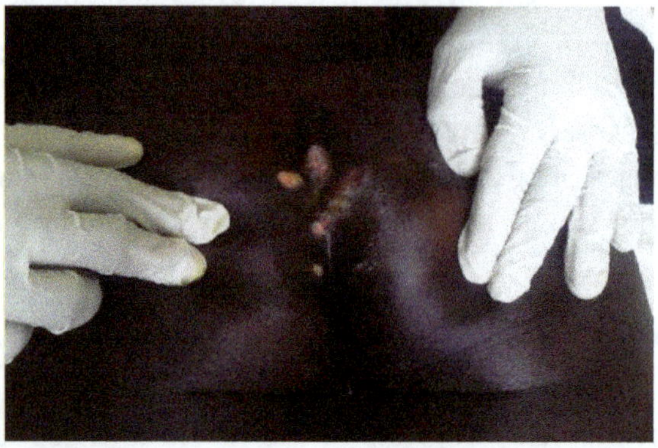

Fig. 2. Ano genital Herpetic Ulcers in a patient with PcP.

#### 4.1.1.4 Pneumocystis pneumonia - Diagnostic tests

**Radiologic imaging**

Patients suspected to have PcP should have a chest radiograph which typically shows bilateral interstitial or alveolar shadows in the mid zones with basal and apical sparing. In some situations PcP may be present without any obvious changes on the chest radiograph. In these situations high resolution chest CT scan may reveal typical abnormalities that may render the performance of a fiberoptic bronchoscopy procedure unwarranted[39]. Radiostopic studies using Gallium 67 scintigraphy, where available may help to distinguish lung infections from neoplastic and other diseases processes[40].

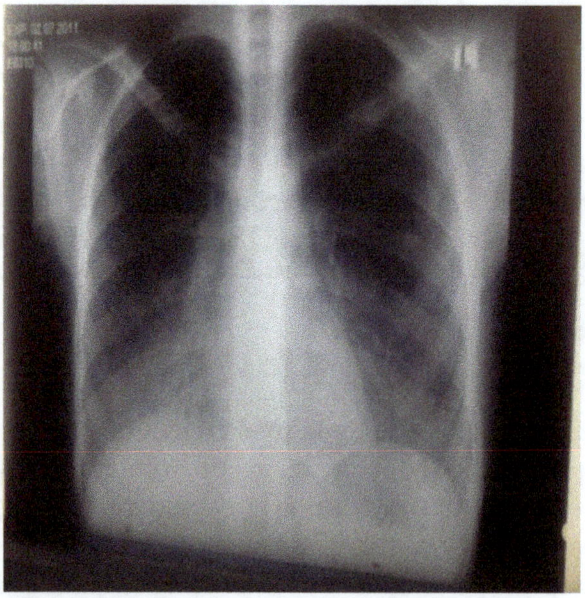

Fig. 3. Chest Radiograph showing shadows typical of PcP.

**Lung function testing**

Patients with PcP typically are hypoxemic and will desaturate further when exercised, an observation that has been used as a diagnostic test to predict the presence of this infection [41],

[42]. The measurement of diffusion capacity has also been found to be a useful diagnostic test[43].

### Microbiological tests

The definitive diagnosis of PcP is based on the identification of the pathogen in lung samples most commonly obtained through induced sputum, fiberoptic bronchoscopy or open lung biopsy. While some controversy still exists, fiberoptic bronchoscopy with lavage is the standard procedure for the detection of Pneumocystis jirovecii[44]. Both bronchial brushings and transbronchial biopsy during the bronchoscopy procedure may offer no added value in the evaluation of patients suspected to have PcP[45]. In general lower respiratory tract specimens are subjected to either cytochemical staining using May-Grünwald-Giemsa (MGG), toluidine blue-O (TOL), Papani-colou (PAP) and Grocott methenamine silver (GRO); immunofluorescent staining with monoclonal antibodies or PCR. However PCR may not distinguish infection from colonization[46] .Examination of expectorated sputum remains a useful procedure for the microbiological diagnosis of PcP especially in low resource settings. When toluidine blue O staining of expectorated sputum is carried out the sensitivity approaches 70% and 35% compared with immunofluorescent staining and PCR respectively while specificity is 100% and thus in these settings examination of expectorated sputum may be a practical procedure for the diagnosis of PcP [47]. The yield from sputum examination may be increased if sputum production is induced following inhalation of hypertonic saline. In a meta analysis of diagnostic procedures for PcP, it was found that, compared with bronchoalvelaor lavage as the gold standard, examination of induced sputum had an overall sensitivity of 55.5% and a specificity of 98.6% with even better sensitivity at 67% versus 43.1% when comparing immunofluorescent staining with cytochemical staining. In settings where the prevalence of PcP is in the range of 25-60%, the positive and negative predictive values ranged from 86-96.7% and 66.2-89.8%, respectively, with immunofluorescent staining , and 79-94.4% and 53-83.5% with cytochemical staining[48].

### Other tests

The diagnosis of PcP may also be aided by the measurement of serum 1-3 beta D -Glucan, a cell wall component of most pathogenic fungi including Pneumocystis jirovecii which has been found to have a sensitivity of nearly 100% and specificity of about 96.4%. Therefore this test may be used as non invasive test for diagnosis of PcP[49,50]. This test may however not correlate with disease severity and should not be used to monitor patients on treatment[87].

### Treatment of Pneumocystis Pneumonia

The drug of first choice for the treatment of PcP remains cotrimoxazole. The recommended dose is 20mg per Kg body weight per day for the trimethoprim and 100 mg per Kg per day for the sulphamethoxazole, given in three or four divided doses. It has been reported, however that lower doses may be used without loss of efficacy and with the added advantage of a reduction in the rate of adverse events[51]. Second line treatment options for patients unable to tolerate high dose cotrimoxazole include clindamycin /primaquine and pentamidine but pentamidine may be associated with a greater risk of death[52]. Trimetrexate with folinic acid is generally well tolerated and has a clinical efficacy of about 70%[53]. Other second line therapies include atovaquone, dapsone, a combination product of trimethoprim and dapsone and eflornithine hydrochloride. A metanalysis of second line therapies, in patients who fail whatever initial treatment is given concluded that the combination of clindamycin plus primaquine appears to be the most effective alternative treatment for patients with PcP who are unresponsive to conventional antipneumocystis agents[54].

**Outcomes**

Pneumocystis pneumonia is a serious life threatening illness in persons living with HIV. The overall in hospital mortality of this illness is in the region of 10-13%. Among the factors that have been associated with death in patients with PcP include older age, recent injection drug use, total bilirubin of greater than 0.6 mg/dl, serum albumin of less than 3 g/dl, alveolar-arterial oxygen gradient of equal or greater than 50 mm Hg, failure of cotrimoxazole treatment and the presence of co- morbidities such as bacterial pneumonia, Kaposis sarcoma and TB[55,56,57]. Patients who need to be admitted to the intensive care unit may suffer very high rates of deaths that could reach 80% within the ICU and up to 34 % three months post ICU admission[58]. The high mortality of patients who need to be mechanically ventilated appears to be associated with high APACHE II scores, high levels of Positive End Expiratory Pressures (PEEP),the presence of co- infection with CMV and lower CD 4 T cell counts [59,60].
In an attempt to lower the mortality of PcP adjunctive systemic steroids are recommended[61] based on the results of clinical trials that documented a reduction in mortality in patients with moderate to severe disease[62,63,64]. Use of adjunctive steroids for the treatment of moderate to severe PcP has not been associated with increased long term mortality after the PcP episode nor with an increase in the incidence of other opportunistic infections[65,66].
There have been concerns that patients infected with Pneumocystis jirovecii that has developed mutations in the dihdropteroate synthase reductase gene may not respond as well to cotrimoxazole as patients whose pathogen does not carry these mutations. The majority of studies however indicate that the development of mutations on the dihdropteroate synthase reductace gene does not have an impact on the efficacy of cotrimoxazole in the treatment of PcP[67,68] However it has been reported that DHPS mutations increase the risk of death in patients with PcP [69].
It has been suggested that measurement of C- Reactive Protein (CRP) may be a useful prognostic marker in patients with PcP. In one study the levels of CRP were negatively correlated with arterial oxygenation ($PaO_2$)[70].

**Prevention**

Pneumocystis pneumonia in HIV infected persons is a preventable disease. The most effective treatment for the prevention of PcP is cART which reconstitutes the immune system and dramatically reduces the incidence of opportunistic infections including PcP[16, 17, 18, 19]. Many HIV infected persons with risk factors for PcP will however require to be protected from this disease even if they have been placed on cART until CD4 T cell recovery has taken place. Although aeroslolized pentamidine and cotrimoxazole may have equal efficacy[71], the preferred drug is cotrimoxazole[72] but if this cannot be tolerated aerosolized pentamidine or atovaquone which have been found to have similar efficacy may be used[73]. Mutation in the dihdrofolate reductase gene may however, lead to prophylaxis failures[74,75]. An alternative drug is dapsone which appears to have an efficacy equal to that of atovaquone but which may be less safe[76]. In patients receiving cART it has been recommended that prophylaxis for PcP be discontinued when the CD 4 T cell count climbs to 200 and above[77] but recent studies suggest that prophylaxis may be discontinued when viral suppression is achieved and before the CD 4 T cell count reaches 200 and above[78,79]. These are reassuring observations because cotrimoxazole treatment may sometimes be associated serious life threatening complications including septic shock like syndrome[80].

### Complications

Pneumocystis pneumonia may result in pneumothorax and pneumomediastinum both of which may be life threatening. These complications are thought to arise from newly formed cysts and bronchiectasis[81]

## 4.1.2 Other fungal pneumonias in HIV infected persons

Pneumonia caused by fungal pathogens, other than Pneumocystis jirovecii, though less common when compared with PcP and bacterial pneumonia is a frequent cause of morbidity and mortality in HIV infected persons. Fungal pathogens have been identified mostly in severely immunocompromised patients with CD 4 T cell count below 200 and the lung is often involved in a disease process that is often disseminated and or where multiple pathogens are causing disease. The mortality of fungal pneumonia in HIV infected persons is thus high.

Of the fungal pathogens that have been associated with lung disease in persons living with HIV Cryptococcus may not only be the commonest pathogen but also the best characterized. This fungus is ubiquitous and is more famous for causing meningitis in severely immunocompromised patients. Lung disease due to Cryptococcus neorformans has been reported in all parts of the world and tends to occur in patients who have CD 4 T cell counts below 200 [82,83,84], The other ubiquitous fungus that has been associated with lung disease in HIV infected persons is Aspergillus spp. Invasive Aspergillosis occurs most commonly in patients who have a severely depressed immune system and often participates in disease in partnership with other pathogens, as a disseminated infection which confers a high mortality[85,86,87]. Other fungal pathogens are mostly confined to specific geographic areas where they have been reported to cause significant morbidity and mortality in HIV infected persons. These fungal pathogens include Histoplasma spp, Coccidioides spp, Paracoccidiodies spp, Pencillium marneffei, Sporotrichosis spp and Blastomycosis[88,89,90,].

### 4.1.2.1 Clinical manifestations

Pneumonia due to fungal pathogens, other than PcP, may follow an acute or sub acute course. The disease may be indistinguishable from pneumonia due to bacterial pathogens and TB. There are no clinical features that distinguish fungal pneumonia from pneumonia due to other pathogens. As in other forms of pneumonia the clinical syndrome is characterized by the presence of a cough, shortness of breath and fever as the primary symptoms. In the presence of disseminated disease or meningitis, headache, malaise, vomiting, confusion and wasting may be present. Specific examination of the chest may reveal tachypnea, signs of consolidation or the presence of a pleural effusion while chest radiography may reveal segmental, lobar or multi lobar consolidation, pleural effusion and or widespread reticular, nodular, reticulo - nodular or mixed alveolar and interstitial shadowing.

### 4.1.2.2 Diagnosis

The diagnosis of fungal pneumonia is based on the identification of fungal pathogens in respiratory specimens mostly obtained at fiberoptic bronchoscopy with bronchoalveolar lavage, bronchial brushings or occasionally through biopsies. To confirm a fungal pathogen the lung specimens are cultured in Sabborauds media or subjected to PCR. For Cryptococcal disease measurement of serum Cryptococal antigen may be yield positive results, especially when the disease is disseminated. Cryptococcal antigen in serum may be negative in isolated pulmonary disease.

#### 4.1.2.3 Treatment

The treatment of fungal pneumonia is dependent on the specific pathogen. Many classes of antifungal agents are now available for the treatment of serious fungal infections such as pneumonia. These include polyene antifungals such as amphotericin B, imidazole, triazole and thiazole antifungals such ketoconazole, fluconazole and itraconazole and echinocandins such as caspofungin, micafungin and anidulafungin

#### 4.1.2.4 Prevention

The most important intervention for the prevention of fungal pneumonia is immune reconstitution using cART. While fluconazole has been used to prevent Cryptococcal infections in HIV infected persons it has not found widespread use and the efficacy may be suboptimal [91].

## 4.2 Community Acquired Bacterial Pneumonia (CABP) in HIV infected persons

### 4.2.1 Epidemiology

Persons living with HIV have a high incidence of community acquired bacterial pneumonia[92]. Often CABP is the index diagnosis for HIV [93,94]. With the advent of cART, the incidence of CABP fell but not as much as that of PcP in high income countries probably as a result of the presence of other risk factors that drive the susceptibility to bacterial pneumonia such as intravenous drugs use, smoking and alcohol abuse among HIV infected individuals[95,96, 97,]. In one French study, CABP was the cause of admission to the intensive care unit in 74% of 147 HIV infected patients admitted to ICU and surpassed PcP as the predominant cause of acute respiratory failure in the era of cART[98]. In African HIV infected patients CABP and in particular pneumococcal disease remains a major cause of morbidity and mortality. Autopsy studies have also documented high rates of bacterial pneumonia in HIV patients dying of lung disease. For example in one Brazilian autopsy study involving 240 HIV infected patients dying of respiratory failure, the cause of death was attributed to CABP in 36 % [99]. In a similar study from one USA centre, 47 patients with a pre mortem diagnosis of TB, CABP was deemed to have been the cause of death in 13 (26%)[100].

The incidence of lower respiratory tract infection increases as the CD4 T cell count declines and in the absence of ART. Acute bronchitis, CABP and PcP will be experienced by more than 80% of patients with a CD 4 T cell count of less than 200 even when these patients are provided with chemoprophylaxis[101]. Injecting drug users have an increased incidence of BP compared with other categories of HIV acquisition as are patients who smoke tobacco, have liver cirrhosis and have suffered a previous episodes of BP[102,103]. Smoking cessation has been found to be beneficial in reducing the incidence of BP in HIV infected persons[104,105,106]. Other factors that increase the risk of BP and in particular pneumococcal pneumonia include age, not being on HAART[107] and neutropenia[108]. On the other hand the major risk factor for nosocomial pneumonia is the duration of hospitalization[109,110]. The pathogens commonly encountered in nosocomial pneumonia include Pseudomonas aeruginosa, Staphylococcus aureus, and Streptococcus pneumoniae.

### 4.2.2 Clinical manifestations

Community acquired bacterial pneumonia is largely an acute illness in which symptoms evolve rapidly over a few days [111].The classical symptoms include cough with or without sputum expectoration, chest pain which is often pleuritic in nature, difficulties in breathing and rapid breathing primarily driven by the chest pain and fever. Clinical examination usually reveals a sickly patient who is febrile, tachypneic but usually not as tachypneic as the patient with PcP and who has a tachycardia. Specific examination of the chest may reveal dullness to percussion, with bronchial breath sounds and pulmonary rales over the affected lobe or lobes of the lungs.

### 4.2.3 Imaging

A plain chest radiograph should be obtained in all patients suspected to have bacterial pneumonia. The plain chest x-ray typically shows alveolar shadows with segmental, lobar or bronchopneumonic distribution and these changes are similar to those seen in HIV sero negative patients[112]. Although diffuse interstitial shadowing is less common this radiographic picture should not be used to exclude BP . Other changes that may be visible on the chest radiograph include the presence of pleural effusions and cavitations. No radiographic appearance is pathognomonic of any specific pathogen. The chest x-ray in BP is largely uninfluenced by cART but patients with CD 4 T cell count less than 200 are likely to have a bronchopneumonic picture. It has also been documented that bacteremic patients were more likely to have a lobar lesion and a higher CD4 T cell count above 200[113,114]. A chest CT scan may be very helpful. It may reveal lesions where the plain chest x-ray does not and have high specificity for certain infections such PcP[115].

### 4.2.4 Laboratory tests

In hospitalized patients with CABP total white blood cell count, should be measured. A total white cell count of below $4x10^9$ /L has been associated with bacteraemia and excess mortality in HIV negative patients with community acquired pneumonia[116] and may carry the same risk in HIV infected persons [117]. Similarly thrombocytopenia (count of less than 100,000 $x10^9/l$) appears to signify severe disease that necessitates aggressive treatment including admission to the intensive care unit[118]. Measurement of the CRP has not been documented to be able to discriminate between PcP and BP[119], however, using the cut off value of 3ng/ml for procalcitonin and 246 mg/l for CRP one group of investigators reported an increased capability to distinguish BP from TB with a sensitivity of 81.8% and a specificity of 82.5% for the procalcitonin and 78.8% and 82.3% respectively for the CRP[120].

In hospitalized patients the measurement of blood urea, creatinine, sugar, albumin, bilirubin, AST and ALT helps to place patients in specific risk groups for poor outcomes using the CURB - 65[121] and or Pneumonia Severity Index criteria[122]

The microbiological diagnosis of CABP is dependent on the detection of the pathogen itself in culture, components of the pathogen (antigen) in body fluids or the antibody response to the pathogen. Relevant samples where the pathogen or its antigen may be identified include sputum, bronchoalveolar lavage fluid, bronchial brushings, lung biopsies or aspirates, blood, urine and pleural fluid. The interpretation of microbiological culture results from sputum and other respiratory secretions is hampered by the contamination of these samples by oropharyngeal bacterial colonizers and precautions must be taken to ensure that not only are good quality specimens obtained but also appropriate and proven methods for interpreting results of bacterial cultures from these specimens are followed. A good quality sputum sample is for example one that has low number of squamous cells and high number of polymorphonuclear cells[123].

### 4.2.5 Sputum microbiologic testing

In hospitalized patients, as far as feasible, sputum samples should be collected for gram staining and bacterial culture. If a sputum gram stain reveals a predominance of a pathogen with specific staining and morphological features (e.g. gram positive diplococci) this is highly predictive of the pathogen that is responsible for that episode of pneumonia. The sensitivity of sputum gram stain may reach 58%[124]. Sputum bacterial culture may be diagnostic in up to 34% of pneumonia episodes and be correlated with the organism isolated from a sterile site[125]. Compared with BAL and TBB the sensitivity and specificity of induced sputum is about 60% and 40% respectively[126]. Using quantitative bacterial culture the cut off for significant bacterial growth is usually considered to be $10^5$ colony forming units per ml of sputum. In settings where PcP incidence may be low the fiberoptic bronchoscopy procedure may add little value to the examination of sputum for other pathogens[127].

### 4.2.6 Urinary antigen testing

Urinary antigen tests are available for two bacterial pathogens: Streptococcus pneumoniae and Legionella pneumophila sero group 1. The urinary pneumococcal antigen test is a rapid test with good test performance parameters including a sensitivity in the region of 81%, specificity 98%, positive (PPV) and negative predictive values (NPV) 98%, and 82%, respectively[137]. The urine pneumococcal antigen test may be positive many weeks after the pneumonia has resolved[128]. The urinary antigen test for Legionella pneumophila sero group 1 has a sensitivity of 70-90% and a specificity of nearly 100% for the detection of this pathogen[129]

### 4.2.7 Serological tests

These tests are used primarily for the detection of atypical pathogens such as Mycoplasma pneumoniae[130], Chlamydophila Spp and Legionella Spp other than Pneumophila Sero group 1. The major draw back is that interpretation often requires comparison of results of acute and convalescent sera and thus may not be useful for clinical decision making.

### 4.2.8 Fiberoptic bronchoscopy

Fiberoptic bronchoscopy is a commonly used procedure for the evaluation of respiratory symptoms in HIV infected persons. Although the diagnostic yield may reach 74% only about 25% of bronchoscopies yield useful results that lead to a change in diagnosis and therapy[131,132,133],. In situations where there are low rates of PcP and Kaposis sarcoma the fiberoptic bronchoscopy procedure may not yield additional results from that obtained through examination of expectorated sputum and other easily obtained body fluids[145, 134], and therefore in such settings this procedure should be used judiciously.

### 4.2.9 Fine needle transthoracic biopsy/aspiration

This may be an underutilized procedure for the evaluation of respiratory symptoms in patients infected with HIV. The suitable patient for this procedure has a peripheral lesion close to the pleural membrane. The common complication with this procedure is pneumothorax which rarely requires pleural drainage[135].

### 4.2.10 The range of pathogens

The range of pathogens involved in CABP in HIV infected persons is wide but the most common pathogens include Streptococcus pneumoniae, Staphylococcus aureus, Klebsiella pneumoniae, Haemophilus influenzae, H. parainfluenzae and Pseudomonas aeruginosa. Streptococcus pneumoniae is the most common pathogen isolated in 40- 60% of bacteriologically confirmed cases [136,137,138]. In TB endemic areas TB is a common cause of acute community acquired pneumonia and should always be screened for in all patients presenting with this condition.

Persons living with HIV are at increased risk of pneumococcal bacteraemia associated with community acquired pneumonia [139,140,141]. However the impact of the bacteraemia on survival appears to be uncertain with some studies suggesting there is no increase in the risk of mortality while others have found an association between pneumococcal bacteraemia and mortality from community acquired pneumonia [142,154,155]. Compared with sero negative patients HIV infected patients may be predisposed to harbouring penicillin resistant pneumococci[155,143].

Other pathogens that have been identified in HIV infected patients with community acquired pneumonia include:

- Rhodococcus equi, a gram-positive, coryneform bacterium that causes zoonotic infection mainly in horses and foals. Most cases have been reported in case reports and or case series[144, 145,146],
- Enterococcus that may be vancomyicn resistant and associated with lung abscess and empyema[147]
- Norcadia asteroides a gram positive filamentous rod which may cause chronic lung infection and may sometimes disseminate with associated high mortality [148,149]. This infection may be difficult to diagnose.
- Legionella pneumophila, although it remains unclear if HIV infected persons are at increased risk of infection or severe disease[150 151]
- Mycoplasma pneumoniae which has been found in up to 17% of patients with community acquired pneumonia in both HIV negative and positive persons[152, 153].
- Moraxella catarrhalis though this pathogen appears to be an uncommon cause of community acquired pneumonia. In one large study only 4 cases among 2123 patients hospitalized over a nine year period were found to have this pathogen[154]
- Community acquired Pseudomonas aeruginosa which has been described as a cause of severe and often fulminant community acquired pneumonia in patients who are severely immune suppressed and who may not have the traditional risk factors for this infection such as central lines and neutropenia[155,156, 157].
- Salmonella which has been described mainly in patients with Salmonella bacteraemia[158].

Often the HIV infected person has multiple pathogens causing the respiratory illness[159, 160, 161, 162] such as fungi, bacterial and viral pathogens.

### 4.2.11 Treatment of community acquired bacterial pneumonia in HIV infected persons

A holistic approach should be adopted to the care of HIV infected patients with community acquired pneumonia. The benefit of targeted anti microbial therapy are likely to accrue if attention is paid to hydration, oxygenation and nutritional needs among other needs of the patient. Control of symptoms such as pain, fever, vomiting and diarrhoea which often are part of the pneumonia syndrome in HIV infected persons will ensure patient comfort as specific antimicrobial treatment takes effect.

The initial antimicrobial treatment will usually be chosen on an empiric basis and this choice should be based on the range of common pathogens isolated in the specific setting, the anti microbial susceptibility patterns of common pathogens, the cost of treatment, co morbid states and to some extent the experience of the treating practitioner. No studies have specifically examined the efficacy of various antibiotics for the management of CABP in HIV infected persons. Thus current practice is based largely on guidelines derived from studies involving HIV sero negative individuals and clinical experience. In TB endemic settings the combination of a beta lactam and a macrolides is preferred over the use of fluoroquinolones to avoid masking TB. The combination of a beta lactam and a macrolide has been associated with better outcomes in HIV sero negative patients, but not in all studies[163], and is recommended by the Infectious Disease Society of America and the American Thoracic Society[164]. Pneumococcal penicillin resistance may be more common in HIV infected persons[165] but outcomes of treatment appear not to be influenced by the presence of intermediate levels of penicillin resistance[166, 167].

In patients with Rhodococcus infection at least two antimicrobial agents should be given simultaneously to treat this infection for a period of up to several months. The combinations of erythromycin and rifampin or imipenem and teicoplanin have been found to be the most effective treatments in Rhodococcus infections[168].

The anti microbial treatment of Nocardia asteroides involves the use of combinations with proven synergy, such as imipenem and amikacin, as the recommended initial therapy.

### 4.2.12 Outcomes of community acquired bacterial pneumonia

Several risk factors may work together to increase the risk of death in HIV infected patients receiving treatment for CABP. These risk factors include not being on ART, presence of pneumococcal antigen in urine for patients with pneumococcal pneumonia[169] and comorbid states such as liver cirrhosis (mostly from alcohol abuse)[170]. Compared with HIV sero negative patients and in situations where health care delivery may be described as optimal HIV infection appears not to increase the mortality risk in hospitalized patients with Community Acquired Pneumonia and neither does it lead to prolongation of hospital stay[171,172].

In patients with acute respiratory failure admitted to the ICU, the risk of death is related to extent of organ failure such as need for mechanical ventilation and use of vasopressor agents rather than HIV parameters such as CD4 T cell count, HIV plasma viral load or use of ART[173].

Bacteremiac pneumococcal disease may confer a higher mortality risk but this has not been a consistent finding [155-159]. Certain pathogens confer a greater risk of death. Compared with Streptococcus pneumoniae for example patients with Legionella, were found to have a higher risk of death probably from a greater prevalence of co morbid conditions[174]. Advancing age and low CD4 T cell count are also risk factors for severe disease and death in HIV infected patients including patients on ART[175,176].

It has been proposed that HIV infected patients be placed in a low risk immunosuppressed group for death and that in this group the Pneumonia Severity Index (PSI) can be used to define patients at risk of death similar with the use of this tool to define groups of patients at risk of death in HIV negative patients[177, 178, 179].

### 4.2.13 Prevention

Vaccination is available for Streptococcus pneumoniae. The 23 valent polysaccharide vaccine appears to be effective in HIV infected persons in North America for reducing all cause pneumonia but those with plasma viral load of greater than 100,000 may not benefit[180],[181],[182], but the results of clinical trials have not always been consistent[183]. On the other hand African patients have not been documented to benefit from the 23 valent pneumoccal vaccine, [184], [185]. To avoid the sub optimal efficacy of the 23 valent pneumococcal vaccine in African HIV infected persons a conjugate vaccine has been developed. A clinical trial of the 7 valent conjugate vaccine among Malawian patients found a protective efficacy of about 74% for the prevention of recurrent pneumococcal pneumonia [186]

The other intervention available for preventing BP in HIV infected persons is cotrimoxazole preventive therapy which is most effective in those with CD 4 T cell count below 200,[187],[188].

### 4.2.14 Other issues

Recent data suggests that recurrent BP may be associated with an increased risk of lung cancer in HIV infected persons probably related to the persistent or recurrent inflammation in the lung[189]. Parapneumonic effusions may be more common in HIV infected patients with community acquired pneumonia and patients with parapneumonic effusions may have more severe disease with higher rates of bacteraemia[190].

## 4.3 Mycobcaterial pneumonia in HIV infected persons

### 4.3.1 Mycobacterium tuberculosis

#### 4.3.1.1 Epidemiology

Tuberculosis is the most common opportunistic infection and the most common cause of death in HIV infected persons. The dramatic increase in the burden of TB in Sub - Saharan Africa has been largely blamed on the HIV epidemic[191]. However, other than for differences in magnitude, TB is the most common opportunistic infection that is observed in the first three months of initiation of cART in both Sub-Saharan Africa and the industrialized world of North America and Europe[192,193]. The TB and HIV epidemics are so intricately intertwined in Sub-Saharan Africa that care and control of one must be linked with the prevention and care of the other[194]. HIV influences TB by increasing the risk of reactivation of latent TB infection, rapid progression of new TB infection to disease and recurrent disease from both re-infection and relapse[195].

#### 4.3.1.2 Clinical manifestations

Pulmonary tuberculosis is characterized by the sub acute onset of cough with or without the production of sputum associated with systemic symptoms of fever, night sweating and loss of weight. The sputum may be stained with blood. These symptoms are not specific for TB. The only symptoms that are significantly more common in TB than in other patients are night sweats and loss of weight[196]. There may also be pleuritic chest pain but shortness of breath is uncommon until the late stages of the disease. The symptoms of TB are largely similar between HIV negative and positive patients, however, depending on the stage of HIV disease, HIV infected persons may have stigmata of the HIV infection such as oro-pharyngeal candidiasis, oral hairy leukoplakia, a non specific skin rash, cutaneous Kaposis sarcoma and peripheral lymph node enlargement.

There may be no significant signs unearthed on specific examination of the chest and even when present these signs are non specific. The chest radiograph is a sensitive but non specific test for detection of TB in both HIV infected and un infected individuals[197]. It may show a variety of lesions which to a large extent depend on the severity of the HIV related immunosuppresesion. When immune function is still relatively well preserved the classical upper lobe fibrocavitary shadows may be seen. With advancing immune dysfunction the radiologic shadows become atypical and include mid and lower zone shadows, intrathoracic lymph node enlargement, pleural effusions, miliary shadowing among others lesions[198, 199].

#### 4.3.1.3 Diagnosis of pulmonary TB

Most TB occurs in middle and low income countries where conventional light microscopic examination of sputum using the Ziehl Nielsen stain is the primary diagnostic test. The test is rapid, relatively simple, inexpensive and highly specific in these settings, however, this test has provided inconsistent sensitivity results ranging from as low as 20%[200] to as high as 80%[201] in comparison to culture confirmed TB and is more commonly negative in HIV infected individuals compared to HIV negative individuals[202]. Currently WHO recommends that two sputum specimens are obtained immediately the patient makes contact with the health care system. The examination of a third sputum specimen has not been found to add much value with the incremental yield of the third specimen not exceeding 4% [203]. Similarly a morning specimen only marginally increases the diagnostic yield of smear microscopy [204] and therefore may not be necessary in the evaluation of patients suspected to have TB. To increase the sensitivity of smear microscopy sputum may treated with bleach or sodium hydroxide and concentrated by centrifugation, or overnight sedimentation preceded by treatment with ammonium sulphate or bleach[205]. However the value of these sputum processes in HIV infected persons is not clear. The yield of sputum microscopy is consistently increased by up to 10% using fluorescence microscopy with auramine O or auramine - rhodamine stains [206] and recently fluorescence microscopy has been simplified by the development of Light Emitting Diode (LED) Fluorescence microscopy[207]. The Gold standard for TB diagnosis remains culture on solid or liquid media. Conventional culture on solid or liquid media for the diagnosis of TB is however a slow process that may take too long to reliably influence clinical decisions. The development of rapid liquid culture systems such as the Mycobaterial Growth Inhibitor Tube (MGIT) has improved the turn around time and thus the clinical utility of culture for the diagnosis of TB[208]. The WHO recently recommended rapid liquid TB culture systems for the diagnosis of TB especially in HIV infected persons[209]. Although recommended by WHO as a bridge to fully automated liquid culture systems for TB diagnosis, non commercial culture systems such Mycobacteria Observation Drug Susceptibility (MODS), Nitrate Reductase Assays (NRAs), Thin layer Agar (TLA) and Colorimetric Redox Indicators (CRIs) systems do not decrease the time to TB diagnosis and drugs susceptibility results[210]. Even though the PCR technique has been used for a long time for the detection of TB, it is the automated cartridge based nucleic acid detection test called the Xpert MTB/Rif test that has the potential to revolutionize the diagnosis of TB especially in HIV infected persons. This test not only provides the diagnosis of TB in under two hours but also is able to indicate if there is likelihood of multi drug resistant TB based on the detection of mutations that confer rifampicin resistance. Diagnostic studies on this test suggest that it has an overall sensitivity of about 92.2% and a specificity of 99% using a single Xpert test. The sensitivity increases to 97.6% using three Xpert tests. Among HIV positive individuals the overall sensitivity of a single Xpert test has been reported to be about 94% compared to 98% in HIV negative individuals. For the detection of rifampicin resistance the sensitivity of this test is about 98%[211,212]. This test is now recommended as the initial test for the detection of pulmonary TB in HIV infected persons[213]. Although several serological tests are commercially available for the detection of TB, none has been found to have a consistently high sensitivity and specificity to replace smear microscopy and their use has recently been discouraged by WHO [214].

#### 4.3.1.4 Treatment of TB in HIV infected persons

Current treatment of pulmonary TB involves the use of combinations of 5 primary drugs: Isoniazid(H), rifampicin(R), ethambutol(E), pyrazinamide(Z),and streptomycin (S). The WHO and the International Standards of TB Care (ISTC) recommends a rifampicin based regimen made of RHZE given daily for two months followed by RH given daily, or two to three times weekly for six months for previously untreated patients[215]. With this regimen most HIV infected patients get cured with a lower risk of failure, relapse and acquired drug resistance[216]. Patients who have been treated previously must be assessed for risk of drug resistance, investigated for drug resistance using the Xpert MTB/Rif test, rapid molecular based line probe assays and culture, and treated with either primary, first line drugs if no drug resistance exists or with second line drugs if drug resistance, especially multi drug resistant TB, is present[238].

#### 4.3.1.5 Drug resistant TB and HIV

The WHO estimated that there were 400,000 cases of multi drug resistant TB, defined as TB bacilli that are resistant to both R and H, in 2009[214]. Although HIV per se appears not to be a risk factor for MDRTB, a link between MDRTB and HIV has been suggested by epidemiologic data from parts of Eastern Europe[217]. Outbreaks of MDRTB in HIV infected persons have been linked to nosocomial transmission of TB and have in general been characterized by high mortality among affected patients[218]. The more recent reports were from Southern Africa where a large majority of the patients were HIV infected, had extensive drug resistance (MDRTB with additional resistance to a fluoroquinolone and an injectable such as kanamycin, amikacin or capreomycin) and died within a few weeks after the diagnosis of XDRTB[219], emphasizing the critical role of implementing robust measures to prevent TB transmission in situations where HIV infected persons receive care.

#### 4.3.1.6 Outcomes

HIV infected PTB patients are at increased risk of death during treatment for TB. Up to 30% of such patients may die during treatment if no life prolonging ART is provided. The risk of death is higher in patients with smear negative disease and those with a lower CD 4 T cell count[220]. Life prolonging ART is able to dramatically reduce the deaths rates in HIV infected TB patients and the earlier it is given the better [221]. Cotrimoxazole preventive therapy is also able to reduce the mortality of HIV associated TB[222].

#### 4.3.1.7 Prevention

HIV associated TB is a preventable disease. Several randomized clinical trials have demonstrated that TB can be effectively prevented using isoniazid given for 6-12 months in HIV infected persons[223]. With the advent of combined ART it was observed that TB incidence fell in persons on ART in North America and Europe. The fall in TB incidence has been observed to be greater in persons with a higher baseline CD4 T cell count, a lower base line viral load and robust immunological and virological responses[224]. Similar observations have been made in South Africa[225]. The combination of ART and Isoniazid Preventive Therapy (IPT) has been observed to confer greater protection against TB[226] and provides further impetus to provide IPT in all HIV infected persons irrespective of whether they are or are not on ART. Currently there is no evidence that appropriately applied IPT leads to the expansion of isoniazid resistance[227].

### 4.3.2 Other Mycobacteria

#### 4.3.2.1 Mycobacterium Avium Complex and other Non Tuberculous Mycobacteria

Mycobacterium avium complex (MAC) is isolated with increasing frequency from respiratory specimens in HIV infected persons, however, the significance of isolating MAC from respiratory specimens is unclear. Criteria have been developed for defining clinical disease in patients who have non Tuberculous Mycobacteria isolated from respiratory samples[228]. HIV infected persons with pulmonary MAC are more likely to have fever, diffuse pulmonary abnormalities, lymphadenopathy and concurrent disease including disseminated MAC, PcP and BP compared with HIV negative individuals [229]. These infections generally occur late in the course of HIV disease and confer a poor long term prognosis [230].

### 4.4 Viral pneumonia

Viral pathogens have also been implicated in HIV associated lung disease. These viruses have included Cytomegalovirus (CMV), Herpes Simplex Virus (HSV) and Influenza including H1N1. For CMV the difficult has been distinguishing infection from colonization. The most important risk factor for viral pneumonia is a CD 4 T cell count below 200. These pneumonias may be difficult to diagnose and carry a high mortality.

### 4.4.1 CMV

This is the most common virus that has been implicated in HIV associated pneumonia. The clinical presentation is similar to pneumonia due to other pathogens and is largely non specific. The symptoms include fever, shortness of breath, and cough. Pneumonia due to CMV may be the initial presentation of HIV disease[231] and in the pre ART era, survival post CMV pneumonia, when successfully treated was short[232, 233]. Often CMV pneumonia is not recognized or diagnosed prior to death[234,235]. Patients with a high plasma viral load may also be at risk of CMV pneumonia[236].

The diagnosis of CMV may be problematic. When isolated in respiratory specimens such as bronchoalveolar lavage this virus may be a colonizer and not necessarily the cause of the lung disease [237]. To diagnose respiratory disease the current consensus is that CMV should be isolated in lung secretions (BAL or brushes), and demonstrated to be available in histological specimens through immunohistochemistry or in situ hybridization in the presence of pulmonary infiltrates on the chest radiograph. The treatment of CMV involves the use of ganciclovir or forscanet.

As with fungal pneumonia the most important intervention for the prevention of CMV pneumonia is immune reconstitution using anti- retroviral treatment. No chemo preventive intervention has been identified. Acyclovir has been tried but was not found to be efficacious[238]

### 4.4.2 Herpes simplex

Herpes simplex virus type 1 and type 2 have both been associated with HIV pneumonia. The pneumonia may occur in association with cutaneous herpes and thus represent disseminated disease[239,240]. Varicella pneumonia has been described and may present as a recurrent pneumonia[241].

### 4.5 Parasitic lung disease in HIV

Lung disease caused by parasites may less common. The most common parasites that have been associated with HIV lung disease are Toxoplasma gondii and Strongyloides stercoralis.

Epidemiological studies to obtain good estimates of the incidence of these parasites in HIV infected persons have not been carried out.

### 4.6 Non infectious HIV associated lung disease

Several non infectious lung diseases have been observed in HIV infected persons. These diseases include pulmonary arterial hypertension, bronchiolitis obliterans organizing pneumonia, sarcoidosis and chronic obstructive pulmonary disease. The incidence of these diseases may be increasing as HIV infected individuals survive longer with cART.

#### 4.6.1 Interstitial pneumonitis

The HIV syndrome is associated with an increased incidence of non specific interstitial pneumonitis and lymphoid interstitial pneumonitis, both of which may result from the chronic inflammatory state induced by HIV[242,243]. Lymphocytic Interstitial pneumonia in HIV infected persons may be associated with respiratory symptoms of cough and dyspnoea and cause lung function abnormalities[244]. The radiological picture is diffuse interstitial shadowing and a lung biopsy procedure is required for the diagnosis. The disease has been thought to be related to the host immune response[245] and directly linked to HIV[246]. There is usually a predominance of CD8 positive T lymphocytes[226]. This entity may also occur as part of the immune reconstitution inflammatory syndrome[247]. It responds to systemic steroids and also resolves with ART[248,249]. The incidence has declined with the widespread use of anti-retroviral treatment[250]

#### 4.6.2 Non specific pneumonitis

A non specific pneumonitis associated with cough and dyspnoea and diffuse interstitial shadowing on the chest x-ray often occurs in HIV infected persons. This disease entity may mimic PcP [251] and even appear to respond to PcP treatment[252]. However a search for Pneumocystis jirovecii is usually negative [253].

#### 4.6.3 Immune reconstitution inflammatory syndrome

The immune reconstitution inflammatory syndrome represents an exaggerated immune response to infectious and non infectious agents as immune recovery occurs. The syndrome is characterized by the appearance of worsening symptoms and signs of specific infections as immune recovery takes place. While most episodes are mild, severe life threatening disease may occur. The syndrome has been described to occur with many infections including Pneumocystis jirovecii, CMV, TB and Cryptococcus [254,255,256,257].

#### 4.6.4 Pulmonary Arterial Hypertension (PAH)

Pulmonary arterial hypertension associated with HIV is a rare clinical entity but when it occurs it leads to significant morbidity and mortality. The available literature is mostly based on case reports. This clinical entity appears to occurs at relatively high CD4 T cell of about 300. The clinical, radiographic and echocardiographic findings are similar to idiopathic PAH in HIV sero negative persons. Highly active antiretroviral therapy, bosentan, and prostaglandin therapy have all been reported to be beneficial in improving hemodynamic and functional status in HIV-related PAH[258]. In a French study the median survival of patients with HIV associated PAH receiving ART and PAH specific therapy was 88% and 72% at 1 and 3 years respectively. There was better survival in patients with CD4 T cell count of greater than 200 and a higher cardiac index. Anti-retroviral therapy did not appear to influence hemodynamic parameters [259].

### 4.6.5 Pulmonary maligancies in HIV infected persons

Both Kaposis sarcoma (KS) and non Hodgkins Lymphoma (NHL), the two AIDS defining malignancies (ADMs) have been associated with lung disease. Of the two malignancies KS has been the more common one. In HIV associated KS, the tumour most often afflicts the lung as part of a disseminated disease process but may also occur as a primary lung disease. Non Hodgikins lymphoma occurring as primary lung disease has been described in several case reports and series[51]. Persons living with HIV appear to be at increased risk of primary lung cancer, a non ADM[52].

Endobronchial Kaposis Sarcoma is seen in about 15% of patients with advanced HIV disease. The clinical presentation is indistinguishable from that of other pulmonary complications of HIV. Thus patients may present with cough, haemoptysis and dyspnoea. Both alveolar and interstitial shadows may be seen on the chest radiograph. Chest CT scans usually reveal the shadows better. The diagnosis requires visual detection of typical cherry red lesions at fiberoptic bronchoscopy. The lesions are usually not biopsied because of the risk of bleeding. Pulmonary KS usually occurs in the setting of disseminated KS and the prognosis is typically poor.

Non Hodgikins lymphoma involving the lung has been reported in case series and cohorts. The clinical presentation is usually non specific and includes fever, weight loss, dyspnea, generalized lymphadenopathy, chest pain and cough. The chest raidiograph reveals nodular lesions or interstitial shadows. The diagnosis of lymphoma is more reliably made on open lung biopsy. In the pre - ART era the diagnosis of NHL carried with it a poor prognosis even with specific lymphoma treatment [260].

The risk of lung cancer in HIV infected persons appears to be increased and this increase may not be fully explained by smoking[261]. Although the data is scanty, recurrent pneumonia, through the promotion of chronic infection has been found to be associated with the increased risk of lung cancer in HIV infected persons[262]. The incidence of lung cancer, may have increased in post HAART era[263]. However the incidence of lung cancer in HIV infected women appears not to be higher that that in HIV un infected women and the driver of the lung cancer risk is tobacco smoking and not the HIV infection[264]. HIV infected patients with primary lung cancer are younger, tend to present with aggressive and advanced disease and have poorer outcomes[265,266].

### 4.6.6 Chronic obstructive pulmonary disease

Respiratory symptoms and functional abnormalities are common in patients infected with HIV including those on combined anti -retroviral therapy. A recent observational study documented respiratory symptoms and functional abnormalities in 47.3% and 64.1% of study participants respectively. Irreversible airways obstruction compatible with COPD, independently associated with pack years smoked, intravenous drug use and the use of anti -retroviral therapy was found in 21% of study participants[267]. In patients with obstructive airways disease, HIV infection appears to confer a higher risk of moderate but not severe dyspnoea[268].

### 4.6.7 Bronchiolitis obliterans organizing pneumonia

Bronchiolitis obliterans organizing pneumonia (BOOP) is a disease of the small airways characterized by intraluminal polyps of myxoid connective tissue. The concomitant occurrence of BOOP with HIV has been described in a few case reports. In the cases reported, the clinical manifestations have included sub acute onset of dyspnoea which progressed to respiratory failure, non productive cough and fever. The most common chest radiographic findings included bilateral mixed interstitial and alveolar shadows. When these patients are investigated for infection, no pathogens are found and empiric antibiotic therapy is not effective. The diagnosis of BOOP is made at open lung biopsy. Patients respond very well to corticosteroids at a dose of about 1 mg/Kg for up to three months[269].

#### 4.6.8 Hypersentivity pneumonitis

Case reports of hypersensivity pneumonitis associated with drugs used in the management of HIV infection including dapsone[270], efavirenz[271] and other anti retrovirals[272] have been published. The burden of illness and or death caused hypersensivity pneumonitis in HIV infected persons is currently unclear.

#### 4.6.9 Sarcoidosis

Sarcoidosis is a multi system disease in which tissues are infiltrated with non caseating granulomas. The lung is a common target of sarcoid lesions. Pulmonary sarcoidosis associated with HIV has been reported in case reports and series[273,274]. Many of the sarcoidosis case reports have appeared in the post HAART era and it is unclear if this entity, in the ART context is related to immune recovery. In patients who use adulterated drugs talc granulamotosis must be considered in the differential diagnosis of interstitial lung disease. This clinical entity is indistinguishable from opportunistic infections and requires examination of lung biopsy specimens which show granulomas with intracellular talc crystals[275].

## 5. References

[1] UNAIDS Report on the Global AIDS Epidemic 2010.

[2] Masur H, Michelis MA, Greene JB, Onorato I, Stouwe RA, Holzman RS, Wormser G, Brettman L, Lange M, Murray HW, Cunningham-Rundles S. An outbreak of community-acquired Pneumocystis carinii pneumonia: initial manifestation of cellular immune dysfunction. N Engl J Med. 1981 Dec 10;305(24):1431-8.

[3] Gottlieb MS, Schroff R, Schanker HM, Weisman JD, Fan PT, Wolf RA, Saxon A. Pneumocystis carinii pneumonia and mucosal candidiasis in previously healthy homosexual men: evidence of a new acquired cellular immunodeficiency. N Engl J Med. 1981 Dec 10;305(24):1425-31.

[4] Centers for Disease Control (CDC). Kaposi's sarcoma and Pneumocystis pneumonia among homosexual men--New York City and California. MMWR Morb Mortal Wkly Rep. 1981 Jul 3;30(25):305-8.

[5] Centers for Disease Control (CDC). A cluster of Kaposi's sarcoma and Pneumocystis carinii pneumonia among homosexual male residents of Los Angeles and Orange Counties, California. MMWR Morb Mortal Wkly Rep. 1982 Jun 18;31(23):305-7.)

[6] Masur H, Michelis MA, Wormser GP, Lewin S, Gold J, Tapper ML, Giron J, Lerner CW, Armstrong D, Setia U, Sender JA, Siebken RS, Nicholas P, Arlen Z, Maayan S, Ernst JA, Siegal FP, Cunningham-Rundles S.Opportunistic infection in previously healthy women. Initial manifestations of a community-acquired cellular immunodeficiency. Ann Intern Med. 1982 Oct;97(4):533-9.

[7] Design of a prospective study of the pulmonary complications of human immunodeficiency virus infection. The Pulmonary Complications of HIV Infection Study Group. J Clin Epidemiol. 1993 Jun;46(6):497-507

[8] Diaz PT, Wewers MD, Pacht E, Drake J, Nagaraja HN, Clanton TL.Respiratory symptoms among HIV-seropositive individuals. Chest. 2003 Jun;123(6):1977-82)

[9] Buchacz K, Baker RK, Palella FJ Jr, Chmiel JS, Lichtenstein KA, Novak RM, Wood KC, Brooks JT; HOPS Investigators. AIDS-defining opportunistic illnesses in US patients, 1994-2007: a cohort study AIDS. 2010 Jun 19;24(10):1549-59

[10] Hanna DB, Gupta LS, Jones LE, Thompson DM, Kellerman SE, Sackoff JE.AIDS-defining opportunistic illnesses in the HAART era in New York City. AIDS Care. 2007 Feb;19(2):264-72.

[11] Bonnet F, Lewden C, May T, Heripret L, Jougla E, Bevilacqua S, Costagliola D, Salmon D, Chêne G, Morlat P Opportunistic infections as causes of death in HIV-infected patients in the HAART era in France.; Mortalité 2000 Study Group.Scand J Infect Dis. 2005;37(6-7):482-7

[12] Crothers K, Huang L, Goulet JL, Goetz MB, Brown ST, Rodriguez-Barradas MC, Oursler KK, Rimland D, Gibert CL, Butt AA, Justice AC. HIV infection and risk for incident pulmonary diseases in the combination antiretroviral therapy era. Am J Respir Crit Care Med. 2011 Feb 1; 183(3):388-95. Epub 2010 Sep 17.

[13] Bonnet F, Chêne G, Thiébaut R, Dupon M, Lawson-Ayayi S, Pellegrin JL, Dabis F, Morlat P; Groupe d'Epidémiologie Clinique du SIDA en Aquitaine (GECSA).Trends and determinants of severe morbidity in HIV-infected patients: the ANRS CO3 Aquitaine Cohort, 2000-2004.HIV Med. 2007 Nov;8(8):547-54.

[14] Phair J, Muñoz A, Detels R, Kaslow R, Rinaldo C, Saah A. The risk of Pneumocystis carinii pneumonia among men infected with human immunodeficiency virus type 1. Multicenter AIDS Cohort Study Group. N Engl J Med. 1990 Jan 18;322(3):161-5.)

[15] The Study on BV in HIV infected women in USA

[16] Dufour V, Cadranel J, Wislez M, Lavole A, Bergot E, Parrot A, Rufat P, Mayaud C.Changes in the pattern of respiratory diseases necessitating hospitalization of HIV-infected patients since the advent of highly active antiretroviral therapy. Lung. 2004;182(6):331-41; 279.

[17] Serraino D, Puro V, Boumis E, Angeletti C, Girardi E, Petrosillo N, Ippolito G.Epidemiological aspects of major opportunistic infections of the respiratory tract in persons with AIDS: Europe, 1993-2000. AIDS. 2003 Sep 26;17(14):2109-16;

[18] Pulvirenti J, Herrera P, Venkataraman P, Ahmed N.Pneumocystis carinii pneumonia in HIV-infected patients in the HAART era. AIDS Patient Care STDS. 2003 Jun;17(6):261-5.

[19] Grant AD, Sidibe K, Domoua K, et al. Spectrum of disease among HIV infected adults hospitalized in a respiratory medicine unit in Abidjan, Cote d'Ivoire. Int J Tuberc Lung Dis 1998; 2: 926-94

[20] Dye C, Scheele S, Dolin P et al. Consensus statement: global burden of tuberculosis: estimated incidence, prevalence and mortality by country; WHO global surveillance and monitoring project. JAMA 1999; 228: 677-686

[21] Range N, Ipuge YA, O'Brien RJ et al. Trend in HIV prevalence among tuberculosis patients in Tanzania, 1991-1998. Int J Tuberc Lung Dis 2001; 5: 405 -412

[22] World Tuberculosis Report 2010, World Health Organization

[23] Stringer JR, Cushion MT, Wakefield AE. New nomenclature for the genus Pneumocytis. J. Eukaryot Microbiol 2001; 48(suppl): 184 S-189S

[24] Batungwanayo J, Taelman H, Lucas S, Bogaerts J, Alard D, Kagame A, Blanche P, Clerinx J, van de Perre P, Allen S. Pulmonary disease associated with the human immunodeficiency virus in Kigali, Rwanda. A fiberoptic bronchoscopic study of 111 cases of undetermined etiology. Am J Respir Crit Care Med. 1994 Jun;149(6):1591-6.

[25] Lucas SB, Hounnou A, Peacock C, Beaumel A, Djomand G, N'Gbichi JM, Yeboue K, Hondé M, Diomande M, Giordano C, et al. The mortality and pathology of HIV infection in a west African city. AIDS. 1993 Dec;7(12):1569-79.

[26] Atzori C, Bruno A, Chichino G, Gatti S, Scaglia M. Pneumocystis carinii pneumonia and tuberculosis in Tanzanian patients infected with HIV. Trans R Soc Trop Med Hyg. 1993 Jan-Feb;87(1):55-6.

[27] Kamanfu G, Mlika-Cabanne N, Girard PM, Nimubona S, Mpfizi B, Cishako A, Roux P, Coulaud JP, Larouzé B, Aubry P, et al. Pulmonary complications of human immunodeficiency virus infection in Bujumbura, Burundi.Am Rev Respir Dis. 1993 Mar;147(3):658-63.

[28] Lucas SB. Missing infections in AIDS. Trans R Soc Trop Med Hyg 1990; 84 Supl 1: 34 -8.

[29] Chakaya JM, Bii C, Ng'ang'a L, Amukoye E, Ouko T, Muita L, Gathua S, Gitau J, Odongo I, Kabanga JM, Nagai K, Suzumura S, Sugiura Y.Pneumocystis carinii pneumonia in HIV/AIDS patients at an urban district hospital in Kenya. East Afr Med J. 2003 Jan;80(1):30-5.

[30] Worodria W, Okot-Nwang M, Yoo SD, Aisu T. Causes of lower respiratory infection in HIV-infected Ugandan adults who are sputum AFB smear-negative. Int J Tuberc Lung Dis. 2003 Feb;7(2):117-23. 322.

[31] Siika AM, Chakaya JM, Revathi G, Mohamed SS, Bhatt KM.Bronchoscopic study on aetiology of chronic cough in HIV-infected adults with negative sputum smears for Mycobacterium tuberculosis at Kenyatta National Hospital, Nairobi. East Afr Med J. 2006 Jun;83(6):295-305.; 321.

[32] van Oosterhout JJ, Laufer MK, Perez MA, Graham SM, Chimbiya N, Thesing PC, Alvarez-Martinez MJ, Wilson PE, Chagomerana M, Zijlstra EE, Taylor TE, Plowe CV, Meshnick SR. Pneumocystis pneumonia in HIV-positive adults, Malawi. Emerg Infect Dis. 2007 Feb;13(2):325-8..

[33] Lockman S, Hone N, Kenyon TA, Mwasekaga M, Villauthapillai M, Creek T, Zell E, Kirby A, Thacker WL, Talkington D, Moura IN, Binkin NJ, Clay L, Tappero JW. Etiology of pulmonary infections in predominantly HIV-infected adults with suspected tuberculosis, Botswana. Int J Tuberc Lung Dis. 2003 Aug;7(8):714-23

[34] Garcia-Jardon M, Bhat VG, Blanco-Blanco E, Stepian A. Postmortem findings in HIV/AIDS patients in a tertiary care hospital in rural South Africa.. Trop Doct. 2010 Apr;40(2):81-4.

[35] Nkinin SW, Daly KR, Walzer PD, Ndzi ES, Asonganyi T, Respaldiza N, Medrano FJ, Kaneshiro ES. Evidence for high prevalence of Pneumocystis jirovecii exposure among Cameroonians Acta Trop. 2009 Nov;112(2):219-24. Epub 2009 Aug 7.

[36] Kaplan JE, Hanson DL, Navin TR, Jones JL. Risk factors for primary Pneumocystis carinii pneumonia in human immunodeficiency virus-infected adolescents and adults in the United States: reassessment of indications for chemoprophylaxis. J Infect Dis. 1998 Oct;178(4):1126-32.

[37] Moorman AC, Von Bargen JC, Palella FJ, Holmberg SD. Pneumocystis carinii pneumonia incidence and chemoprophylaxis failure in ambulatory HIV-infected patients. HIV Outpatient Study (HOPS) Investigators. J Acquir Immune Defic Syndr Hum Retrovirol. 1998 Oct 1;19(2):182-8.

[38] Stansell JD, Osmond DH, Charlebois E, LaVange L, Wallace JM, Alexander BV, Glassroth J, Kvale PA, Rosen MJ, Reichman LB, Turner JR, Hopewell PC. Predictors of Pneumocystis carinii pneumonia in HIV-infected persons. Pulmonary Complications of HIV Infection Study Group. Am J Respir Crit Care Med. 1997 Jan;155(1):60-6.

[39] Richards PJ, Riddell L, Reznek RH, Armstrong P, Pinching AJ, Parkin JM. High resolution computed tomography in HIV patients with suspected Pneumocystis carinii pneumonia and a normal chest radiograph. Clin Radiol. 1996 Oct;51(10):689-93.

[40] Moser E, Tatsch K, Kirsch CM, Küffer G, Goebel FD. Value of 67gallium scintigraphy in primary diagnosis and follow-up of opportunistic pneumonia in patients with AIDS. Lung. 1990;168 Suppl:692-703.

[41] Chouaid C, Maillard D, Housset B, Febvre M, Zaoui D, Lebeau B. Cost effectiveness of noninvasive oxygen saturation measurement during exercise for the diagnosis of Pneumocystis carinii pneumonia. Am Rev Respir Dis. 1993 Jun;147(6 Pt 1):1360-3.

[42] Stover DE, Greeno RA, Gagliardi AJ. The use of a simple exercise test for the diagnosis of Pneumocystis carinii pneumonia in patients with AIDS. Am Rev Respir Dis. 1989 Jun;139(6):1343-6.

[43] Huang L, Stansell J, Osmond D, Turner J, Shafer KP, Fulkerson W, Kvale P, Wallace J, Rosen M, Glassroth J, Reichman L, Hopewell P. Performance of an algorithm to detect Pneumocystis carinii pneumonia in symptomatic HIV-infected persons. Pulmonary Complications of HIV Infection Study Group. Chest. 1999 Apr;115(4):1025-32.

[44] Lewin SR, Hoy J, Crowe SM, McDonald CF.The role of bronchoscopy in the diagnosis and treatment of pulmonary disease in HIV-infected patients. Aust N Z J Med. 1995 Apr;25(2):133-9

[45] Djamin RS, Drent M, Schreurs AJ, Groen EA, Wagenaar SS.Diagnosis of Pneumocystis carinii pneumonia in HIV-positive patients. Bronchoalveolar lavage versus bronchial brushing. Acta Cytol. 1998 Jul-Aug;42(4):933-8.

[46] Morris A, Kingsley LA, Groner G, Lebedera IP, Beard CB, Norrisk A. Prevelance and clinical predictors of Pneumocytis colonization among HIV infected men. AIDS 2004; 18(5): 793-798

[47] Aderaye G, Woldeamanuel Y, Asrat D, Lebbad M, Beser J, Worku A, Fernandez V, Lindquist L. Evaluation of Toluidine Blue O staining for the diagnosis of Pneumocystis jiroveci in expectorated sputum sample and bronchoalveolar lavage from HIV-infected patients in a tertiary care referral center in Ethiopia. Infection. 2008 Jun;36(3):237-43. Epub 2008 May 15.

[48] Cruciani M, Marcati P, Malena M, Bosco O, Serpelloni G, Mengoli C.Meta-analysis of diagnostic procedures for Pneumocystis carinii pneumonia in HIV-1-infected patients. Eur Respir J. 2002 Oct;20(4):982-9.

[49] Desmet S, Van Wijngaerden E, Maertens J, Verhaegen J, Verbeken E, De Munter P, Meersseman W, Van Meensel B, Van Eldere J, Lagrou K. Serum (1-3)-beta-D-glucan as a tool for diagnosis of Pneumocystis jirovecii pneumonia in patients with human

immunodeficiency virus infection or hematological malignancy. J Clin Microbiol. 2009 Dec;47(12):3871-4. Epub 2009 Oct 21.

[50] Watanabe T, Yasuoka A, Tanuma J, Yazaki H, Honda H, Tsukada K, Honda M, Gatanaga H, Teruya K, Kikuchi Y, Oka S. Serum (1-->3) beta-D-glucan as a noninvasive adjunct marker for the diagnosis of Pneumocystis pneumonia in patients with AIDS. Clin Infect Dis. 2009 Oct 1;49(7):1128-31.

[51] Thomas M, Rupali P, Woodhouse A, Ellis-Pegler R. Good outcome with trimethoprim 10 mg/kg/day-sulfamethoxazole 50 mg/kg/day for Pneumocystis jirovecii pneumonia in HIV infected patients. Scand J Infect Dis. 2009;41(11-12):862-8.

[52] Helweg-Larsen J, Benfield T, Atzori C, Miller RF. Clinical efficacy of first- and second-line treatments for HIV-associated Pneumocystis jirovecii pneumonia: a tri-centre cohort study. J Antimicrob Chemother. 2009 Dec;64(6):1282-90. Epub 2009 Oct 26

[53] Short CE, Gilleece YC, Fisher MJ, Churchill DR. Trimetrexate and folinic acid: a valuable salvage option for Pneumocystis jirovecii pneumonia. AIDS. 2009 Jun 19;23(10):1287-90.

[54] Smego RA Jr, Nagar S, Maloba B, Popara M. A meta-analysis of salvage therapy for Pneumocystis carinii pneumonia. Arch Intern Med. 2001 Jun 25;161(12):1529-33.)

[55] Fei MW, Kim EJ, Sant CA, Jarlsberg LG, Davis JL, Swartzman A, Huang L. Predicting mortality from HIV-associated Pneumocystis pneumonia at illness presentation: an observational cohort study. Thorax. 2 009 Dec;64(12):1070-6. Epub 2009 Oct 12.

[56] Walzer PD, Evans HE, Copas AJ, Edwards SG, Grant AD, Miller RF. Early predictors of mortality from Pneumocystis jirovecii pneumonia in HIV-infected patients: 1985-2006. Int J STD AIDS. 2009 Sep;20(9):652-3.

[57] Fisk M, Sage EK, Edwards SG, Cartledge JD, Miller RF. Outcome from treatment of Pneumocystis jirovecii pneumonia with co-trimoxazole. Clin Infect Dis. 2008 Feb 15;46(4):625-33

[58] Bédos JP, Dumoulin JL, Gachot B, Veber B, Wolff M, Régnier B, Chevret S. Pneumocystis carinii pneumonia requiring intensive care management: survival and prognostic study in 110 patients with human immunodeficiency virus. Crit Care Med. 1999 Jun;27(6):1109-15.

[59] Boonsarngsuk V, Sirilak S, Kiatboonsri S. Acute respiratory failure due to Pneumocystis pneumonia: outcome and prognostic factors. Int J Infect Dis. 2009 Jan;13(1):59-66. Epub 2008 Jun 24

[60] Forrest DM, Zala C, Djurdjev O, Singer J, Craib KJ, Lawson L, Russell JA, Montaner JS.Determinants of short- and long-term outcome in patients with respiratory failure caused by AIDS-related Pneumocystis carinii pneumonia. Arch Intern Med. 1999 Apr 12;159(7):741-7

[61] National Institutes of Health - University of Carlifonia Expert panel for corticosteroids as adjunctive therapy for Pneumocytis pneumonia in the acquired immunodeficiency syndrome. N Eng J med 1990; 323: 1500-1504

[62] Bozette SA, Sattler FR, Chiu J et al. A controlled trial of early adjunctive treatment with corticosteroids for Pneumocytis carinii pneumonia in the acquired immunodeficiency syndrome. N Eng J Med 1990; 323: 1441 -1457

[63] Gagnon S, Boota AM, Fischl MA et al. Corticosteroids as adjunctive therapy for severe Pneumocystis pneumonia in the acquired immunodeficiency syndrome: a double blind placebo controlled trial. N Eng J Med 1990; 1990: 1444-1450

[64] Montaner JSG, Lawson LM, Levitt N et al. Corticosteroids prevent early deterioration in patients with moderately severe Pneumocystis carinii pneumonia and the acquired immunodeficiency syndrome (AIDS). Ann Intern Med 1990; 113: 14-20

[65] Gallant JE, Chaisson RE, Moore RD. The effect of adjunctive corticosteroids for the treatment of Pneumocystis carinii pneumonia on mortality and subsequent complications. Chest. 1998 Nov;114(5):1258-63.

[66] Walmsley S, Levinton C, Brunton J, Muradali D, Rappaport D, Bast M, Spence D, Salit I. A multicenter randomized double-blind placebo-controlled trial of adjunctive corticosteroids in the treatment of Pneumocystis carinii pneumonia complicating the acquired immune deficiency syndrome. J Acquir Immune Defic Syndr Hum Retrovirol. 1995 Apr 1;8(4):348-57.

[67] Crothers K, Beard CB, Turner J, Groner G, Fox M, Morris A, Eiser S, Huang L. Severity and outcome of HIV-associated Pneumocystis pneumonia containing Pneumocystis jirovecii dihydropteroate synthase gene mutations. AIDS. 2005 May 20;19(8):801-5.

[68] Navin TR, Beard CB, Huang L, del Rio C, Lee S, Pieniazek NJ, Carter JL, Le T, Hightower A, Rimland D. Effect of mutations in Pneumocystis carinii dihydropteroate synthase gene on outcome of P carinii pneumonia in patients with HIV-1: a prospective study. Lancet. 2001 Aug 18;358(9281):545-9.

[69] Helweg-Larsen J, Benfield TL, Eugen-Olsen J, Lundgren JD, Lundgren B.Effects of mutations in Pneumocystis carinii dihydropteroate synthase gene on outcome of AIDS-associated P. carinii pneumonia. Lancet.1999 Oct 16;354(9187):1347-51.

[70] Sage EK, Noursadeghi M, Evans HE, Parker SJ, Copas AJ, Edwards SG, Miller RF. Prognostic value of C-reactive protein in HIV-infected patients with Pneumocystis jirovecii pneumonia. Int J STD AIDS. 2010 Apr;21(4):288-92.

[71] Rizzardi GP, Lazzarin A, Musicco M, Frigerio D, Maillard M, Lucchini M, Moroni M. Risks and benefits of aerosolized pentamidine and cotrimoxazole in primary prophylaxis of Pneumocystis carinii pneumonia in HIV-1-infected patients: a two-year Italian multicentric randomized controlled trial. The Italian PCP Study Group. J Infect. 1996 Mar;32(2):123-31

[72] Warnock AC, Rimland D. Comparison of trimethoprim-sulfamethoxazole, dapsone, and pentamidine in the prophylaxis of Pneumocystis carinii pneumonia. Pharmacotherapy. 1996 Nov-Dec;16(6):1030-8.

[73] Chan C, Montaner J, Lefebvre EA, Morey G, Dohn M, McIvor RA, Scott J, Marina R, Caldwell P.Atovaquone suspension compared with aerosolized pentamidine for prevention of Pneumocystis carinii pneumonia in human immunodeficiency virus-infected subjects intolerant of trimethoprim or sulfonamides. J Infect Dis. 1999 Aug;180(2):369-76.

[74] Kazanjian P, Locke AB, Hossler PA, Lane BR, Bartlett MS, Smith JW, Cannon M, Meshnick SR.Pneumocystis carinii mutations associated with sulfa and sulfone prophylaxis failures in AIDS patients. AIDS. 1998 May 28;12(8):873-8

[75] Nahimana A, Rabodonirina M, Bille J, Francioli P, Hauser PM. Mutations of Pneumocystis jirovecii dihydrofolate reductase associated with failure of prophylaxis. Antimicrob Agents Chemother. 2004 Nov;48(11):4301-5.

[76] El-Sadr WM, Murphy RL, Yurik TM, Luskin-Hawk R, Cheung TW, Balfour HH Jr, Eng R, Hooton TM, Kerkering TM, Schutz M, van der Horst C, Hafner R.Atovaquone compared with dapsone for the prevention of Pneumocystis carinii pneumonia in patients with HIV infection who cannot tolerate trimethoprim, sulfonamides, or

both. Community Program for Clinical Research on AIDS and the AIDS Clinical Trials Group. N Engl J Med. 1998 Dec 24;339(26):1889-95.

[77] Lopez Bernaldo de Quiros JC, Miro JM, Peña JM, Podzamczer D, Alberdi JC, Martínez E, Cosin J, Claramonte X, Gonzalez J, Domingo P, Casado JL, Ribera E; Grupo de Estudio del SIDA 04/98. A randomized trial of the discontinuation of primary and secondary prophylaxis against Pneumocystis carinii pneumonia after highly active antiretroviral therapy in patients with HIV infection. Grupo de Estudio del SIDA 04/98. N Engl J Med. 2001 Jan 18;344(3):159-67.

[78] Cheng CY, Chen MY, Hsieh SM, Sheng WH, Sun HY, Lo YC, Liu WC, Hung CC. May 21;10:126.Risk of pneumocystosis after early discontinuation of prophylaxis among HIV-infected patients receiving highly active antiretroviral therapy.BMC Infect Dis. 2010

[79] D'Egidio GE, Kravcik S, Cooper CL, Cameron DW, Fergusson DA, Angel JB. Pneumocystis jiroveci pneumonia prophylaxis is not required with a CD4+ T-cell count < 200 cells/microl when viral replication is suppressed. AIDS. 2007 Aug 20;21(13):1711-5.

[80] Scourfield A, Tan LK, Nelson M. Severe septic-shock like reaction to co-trimoxazole in an HIV-positive man Int J STD AIDS. 2010 Jul;21(7):521-3.

[81] Cho JY, Kim DM, Kwon YE, Yoon SH, Lee SI Newly formed cystic lesions for the development of pneumomediastinum in Pneumocystis jirovecii pneumonia BMC Infect Dis. 2009 Oct 18;9:171.

[82] Batungwanayo J, Taelman H, Bogaerts J, Allen S, Lucas S, Kagame A, Clerinx J, Montané J, Saraux A, Mühlberger F, et al. Pulmonary cryptococcosis associated with HIV-1 infection in Rwanda: a retrospective study of 37 cases. AIDS. 1994 Sep;8(9):1271-6.

[83] Lee KH, Chang UI, Kim HW, Kim G, Kim SK, Yoo J, Wie SH. Acute respiratory failure associated with cryptococcal pneumonia and disseminated cryptococcosis in an AIDS patient Korean J Intern Med. 2006 Mar;21(1):39-42

[84] Baddley JW, Perfect JR, Oster RA, Larsen RA, Pankey GA, Henderson H, Haas DW, Kauffman CA, Patel R, Zaas AK, Pappas PG. Pulmonary cryptococcosis in patients without HIV infection: factors associated with disseminated disease. Eur J Clin Microbiol Infect Dis. 2008 Oct;27(10):937-43. Epub 2008 May 1.

[85] Denning DW, Follansbee SE, Scolaro M, Norris S, Edelstein H, Stevens DA. Pulmonary aspergillosis in the acquired immunodeficiency syndrome.N Engl J Med. 1991 Mar 7;324(10):654-62.

[86] Klapholz A, Salomon N, Perlman DC, Talavera W. Aspergillosis in the acquired immunodeficiency syndrome. Chest. 1991 Dec;100(6):1614-8.

[87] Klapholz A, Salomon N, Perlman DC, Talavera W. Aspergillosis in the acquired immunodeficiency syndrome. Chest. 1991 Dec;100(6):1614-8.

[88] Vathesatogkit P, Goldenberg R, Parsey M. A 27-year-old HIV-infected woman with severe sepsis and pulmonary infiltrates. Disseminated histoplasmosis with severe sepsis and acute respiratory failure.Chest. 2003 Jan;123(1):272-3, 274-6.

[89] Mora DJ, dos Santos CT, Silva-Vergara ML. Disseminated histoplasmosis in acquired immunodeficiency syndrome patients in Uberaba, MG, Brazil. Mycoses. 2008 Mar;51(2):136-40.

[90] Pappas PG, Pottage JC, Powderly WG, Fraser VJ, Stratton CW, McKenzie S, Tapper ML, Chmel H, Bonebrake FC, Blum R, et al. Blastomycosis in patients with the acquired immunodeficiency syndrome Ann Intern Med. 1992 May 15;116(10):847-53.

[91] Limper AH, Knox KS, Sarosi GA, Ampel NM, Bennett JE, Catanzaro A, Davies SF, Dismukes WE, Hage CA, Marr KA, Mody CH, Perfect JR, Stevens DA; American Thoracic Society Fungal Working Group. An official american thoracic society statement: treatment of fungal infections in adult pulmonary and critical care patients.Am J Respir Crit Care Med. 2011 Jan 1;183(1):96-128

[92] Charalambous S, Day JH, Fielding K, De Cock KM, Churchyard GJ, Corbett EL.HIV infection and chronic chest disease as risk factors for bacterial pneumonia: a case-control study.AIDS. 2003 Jul 4;17(10):1531-7.

[93] Falguera M, Martín M, Ruiz-González A, Pifarré R, García M. Community-acquired pneumonia as the initial manifestation of serious underlying diseases.Am J Med. 2005 Apr;118(4):378-83.

[94] Inverarity D, Bradshaw Q, Wright P, Grant A. The spectrum of HIV-related disease in rural Central Thailand.Southeast Asian J Trop Med Public Health. 2002 Dec;33(4):822-31

[95] Sullivan JH, Moore RD, Keruly JC, Chaisson RE. Effect of antiretroviral therapy on the incidence of bacterial pneumonia in patients with advanced HIV infection Am J Respir Crit Care Med. 2000 Jul;162(1):64-7

[96] Madeddu G, Porqueddu EM, Cambosu F, Saba F, Fois AG, Pirina P, Mura MS. Bacterial community acquired pneumonia in HIV-infected inpatients in the highly active antiretroviral therapy era. Infection. 2008 Jun;36(3):231-6. Epub 2008 May 10.

[97] Saindou M, Chidiac C, Miailhes P, Voirin N, Baratin D, Amiri M, Livrozet JM, Touraine JL, Trepo C, Peyramond D, Vanhems P. Pneumococcal pneumonia in HIV-infected patients by antiretroviral therapy periods HIV Med. 2008 Apr;9(4):203-7. Epub 2008 Feb 21

[98] Barbier F, Coquet I, Legriel S, Pavie J, Darmon M, Mayaux J, Molina JM, Schlemmer B, Azoulay E. Etiologies and outcome of acute respiratory failure in HIV-infected patients Intensive Care Med. 2009 Oct;35(10):1678-86. Epub 2009 Jul 3

[99] Soeiro Ade M, Hovnanian AL, Parra ER, Canzian M, Capelozzi VL. Post-mortem histological pulmonary analysis in patients with HIV/AIDS. Clinics (Sao Paulo). 2008 Aug;63(4):497-502.

[100] Martinson NA, Karstaedt A, Venter WD, Omar T, King P, Mbengo T, Marais E, McIntyre J, Chaisson RE, Hale M. Causes of death in hospitalized adults with a premortem diagnosis of tuberculosis: an autopsy study AIDS. 2007 Oct 1;21(15):2043-50.

[101] Wallace JM, Hansen NI, Lavange L, Glassroth J, Browdy BL, Rosen MJ, Kvale PA, Mangura BT, Reichman LB, Hopewell PC. Pulmonary Complications of HIV Infection Study Group. Respiratory disease trends in the Pulmonary Complications of HIV Infection Study cohort. Am J Respir Crit Care Med. 1997 Jan;155(1):72-80.

[102] Burns DN, Hillman D, Neaton JD, Sherer R, Mitchell T, Capps L, Vallier WG, Thurnherr MD, Gordin FM. Cigarette smoking, bacterial pneumonia, and other clinical outcomes in HIV-1 infection. Terry Beirn Community Programs for Clinical Research on AIDS. J Acquir Immune Defic Syndr Hum Retrovirol. 1996 Dec 1;13(4):374-83.

[103] Tumbarello M, Tacconelli E, de Gaetano K, Ardito F, Pirronti T, Cauda R, Ortona L. Bacterial pneumonia in HIV-infected patients: analysis of risk factors and prognostic indicators.J Acquir Immune Defic Syndr Hum Retrovirol. 1998 May 1;18(1):39-45.

[104] Bénard A, Mercié P, Alioum A, Bonnet F, Lazaro E, Dupon M, Neau D, Dabis F, Chêne G; Groupe d'Epidémiologie Clinique du Sida en Aquitaine.Bacterial pneumonia among HIV-infected patients: decreased risk after tobacco smoking cessation. ANRS CO3 Aquitaine Cohort, 2000-2007. PLoS One. 2010 Jan 26;5(1):e8896

[105] Gordin FM, Roediger MP, Girard PM, Lundgren JD, Miro JM, Palfreeman A, Rodriguez-Barradas MC, Wolff MJ, Easterbrook PJ, Clezy K, Slater LN. Pneumonia in HIV-infected persons: increased risk with cigarette smoking and treatment interruption. Am J Respir Crit Care Med. 2008 Sep 15;178(6):630-6. Epub 2008 Jul 10

[106] Crothers K, Griffith TA, McGinnis KA, Rodriguez-Barradas MC, Leaf DA, Weissman S, Gibert CL, Butt AA, Justice AC.J Gen The impact of cigarette smoking on mortality, quality of life, and comorbid illness among HIV-positive veterans. Intern Med. 2005 Dec;20(12):1142-5.)

[107] Saindou M, Chidiac C, Miailhes P, Voirin N, Baratin D, Amiri M, Livrozet JM, Touraine JL, Trepo C, Peyramond D, Vanhems P.Pneumococcal pneumonia in HIV-infected patients by antiretroviral therapy periods. HIV Med. 2008 Apr;9(4):203-7. Epub 2008 Feb 21

[108] Moore RD, Keruly JC, Chaisson RE. Neutropenia and bacterial infection in acquired immunodeficiency syndrome. Arch Intern Med. 1995 Oct 9;155(18):1965-70.

[109] Franzetti F, Grassini A, Piazza M, Degl'innocenti M, Bandera A, Gazzola L, Marchetti G, Gori A. Nosocomial bacterial pneumonia in HIV-infected patients: risk factors for adverse outcome and implications for rational empiric antibiotic therapy. Infection. 2006 Feb;34(1):9-16.

[110] Tumbarello M, Tacconelli E, de Gaetano Donati K, Bertagnolio S, Cataldo M, Pirronti T, Ardito F, Cauda R. Nosocomial bacterial pneumonia in human immunodeficiency virus infected subjects: incidence, risk factors and outcome Eur Respir J. 2001 Apr;17(4):636-40.

[111] Chave JP, Bille J, Glauser MP, Francioli P. Diagnosis of pulmonary infections in patients infected with the human immunodeficiency virus. Eur J Clin Microbiol Infect Dis. 1989 Feb;8(2):123-6.

[112] French N, Williams G, Williamson V, Bhatt SM, Gilks CF. The radiographic appearance of pneumococcal pneumonia in adults is unaltered by HIV-1-infection in hospitalized Kenyans. Br J Radiol. 2007 May;80(953):302-6. Epub 2006 Sep 27

[113] Rizzi EB, Schininá V, Rovighi L, Cristofaro M, Bordi E, Narciso P, Bibbolino C. HIV-related pneumococcal lung disease: does highly active antiretroviral therapy or bacteremia modify radiologic appearance? AIDS Patient Care STDS. 2008 Feb;22(2):105-11.

[114] Shah RM, Gupta S, Angeid-Backman E, O'Donnell J. Pneumococcal pneumonia in patients requiring hospitalization: effects of bacteremia and HIV seropositivity on radiographic appearance.AJR Am J Roentgenol. 2000 Dec;175(6):1533-6.

[115] Nyamande K, Lalloo UG, Vawda F. Comparison of plain chest radiography and high-resolution CT in human immunodeficiency virus infected patients with community-acquired pneumonia: a sub-Saharan Africa study. AIDS. 2002 Oct 18;16(15):2095-6

[116] Mark PE. The clinical features of severe community acquired pneumonis presenting as septic shock. Norasept II study investigators. J. Crit Care 2000; 15: 85-90

[117] JAG Scott, AJ Hall, C Muyodi et al. Aetiology, outcome and risk factors for mortality among adults with acute pneumonia in Kenya. Lancet 200; 355(9211): 1225-1230

[118] Watanakunakorn C, Bailey TA. Adult bacteremic pneumococcal pneumonia in a community teaching hospital 1992-1996: a detailed analysis of 108 cases. Arch. Intern Med 1997; 157: 1965-71

[119] Storgaard M, Laursen AL, Andersen PL. The C-reactive protein responses in HIV-infected patients with pneumonia.Scand J Infect Dis. 1993;25(3):305-9.

[120] Schleicher GK, Herbert V, Brink A, Martin S, Maraj R, Galpin JS, Feldman C. Procalcitonin and C-reactive protein levels in HIV-positive subjects with tuberculosis and pneumonia. Eur Respir J. 2005 Apr;25(4):688-92.

[121] Lim WS, Vander Eerden MM, Laing R et al. Defining community acquired pneumonia severity on presentation to hospital. An international derivation and validation study. Thorax 2003; 58: 377-82

[122] Fine MJ, Auble TE, Yealy DM et al. A prediction rule to identify low risk patients with community acquired pneumonia. N. Eng J Med 1997; 336: 243-50

[123] Murray PR, Washington JA. Microscopic and bacteriologic analysis of expectorated sputum. Mayo Clin Proc 1975; 50(6): 339-44.

[124] Boulware DR, Daley CL, Merrifield C, Hopewell PC, Janoff EN. Rapid diagnosis of pneumococcal pneumonia among HIV-infected adults with urine antigen detection J Infect. 2007 Oct;55(4):300-9. Epub 2007 Aug 10.

[125] Cordero E, Pachón J, Rivero A, Girón-González JA, Gómez-Mateos J, Merino MD, Torres-Tortosa M, González-Serrano M, Aliaga L, Collado A, Hernández-Quero J, Barrera A, Nuño E Usefulness of sputum culture for diagnosis of bacterial pneumonia in HIV-infected patients. Eur J Clin Microbiol Infect Dis. 2002 May;21(5):362-7. Epub 2002 May 7.

[126] da Silva RM, Teixeira PJ, Moreira Jda S. The clinical utility of induced sputum for the diagnosis of bacterial community-acquired pneumonia in HIV-infected patients: a prospective cross-sectional study.Braz J Infect Dis. 2006 Apr;10(2):89-93.

[127] Daley CL, Mugusi F, Chen LL, Schmidt DM, Small PM, Bearer E, Aris E, Mtoni IM, Cegielski JP, Lallinger G, Mbaga I, Murray JF.Pulmonary complications of HIV infection in Dar es Salaam, Tanzania. Role of bronchoscopy and bronchoalveolar lavage. Am J Respir Crit Care Med. 1996 Jul;154(1):105-10.

[128] Marcos MA, Jiménez de Anta MT, de la Bellacasa JP, González J, Martínez E, García E, Mensa J, de Roux A, Torres A. Rapid urinary antigen test for diagnosis of pneumococcal community-acquired pneumonia in adults. Eur Respir J. 2003 Feb;21(2):209-14.

[129] Yzerman EP, den Boer JW, Lettinga KD, Schellekens J, Dankert J, Peeters M. Sensitivity of three urinary antigen tets associated with clinical severity in large outbreak of legionnaires disease in the Netherlands. J clin Microbiol 2002; 40: 3232-6

[130] Shankar EM, Kumarasamy N, Balakrishnan P, Solomon S, Lejith R, Vengatesan A, Anand Rao U. Serosurveillance of acute Mycoplasma pneumoniae infection among HIV infected patients with pulmonary complaints in Chennai, Southern India. J Infect. 2006 Nov;53(5):325-30. Epub 2006 Jan 25.

[131] Jiménez ML, Aspa J, Padilla B, Ancochea J, González A, Fraga J, Santos I, Martínez R, Gómez Herruz P, López-Brea M. Fiberoptic bronchoscopic diagnosis of pulmonary

disease in 151 HIV-infected patients with pneumonitis. Eur J Clin Microbiol Infect Dis. 1991 Jun;10(6):491-6.

[132] Heurlin N, Brattström C, Lönnqvist B, Westman L, Lidman C, Andersson J Aetiology of pulmonary diseases in immunocompromised patients. Eur Respir J. 1991 Jan;4(1):10-8.

[133] Taylor IK, Coker RJ, Clarke J, Moss FM, Nieman R, Evans DJ, Veale D, Shaw RJ, Robinson DS, Mitchell DM. Pulmonary complications of HIV disease: 10 year retrospective evaluation of yields from bronchoalveolar lavage, 1983-93. Thorax. 1995 Dec;50(12):1240-5.

[134] Daley CL, Mugusi F, Chen LL, Schmidt DM, Small PM, Bearer E, Aris E, Mtoni IM, Cegielski JP, Lallinger G, Mbaga I, Murray JF. Pulmonary complications of HIV infection in Dar es Salaam, Tanzania. Role of bronchoscopy and bronchoalveolar lavage Am J Respir Crit Care Med. 1996 Jul;154(1):105-10.

[135] Falguera M, Nogues A, Ruiz-González A, García M, Puig T, Rubio-Caballero M. Transthoracic needle aspiration in the study of pulmonary infections in patients with HIV. Chest. 1994 Sep;106(3):697-702.

[136] McLeod DT, Neill P, Robertson VJ, Latif AS, Emmanuel JC, Els JE, Gwanzura LK, Trijssenaar FE, Nziramasanga P, Jongeling GR, et al. Pulmonary diseases in patients infected with the human immunodeficiency virus in Zimbabwe, Central Africa. Trans R Soc Trop Med Hyg. 1989 Sep-Oct;83(5):694-7.

[137] Jensen BN, Gerstoft J, Højlyng N, Backer V, Paaske M, Gomme G, Skinhøj P. Pulmonary pathogens in HIV-infected patients. Scand J Infect Dis. 1990;22(4):413-20.

[138] McLoughlin P, Mulcahy F, O'Briain DS, Kane B, Mulvihill E, Prichard JS. Lung pathology in HIV positive patients. Ir Med J. 1990 Sep;83(3):109-11.

[139] Redd SC, Rutherford GW 3rd, Sande MA, Lifson AR, Hadley WK, Facklam RR, Spika JS. The role of human immunodeficiency virus infection in pneumococcal bacteremia in San Francisco residents. J Infect Dis. 1990 Nov;162(5):1012-7.

[140] Feldman C, Glatthaar M, Morar R, Mahomed AG, Kaka S, Cassel M, Klugman KP. Bacteremic pneumococcal pneumonia in HIV-seropositive and HIV-seronegative adults. Chest. 1999 Jul;116(1):107-14.

[141] Koulla-Shiro S, Kuaban C, Belec L. Acute community-acquired bacterial pneumonia in Human Immunodeficiency Virus (HIV) infected and non-HIV-infected adult patients in Cameroon: aetiology and outcome. Tuber Lung Dis. 1996 Feb;77(1):47-51.

[142] Pesola GR, Charles A. Pneumococcal bacteremia with pneumonia. Mortality in acquired immunodeficiency syndrome. Chest. 1992 Jan;101(1):150-5.

[143] Falcó V, Fernández de Sevilla T, Alegre J, Barbé J, Ferrer A, Ocaña I, Ribera E, Martínez-Vázquez JM. Bacterial pneumonia in HIV-infected patients: a prospective study of 68 episodes. Eur Respir J. 1994 Feb;7(2):235-9.

[144] Topino S, Galati V, Grilli E, Petrosillo N Rhodococcus equi infection in HIV-infected individuals: case reports and review of the literature..AIDS Patient Care STDS. 2010 Apr;24(4):211-22

[145] Hulsewé-Evers HP, Jansveld CA, Jansz AR, Schneider MM, Bravenboer B. HIV-infected patient with a Rhodococcus equi pneumonia. Neth J Med. 2000 Jul;57(1):25-9.

[146] Frame BC, Petkus AF. Rhodococcus equi pneumonia: case report and literature review. Ann Pharmacother. 1993 Nov;27(11):1340-2

[147] Vanschooneveld T, Mindru C, Madariaga MG, Kalil AC, Florescu DF. Enterococcus pneumonia complicated with empyema and lung abscess in an HIV-positive patient. Case report and review of the literature. Int J STD AIDS. 2009 Sep;20(9):659-6

[148] Unkle DW, Ricketti AJ, Cleri DJ, Moser RL, Vernaleo JR. An HIV-infected patient with Nocardia asteroides bilateral pneumonia. AIDS Read. 2008 Nov;18(11):566-8.

[149] Menéndez R, Cordero PJ, Santos M, Gobernado M, Marco V. Pulmonary infection with Nocardia species: a report of 10 cases and review. Eur Respir J. 1997 Jul;10(7):1542-6.

[150] Sandkovsky U, Sandkovsky G, Suh J, Smith B, Sharp V, Polsky B. Legionella pneumonia and HIV: case reports and review of the literature. AIDS Patient Care STDS. 2008 Jun;22(6):473-81.

[151] Bangsborg JM, Jensen BN, Friis-Møller A, Bruun B. Legionellosis in patients with HIV infection. I nfection. 1990 Nov-Dec;18(6):342-6.

[152] Shankar EM, Kumarasamy N, Vignesh R, Balakrishnan P, Solomon SS, Murugavel KG, Saravanan S, Velu V, Farooq SM, Hayath K, Muthu S, Solomon S, Rao UA. Epidemiological studies on pulmonary pathogens in HIV-positive and -negative subjects with or without community-acquired pneumonia with special emphasis on Mycoplasma pneumoniae. Jpn J Infect Dis. 2007 Nov;60(6):337-41.

[153] Lockman S, Hone N, Kenyon TA, Mwasekaga M, Villauthapillai M, Creek T, Zell E, Kirby A, Thacker WL, Talkington D, Moura IN, Binkin NJ, Clay L, Tappero JW. Etiology of pulmonary infections in predominantly HIV-infected adults with suspected tuberculosis, Botswana. Int J Tuberc Lung Dis. 2003 Aug;7(8):714-23

[154] Manfredi R, Nanetti A, Valentini R, Chiodo F. Moraxella catarrhalis pneumonia during HIV disease. J Chemother. 2000 Oct;12(5):406-11.

[155] Schuster MG, Norris AH Community-acquired Pseudomonas aeruginosa pneumonia in patients with HIV infection. AIDS. 1994 Oct;8(10):1437-41.

[156] Ali NJ, Kessel D, Miller RF Bronchopulmonary infection with Pseudomonas aeruginosa in patients infected with human immunodeficiency virus. Genitourin Med. 1995 Apr;71(2):73-7.

[157] Dropulic LK, Leslie JM, Eldred LJ, Zenilman J, Sears CL Clinical manifestations and risk factors of Pseudomonas aeruginosa infection in patients with AIDS. J Infect Dis. 1995 Apr;171(4):930-7.

[158] Casado JL, Navas E, Frutos B, Moreno A, Martín P, Hermida JM, Guerrero A. Salmonella lung involvement in patients with HIV infection. Chest. 1997 Nov 5;112(5):1197-201.

[159] Watanabe H, Asoh N, Kobayashi S, Watanabe K, Oishi K, Kositsakulchai W, Sanchai T, Khantawa B, Tharavichitkul P, Sirisanthana T, Nagatake T. Clinical and microbiological characteristics of community-acquired pneumonia among human immunodeficiency virus-infected patients in northern Thailand. J Infect Chemother. 2008 Apr;14(2):105-9. Epub 2008 Apr 30

[160] Vray M, Germani Y, Chan S, Duc NH, Sar B, Sarr FD, Bercion R, Rahalison L, Maynard M, L'Her P, Chartier L, Mayaud C. Clinical features and etiology of pneumonia in acid-fast bacillus sputum smear-negative HIV-infected patients hospitalized in Asia and Africa. AIDS. 2008 Jul 11;22(11):1323-32.

[161] Castro JG, Manzi G, Espinoza L, Campos M, Boulanger C. Concurrent PCP and TB pneumonia in HIV infected patients. Scand J Infect Dis. 2007;39(11-12):1054-8. Epub 2007 Jun 21.

[162] Soubani AO, Ibrahim I, Forlenza S. Simultaneous nocardial empyema and Pneumocystis carinii pneumonia as an initial manifestation of HIV infection. South Med J. 1993 Nov;86(11):1318-9.
[163] Aspa J, Rajas O, Rodriguez de Castro F, Huertas MC, Borderías L, Cabello FJ, Tábara J, Hernández-Flix S, Martinez-Sanchis A, Torres A; Pneumococcal Pneumonia in Spain Study Group. Impact of initial antibiotic choice on mortality from pneumococcal pneumonia. Eur Respir J. 2006 May;27(5):1010-9. Epub 2006 Feb 2.
[164] Mandell CA, Wunderink RG, Anzueto A et al. Infectious Diseases Society of America/American Thoracic Society consensus guidelines on the management of community acquired pneumonia in adults. Clin Infect Dis 2007; 44(Suppl 2): S27-72
[165] Gwanzura L, Pasi C, Nathoo KJ, Hakim J, Gangaidzo I, Mielke J, Robertson VJ, Heyderman RS, Mason PR. Rapid emergence of resistance to penicillin and trimethoprim-sulphamethoxazole in invasive Streptococcus pneumoniae in Zimbabwe. Int J Antimicrob Agents. 2003 Jun;21(6):557-61.
[166] Falcó V, Almirante B, Jordano Q, Calonge L, del Valle O, Pigrau C, Planes AM, Gavaldà J, Pahissa A. Influence of penicillin resistance on outcome in adult patients with invasive pneumococcal pneumonia: is penicillin useful against intermediately resistant strains?; J Antimicrob Chemother. 2004 Aug;54(2):481-8. Epub 2004 Jun 23.
[167] Yoshimine H, Oishi K, Mubiru F, Nalwoga H, Takahashi H, Amano H, Ombasi P, Watanabe K, Joloba M, Aisu T, Ahmed K, Shimada M, Mugerwa R, Nagatake T. Community-acquired pneumonia in Ugandan adults: short-term parenteral ampicillin therapy for bacterial pneumonia. Am J Trop Med Hyg. 2001 Mar-Apr;64(3-4):172-7.
[168] Arlotti M, Zoboli G, Moscatelli GL, Magnani G, Maserati R, Borghi V, Andreoni M, Libanore M, Bonazzi L, Piscina A, Ciammarughi R. Rhodococcus equi infection in HIV-positive subjects: a retrospective analysis of 24 cases. Scand J Infect Dis. 1996;28(5):463-7.
[169] Perelló R, Miró O, Marcos MA, Almela M, Bragulat E, Sánchez M, Agustí C, Miro JM, Moreno A. Predicting bacteremic pneumonia in HIV-1-infected patients consulting the ED. Am J Emerg Med. 2010 May;28(4):454-9. Epub 2010 Mar 25.
[170] Manno D, Puoti M, Signorini L, Lapadula G, Cadeo B, Soavi L, Paraninfo G, Allegri R, Cristini G, Viale P, Carosi G. Risk factors and clinical characteristics associated with hospitalization for community-acquired bacterial pneumonia in HIV-positive patients according to the presence of liver cirrhosis. Infection. 2009 Aug;37(4):334-9. Epub 2009 Jul 23
[171] Malinis M, Myers J, Bordon J, Peyrani P, Kapoor R, Nakamatzu R, Lopardo G, Torres A, Feldman C, Allen M, Arnold F, Ramirez J. Clinical outcomes of HIV-infected patients hospitalized with bacterial community-acquired pneumonia. Int J Infect Dis. 2010 Jan;14(1):e22-7. Epub 2009 Jul 7.
[172] Mwachari CW, Nduba VN, Park DR, Meier AS, Kariuki JN, Muyodi JA, Karimi F, Kigo A, Holmes KK, Cohen CR. Clinical presentation among HIV-infected and non-infected adults with community acquired pneumonia in Nairobi. Int J Tuberc Lung Dis. 2006 May;10(5):516-22.
[173] Barbier F, Coquet I, Legriel S, Pavie J, Darmon M, Mayaux J, Molina JM, Schlemmer B, Azoulay E. Etiologies and outcome of acute respiratory failure in HIV-infected patients. Intensive Care Med. 2009 Oct;35(10):1678-86. Epub 2009 Jul 3.

[174] Pedro-Botet ML, Sopena N, García-Cruz A, Mateu L, García-Núñez M, Rey-Joly C, Sabrià M. Streptococcus pneumoniae and Legionella pneumophila pneumonia in HIV-infected patients. Scand J Infect Dis. 2007;39(2):122-8.

[175] Sureka A, Parada JP, Deloria-Knoll M, Chmiel JS, Phan L, Lyons TM, Ali S, Yarnold PR, Weinstein RA, Dehovitz JA, Jacobson JM, Goetz MB, Campo RE, Berland D, Bennett CL, Uphold CR. HIV-related pneumonia care in older patients hospitalized in the early HAART era Eur Respir J. AIDS Patient Care STDS. 2004 Feb;18(2):99-107.

[176] Madeddu G, Porqueddu EM, Cambosu F, Saba F, Fois AG, Pirina P, Mura MS. Bacterial community acquired pneumonia in HIV-infected inpatients in the highly active antiretroviral therapy era. Infection. 2008 Jun;36(3):231-6. Epub 2008 May 10.

[177] Sanders KM, Marras TK, Chan CK. Pneumonia severity index in the immunocompromised. Can Respir J. 2006 Mar;13(2):89-93.

[178] Cordero E, Pachón J, Rivero A, Girón JA, Gómez-Mateos J, Merino MD, Torres-Tortosa M, González-Serrano M, Aliaga L, Collado A, Hernández-Quero J, Barrera A, Nuño E. The Grupo Andaluz para el Estudio de las Enfermedades Infecciosas. Community-acquired bacterial pneumonia in human immunodeficiency virus-infected patients: validation of severity criteria. Am J Respir Crit Care Med. 2000 Dec;162(6):2063-8.

[179] Curran A, Falcó V, Crespo M, Martinez X, Ribera E, Villar del Saz S, Imaz A, Coma E, Ferrer A, Pahissa A. Bacterial pneumonia in HIV-infected patients: use of the pneumonia severity index and impact of current management on incidence, aetiology and outcome. HIV Med. 2008 Oct;9(8):609-15. Epub 2008 Jun 28.

[180] Teshale EH, Hanson D, Flannery B, Phares C, Wolfe M, Schuchat A, Sullivan P. Effectiveness of 23-valent polysaccharide pneumococcal vaccine on pneumonia in HIV-infected adults in the United States, 1998--2003. Vaccine. 2008 Oct 29;26(46):5830-4. Epub 2008 Sep 9.

[181] Breiman RF, Keller DW, Phelan MA, Sniadack DH, Stephens DS, Rimland D, Farley MM, Schuchat A, Reingold AL. Evaluation of effectiveness of the 23-valent pneumococcal capsular polysaccharide vaccine for HIV-infected patients. Arch Intern Med. 2000 Sep 25;160(17):2633-8.

[182] Rodriguez-Barradas MC, Goulet J, Brown S, Goetz MB, Rimland D, Simberkoff MS, Crothers K, Justice AC. Impact of pneumococcal vaccination on the incidence of pneumonia by HIV infection status among patients enrolled in the Veterans Aging Cohort 5-Site Study. Clin Infect Dis. 2008 Apr 1;46(7):1093-100.

[183] López-Palomo C, Martín-Zamorano M, Benítez E, Fernández-Gutiérrez C, Guerrero F, Rodríguez-Iglesias M, Girón-González JA. Pneumonia in HIV-infected patients in the HAART era: incidence, risk, and impact of the pneumococcal vaccination. J Med Virol. 2004 Apr;72(4):517-24.

[184] French N, Gilks CF, Mujugira A, Fasching C Pneumococcal vaccination in HIV-1-infected adults in Uganda: humoral response and two vaccine failures AIDS. 1998 Sep 10;12(13):1683-9.

[185] French N, Nakiyingi J, Carpenter LM, Lugada E, Watera C, Moi K, Moore M, Antvelink D, Mulder D, Janoff EN, Whitworth J, Gilks CF 23-valent pneumococcal polysaccharide vaccine in HIV-1-infected Ugandan adults: double-blind, randomised and placebo controlled trial. Lancet. 2000 Jun 17;355(9221):2106-11.

[186] French N, Gordon SB, Mwalukomo T, White SA, Mwafulirwa G, Longwe H, Mwaiponya M, Zijlstra EE, Molyneux ME, Gilks CF. A trial of a 7-valent

pneumococcal conjugate vaccine in HIV-infected adults. N Engl J Med. 2010 Mar 4;362(9):812-22.

[187] Maynart M, Lièvre L, Sow PS, Kony S, Gueye NF, Bassène E, Metro A, Ndoye I, Ba DS, Coulaud JP, Costagliola D; SIDAK Study Group. Primary prevention with cotrimoxazole for HIV-1-infected adults: results of the pilot study in Dakar, Senegal J Acquir Immune Defic Syndr. 2001 Feb 1;26(2):130-6.

[188] DiRienzo AG, van Der Horst C, Finkelstein DM, Frame P, Bozzette SA, Tashima KT. Efficacy of trimethoprim-sulfamethoxazole for the prevention of bacterial infections in a randomized prophylaxis trial of patients with advanced HIV infection. AIDS Res Hum Retroviruses. 2002 Jan 20;18(2):89-94.

[189] Shebl FM, Engels EA, Goedert JJ, Chaturvedi AK. Pulmonary infections and risk of lung cancer among persons with AIDS. J Acquir Immune Defic Syndr. 2010 Nov 1;55(3):375-9.

[190] Gil Suay V, Cordero PJ, Martínez E, Soler JJ, Perpiñá M, Greses JV, Sanchis J. Parapneumonic effusions secondary to community-acquired bacterial pneumonia in human immunodeficiency virus-infected patients. Eur Respir J. 1995 Nov;8(11):1934-9.

[191] Richard E Chaisson, Neil Martinson. Tuberculsosis in Africa- Combating an HIV driven crisis. NEJM 2008;358(11): 1089-1092

[192] The changing incidence of AIDS events in patients receiving highly active antiretroviral therapy. *The antiretroviral therapy collaboration.* Arch Intern Med 2005; 165: 416-423

[193] Grabar S, Lanoy E, Allavena C, Mary-Krause M, Bentata M, Fischer P, Mahamat A, Rabaud C, Costagliola D; on behalf of the Clinical Epidemiology Group of the French Hospital Database on HIV. Causes of the first AIDS-defining illness and subsequent survival before and after the advent of combined antiretroviral therapy. HIV Med. 2008 Apr;9(4):246-256.

[194] De Cock KM, Chairsson RE. Will DOTS do it? A reappraisal of tuberculosis control in countries with high rates of HIV infection. Int J Tuberc Lung Dis 1999; 3: 457-465

[195] Harries AD. Tuberculosis and human immunodeficiency infection in developing countries. Lancet 1990; 335: 387-390

[196] *Brandli O, The clinical presentation of tuberculosis. Respiration 1998;65: 97-105*

[197] Koppaka R, Bock N. How reliable is chest radiography? In Frieden TR ed. Tomans tuberculsosis, case detection, treatment and monitoring, 2nd edition WHO, 2004: 51-60

[198] Post F, Wood R, Pillay GP. Pulmonary tuberculosis in HIV infection: radiographic appearance is related to CD + T cell count. Tuberc Lung Dis 1995; 76(6): 518-521

[199] Perlman DC, El-Sadr W, Nelson ET et al. Variation of chest radiopgraphic patterns in pulmonary tuberculosis by degree of human immunodeficiency virus related immunosuppresion. The Terry Beirn Community Programs for Clinical Research in AIDS (CPCRA). The AIDS Clinical Trials Group (ACTG). Clin Infect Dis 1997; 25(2): 242-246

[200] Behr MA, Warren SA, Salaon H. Transmission of Mycobacterium tuberculosis from patients smear negative for acid fast bacilli. Lance 1999; 353: 444-49

[201] Grzbowski S, Barnett GD, Styblo K. Contacts of active pulmonary tuberculosis. Bull Int Union Tuber 1975; 50: 90-106

[202] Elliot AM, Namaambo K, Allen BW et al. Negative sputum smear results in HIV positive patients with pulmonary tuberculosis in Lusaka, Zambia. Tubervc Lung Dis 1993; 74: 191-94

[203] *Mase SR, Ramsay A, Ng V et al. Yield of serial sputum specimen examinations in the diagnosis of pulmonary tuberculosis: a systematic review. Int J tuberc Lung Dis 2007;11(5): 485-95*

[204] Rawat J, Biswas D, Sindhwani G, Masih V. An alternative 1-day smear microscopy protocol for the diagnosis of pulmonary tuberculosis.Respirology. 2010 Oct;15(7):1127-30. doi: 10.1111/j.1440-1843.2010.01827.x.

[205] Steingart KR, Ng V, Henry M et al. Sputum processing methods to improved the sensitivity of smear microscopy for tuberculosis: a systematic review. Lancet Infect Dis 2006; 6: 664-674

[206] Steingart KR, Henry M, Ng V et al. Fluorescence versus conventional sputum smear microscopy for tuberculsosis: a systematic review. Lancet Infect Dis 2006; 6: 571 -81

[207] Luis Eduardo Cuevas, Najila Al –Sonboli, Lovett Lawson et al. LED Fluorescence microscopy for the diagnosis of pulmonary tuberculosis: a multi country cross sectional evaluation. Plos Medicine 2011; 8(7): e 1001057.doi e10.1371/ journal.pmed.1001057

[208] Crucian M, Scarparo C, Malena M et al. Meta analysis of BACTEC MGIT 960 and BACTEC 460 TB with or without solid media for the detection of Mycobacteria. J Clin Micobiol 2004; 42: 2321 – 2325

[209] Madhukar Pai, Jessica Minion, Karen Steingart and Andrew Ramsay. New and improved tuberculosis diagnostics : evidence, policy, practice and impact. Current Opinion in Pul Med 2010; 16: 271 -284

[210] World Health Organization. Report of the 9th meeting of the Strategic and Technical Advisory Group on TB (STAG –TB) Geneva: World Health Organization; 2009. http://www.who.int/tb/advisory-bodies/stag/en/index.html

[211] Catharina Boehme, Pamela Nabeta, Doris Hilleman et al. Rapid molecular detection of tuberculosis and rifampicin resistance. NEJM 2010 Sept 9; 363 (11): 1005 -15

[212] Boehme CC, Nicol MP, Nabeta P, Michael JS, Gotuzzo E, Tahirli R, Gler MT, Blakemore R, Worodria W, Gray C, Huang L, Caceres T, Mehdiyev R, Raymond L, Whitelaw A, Sagadevan K, Alexander H, Albert H, Cobelens F, Cox H, Alland D, Perkins MD. Feasibility, diagnostic accuracy, and effectiveness of decentralised use of the Xpert MTB/RIF test for diagnosis of tuberculosis and multidrug resistance: a multicentre implementation study.Lancet. 2011 Apr 30;377(9776):1495-505. Epub 2011 Apr 18.

[213] World Health Organization, Strategic and Technical Advisory Group for TB, Meeting report 2010

[214] Steingart KR, Henry M, Laal S et al. Commercial serological antibody detection tests for the diagnosis of of pulmonary tuberculosis: a systematic review. Plos Med 2007; 4: e202

[215] Treatment of Tuberculosis: Guidelines for National Programmes. WHO. WHO/HTM/2009.420

[216] Faiz A Khan, Jessica Minion, Madhular Pai et al. Treatment of active tuberculosis in HIV co-infected patients: a systematic review and meta- analysis. Clin Infect Dis 2010; 50(9): 1288-1299

[217] I. Dubrovina, K. Miskinis, S. Lyepshina et al. Drug resistant tuberculosis and HIV in Ukraine: a threatening convergence of two epidemics. Int J Tuberc Lung Dis 2008; 12(7): 758-762.

[218] Charles D. Wells, J.Peter Cegielski, Lisa J. Nelson et al. HIV Infection and Multi drug resistant tuberculosis - the perfect storm. Journal of Infectious Diseases 2007; 196: S86-107

[219] Gandhi NR, Moll A, Sturm AW et al. Extensively drug-resistant tuberculosis as a cause of death in patients co-infected with tuberculosis and HIV in a rural area of South Africa. Lancet 2006 Nov 4;368(9547):1575-80.

[220] Kangombe CT, Harries AD, Ito K et al. Long term outcome in patients registered with tuberculosis in Zomba, Malawi : mortality at 7 years according to initial HIV status and type of TB. Int J. Tuberc Lung Dis 2004; 8: 829 -836

[221] Salim S. Abdool Karim, Kogieleum Naidoo, Anneke Grobler et al. Timing of initiation of anti –retroviral drugs during tuberculosis therapy. N Eng J Med 2010; 362: 697 -706.

[222] Wiktor SZ, Sassan Maroko M, Grant AD et al. Efficacy of trimethoprim sulphamethoxazole prophylaxis to decrease morbidity and mortality in HIV1 infected patients with tuberculosis in Abidjan, Cote d'Ivoire: a randomized controlled trial. Lancet 1999; 353: 1469-1475

[223] Woldehanna S, Volmink J. Treatment of latent tuberculosis infection in HIV infected persons(Review). Cochrane Database of Systematic Reviews 2004, Issue 1. Art. No.: CD 000171.DOI:10. 1002/14651858.CD000172.pub2

[224] Enrico Girardi, Caroline A Sabin, Antonell d' Amino Montarte et al Incidence of tuberculosis among HIV infected patients receiving highly active antiretroviral therapy in Europe and North America. Clinical Infectious Diseases 2005; 41: 1772-82

[225] Badri M, Wilson D, Wood R. Effect of highly active anti-retroviral therapy on the incidence of tuberculosis in South Africa: a cohort study. Lancet 2002; 359(9323): 2059-2064.

[226] Jonathan E Golub, Valeria Saracen, Solange C Covalcante et al. The impact of antiretroviral therapy and Isoniazid preventive therapy on tuberculosis incidence in HIV infected patients in Rio de Janeiro, Brazil. AIDS 2007, 21: 1441-144

[227] World Health Organization. Policy on Collaborative TB/HIV Activities, 2011.

[228] Diagnosis and treatment of disease caused by non tuberculous mycobacteria. Offficial statement of the American Thoracic Society. Am J Respir Crit Care Med 1997; 156: S1-S25

[229] Raju B, Schluger NW. Significance of respiratory isolates of Mycobacterium avium complex in HIV-positive and HIV-negative patients. Int J Infect Dis. 2000;4(3):134-9.

[230] MacDonell KB, Glassroth J. Mycobacterium avium complex and other nontuberculous mycobacteria in patients with HIV infection.Semin Respir Infect. 1989 Jun;4(2):123-32.

[231] Zhao GG, Li JY, Atlas E, Cleary JP. Cytomegalovirus pneumonitis as an initial presentation in an HIV-infected patient. Conn Med. 1999 Oct;63(10):585-8.

[232] Rodriguez-Barradas MC, Stool E, Musher DM, Gathe J Jr, Goldstein J, Genta RM, Yoffe B. Diagnosing and treating cytomegalovirus pneumonia in patients with AIDS Clin Infect Dis. 1996 Jul;23(1):76-81.

[233] Salomon N, Gomez T, Perlman DC, Laya L, Eber C, Mildvan D. Clinical features and outcomes of HIV-related cytomegalovirus pneumonia. AIDS. 1997 Mar;11(3):319-24.

[234] Dore GJ, Marriott DJ, Duflou JA. Clinico-pathological study of cytomegalovirus (CMV) in AIDS autopsies: under-recognition of CMV pneumonitis and CMV adrenalitis. Aust N Z J Med. 1995 Oct;25(5):503-6.

[235] d'Arminio Monforte A, Vago L, Lazzarin A, Boldorini R, Bini T, Guzzetti S, Antinori S, Moroni M, Costanzi G.. AIDS-defining diseases in 250 HIV-infected patients; a comparative study of clinical and autopsy diagnoses. AIDS. 1992 Oct;6(10):1159-64.

[236] Lyles RH, Chu C, Mellors JW, Margolick JB, Detels R, Giorgi JV, Al-Shboul Q, Phair JP. Prognostic value of plasma HIV RNA in the natural history of Pneumocystis carinii pneumonia, cytomegalovirus and Mycobacterium avium complex. Multicenter AIDS Cohort Study. AIDS. 1999 Feb 25;13(3):341-9.

[237] de la Hoz RE, Byrne SK, Hayashi S, Sherlock C, Cook D, Hogg JC. Diagnosis of cytomegalovirus infection in HIV-infected patients with respiratory disease. Clin Diagn Virol. 1998 May 1;10(1):1-7.

[238] Youle MS, Gazzard BG, Johnson MA, Cooper DA, Hoy JF, Busch H, Ruf B, Griffiths PD, Stephenson SL, Dancox M, et al. Effects of high-dose oral acyclovir on herpesvirus disease and survival in patients with advanced HIV disease: a double-blind, placebo-controlled study. European-Australian Acyclovir Study Group. AIDS. 1994 May;8(5):641-9.

[239] Umar SH, Kanth A. Disseminated cutaneous herpes simplex virus type-1 with interstitial pneumonia as a first presentation of AIDS. J Natl Med Assoc. 1999 Aug;91(8):471-4.

[240] Calore EE. Herpes simplex type 2 pneumonia. Braz J Infect Dis. 2002 Dec;6(6):305-8. Epub 2003 Nov 3.

[241] Fraisse P, Faller M, Rey D, Labouret N, Partisani M, Stoll-Keller F, Lang JM, Weitzenblum E. Recurrent varicella pneumonia complicating an endogenous reactivation of chickenpox in an HIV-infected adult patient. Eur Respir J. 1998 Mar;11(3):776-8..

[242] Resnick L, Pitchenik AE, Fisher E, Croney R. Detection of HTLV-III/LAV - Specific IgG and antigen in bronchoalveolar lavage fluid from two patients with Lympocytic interstitial pneumonitis associated AIDS related complex. AM J Med 1987 Mar; 82(3): 553-6

[243] Travis WD, Fox CG, Devaney KO et al. Lymphoid pneumonitis in 50 adult patients infected with the human immunodeficiency virus: lymphocytic interstitial pneumonitis versus non specific interstitial pneumonitis. Hum Pathol 1992; 23: 529-41

[244] Guillon JM, Autran B, Denis M, Fouret P, Plata F, Mayaud CM, Akoun GM. Human immunodeficiency virus-related lymphocytic alveolitis. Chest. 1988 Dec;94(6):1264-70.

[245] response Itescu S, Brancato LJ, Buxbaum J, Gregersen PK, Rizk CC, Croxson TS, Solomon GE, Winchester R. A diffuse infiltrative CD8 lymphocytosis syndrome in human immunodeficiency virus (HIV) infection: a host immune response associated with HLA-DR5. Ann Intern Med. 1990 Jan 1;112(1):3-10.

[246] Detection of HTLV-III/LAV-specific IgG and antigen in bronchoalveolar lavage fluid from two patients with lymphocytic interstitial pneumonitis associated with AIDS-related complex.

[247] Ingiliz P, Appenrodt B, Gruenhage F, Vogel M, Tschampa H, Tasci S, Rockstroh JK. Lymphoid pneumonitis as an immune reconstitution inflammatory syndrome in a patient with CD4 cell recovery after HAART initiation. HIV Med. 2006 Sep;7(6):411-4.

[248] Ripamonti D, Rizzi M, Maggiolo F, Arici C, Suter F. Resolution of lymphocytic interstitial pneumonia in a human immunodeficiency virus-infected adult following the start of highly active antiretroviral therapy. Scand J Infect Dis. 2003;35(5):348-51.

[249] Dufour V, Wislez M, Bergot E, Mayaud C, Cadranel J. Improvement of symptomatic human immunodeficiency virus-related lymphoid interstitial pneumonia in patients receiving highly active antiretroviral therapy. Case reports and series indicate good responses to treatment with HAART. Clin Infect Dis. 2003 May 15;36(10):e127-30. Epub 2003 May 6.

[250] Basu D, Williams FM, Ahn CW, Reveille JD. Changing spectrum of the diffuse infiltrative lymphocytosis syndrome. Arthritis Rheum. 2006 Jun 15;55(3):466-72.

[251] Sattler F, Nichols L, Hirano L, Hiti A, Hofman F, Hughlett C, Zeng L, Boylen CT, Koss M. Nonspecific interstitial pneumonitis mimicking Pneumocystis carinii pneumonia. Am J Respir Crit Care Med. 1997 Sep;156(3 Pt 1):912-7.

[252] Griffiths MH, Miller RF, Semple SJ. Interstitial pneumonitis in patients infected with the human immunodeficiency virus. Thorax. 1995 Nov;50(11):1141-6.

[253] Ognibene FP, Masur H, Rogers P, Travis WD, Suffredini AF, Feuerstein I, Gill VJ, Baird BF, Carrasquillo JA, Parrillo JE, et al. Nonspecific interstitial pneumonitis without evidence of Pneumocystis carinii in asymptomatic patients infected with human immunodeficiency virus (HIV). Ann Intern Med. 1988 Dec 1;109(11):874-9.

[254] Rodríguez-Rosado R, Soriano V, Dona C, González-Lahoz Opportunistic infections shortly after beginning highly active antiretroviral therapy. J.Antivir Ther. 1998;3(4):229-31.

[255] Mori S, Polatino S, Estrada-Y-Martin RM. Pneumocystis-associated organizing pneumonia as a manifestation of immune reconstitution inflammatory syndrome in an HIV-infected individual with a normal CD4+ T-cell count following antiretroviral therapy. Int J STD AIDS. 2009 Sep;20(9):662-5.

[256] Jagannathan P, Davis E, Jacobson M, Huang L Life-threatening immune reconstitution inflammatory syndrome after Pneumocystis pneumonia: a cautionary case series. AIDS. 2009 Aug 24;23(13):1794-6

[257] Jenny-Avital ER, Abadi M. mmune reconstitution cryptococcosis after initiation of successful highly active antiretroviral therapy. Clin Infect Dis. 2002 Dec 15;35(12):e128-33. Epub 2002 Nov 20.

[258] Janda S, Quon BS, Swiston J. HIV and pulmonary arterial hypertension: a systematic review.HIV Med. 2010 Nov;11(10):620-34. doi: 10.1111/j.1468-1293.2010.00829.x.

[259] Degano B, Guillaume M, Savale L, Montani D, Jaïs X, Yaici A, Le Pavec J, Humbert M, Simonneau G, Sitbon O. HIV-associated pulmonary arterial hypertension: survival and prognostic factors in the modern therapeutic era. AIDS. 2010 Jan 2;24(1):67-75.

[260] Polish LB, Cohn DL, Ryder JW, Myers AM, O'Brien RF. Pulmonary non-Hodgkin's lymphoma in AIDS. Chest. 1989 Dec;96(6):1321-6.

[261] Shiels MS, Cole SR, Mehta SH, Kirk GD. Lung cancer incidence and mortality among HIV-infected and HIV-uninfected injection drug users. J Acquir Immune Defic Syndr. 2010 Dec 1;55(4):510-5.

[262] Shebl FM, Engels EA, Goedert JJ, Chaturvedi AK. Pulmonary infections and risk of lung cancer among persons with AIDS. J Acquir Immune Defic Syndr. 2010 Nov 1;55(3):375-9.

[263] Nutankalva L, Wutoh AK, McNeil J, Frederick WR, Reddy RB, Daftary M, Gentles A, Addae-Afoakwa K. Malignancies in HIV: pre- and post-highly active antiretroviral therapy. J Natl Med Assoc. 2008 Jul;100(7):817-20.

[264] Levine AM, Seaberg EC, Hessol NA, Preston-Martin S, Silver S, Cohen MH, Anastos K, Minkoff H, Orenstein J, Dominguez G, Watts DH. HIV as a risk factor for lung cancer in women: data from the Women's Interagency HIV Study. J Clin Oncol. 2010 Mar 20;28(9):1514-9. Epub 2010 Feb 22.

[265] D'Jaen GA, Pantanowitz L, Bower M, Buskin S, Neil N, Greco EM, Cooley TP, Henry D, Stem J, Dezube BJ, Stebbing J, Aboulafia DM. Human immunodeficiency virus-associated primary lung cancer in the era of highly active antiretroviral therapy: a multi-institutional collaboration. Clin Lung Cancer. 2010 Nov 1;11(6):396-404.

[266] Tirelli U, Spina M, Sandri S, Serraino D, Gobitti C, Fasan M, Sinicco A, Garavelli P, Ridolfo AL, Vaccher E. Lung carcinoma in 36 patients with human immunodeficiency virus infection. The Italian Cooperative Group on AIDS and Tumors. Cancer. 2000 Feb 1;88(3):563-9.

[267] Gingo MR, George MP, Kessinger CJ, Lucht L, Rissler B, Weinman R, Slivka WA, McMahon DK, Wenzel SE, Sciurba FC, Morris A. Pulmonary function abnormalities in HIV-infected patients during the current antiretroviral therapy era. Am J Respir Crit Care Med. 2010 Sep 15;182(6):790-6. Epub 2010 Jun 3.

[268] Drummond MB, Kirk GD, Ricketts EP, McCormack MC, Hague JC, McDyer JF, Mehta SH, Engels EA, Wise RA, Merlo CA. Cross sectional analysis of respiratory symptoms in an injection drug user cohort: the impact of obstructive lung disease and HIV. BMC Pulm Med. 2010 May 11;10:27.

[269] Sanito NJ, Morley TF, Condoluci DV. Bronchiolitis obliterans organizing pneumonia in an AIDS patient.Eur Respir J. 1995 Jun;8(6):1021-4

[270] Tobin-D'Angelo MJ, Hoteit MA, Brown KV, Ray SM, King MD. Dapsone-induced hypersensitivity pneumonitis mimicking Pneumocystis carinii pneumonia in a patient with AIDS. Am J Med Sci. 2004 Mar;327(3):163-5.

[271] Behrens GM, Stoll M, Schmidt RE. Pulmonary hypersensitivity reaction induced by efavirenz. Lancet. 2001 May 12;357(9267):1503-4.

[272] Morris AM, Nishimura S, Huang L Subacute hypersensitivity pneumonitis in an HIV infected patient receiving antiretroviral therapy. Thorax. 2000 Jul;55(7):625-7.

[273] Naccache JM, Antoine M, Wislez M, Fleury-Feith J, Oksenhendler E, Mayaud C, Cadranel. Sarcoid-like pulmonary disorder in human immunodeficiency virus-infected patients receiving antiretroviral therapy.JAm J Respir Crit Care Med. 1999 Jun;159(6):2009-13.

[274] Lenner R, Bregman Z, Teirstein AS, DePalo L. Recurrent pulmonary sarcoidosis in HIV-infected patients receiving highly active antiretroviral therapy.Chest. 2001 Mar;119(3):978-81.

[275] Nan DN, Fernández-Ayala M, Iglesias L, García-Palomo D, Parra JA, Fariñas MC. Talc granulomatosis. A differential diagnosis of interstitial lung disease in HIV patients. Chest. 2000 Jul;118(1):258-60.

7

# Acute Abdomen and HIV Infection

Christophoros Kosmidis, Georgios Anthimidis and Kalliopi Vasiliadou
*Interbalkan European Medical Center, Department of Surgery, Thessaloniki*
*Greece*

## 1. Introduction

Abdominal pain in the HIV-infected patient is a common complaint which constitutes a complicated diagnostic and therapeutic problem. Even though the need for surgical intervention in the HIV/AIDS patient with abdominal complaints is low, the general surgeon will often be called upon to evaluate HIV-infected patients, as a result of the complexity in the interpretation of clinical findings. Once consulted, the surgeon's dilemma is in distinguishing conditions which do not require surgery from surgically treatable pathology and, above all, the true surgical emergencies.

Emergent abdominal operation by itself predisposes the AIDS patient to an increased mortality risk [1,2,3,4]. On the other hand, delayed diagnosis and late surgical exploration result in increased morbidity and mortality [5]. Although profound immunodeficiency is associated with poor prognosis, asymptomatic HIV-infected patients recover well from surgery and do not appear to suffer delayed healing [6,7]. Yet, with new antiviral therapy the operative mortality has dropped as much as necessary for emergency abdominal surgery and the risk-benefit analysis is now more in favour of laparotomy [5,8,9].

## 2. Clinical assessment

A careful medical history is the key component in the evaluation of the HIV/AIDS patient's symptoms. Attention should be directed towards identifying diarrhea, prior opportunistic infections or neoplasms.

Most patients nowadays are aware of their HIV status. However, undiagnosed HIV-related illness may be identified during evaluation of an acute abdomen [1]. A history of risk factors, including intravenous drug abuse and male homosexual practices may alert the physician for an increased possibility of HIV infection; still, the infection rate is elevated in heterosexual patients as well. Hepatitis B (HBV) and C (HCV) viruses are common coinfections [10].

A complete history of medications may lead to possible diagnosis, given that certain antiviral drugs are recognized as causes of pancreatitis (didanosine) and kidney stones (indivar) [11,12]. Patients well informed of their HIV status can relate CD4 counts, which help in the determination of the grade of immunosuppression. This is vital in estimating risks and benefits of surgery in addition to the possibility of opportunistic infections, which may not present until CD4 counts are less than 200 cells/mm$^3$ [13]. In general, CD4 counts are currently recognized as the main prognostic indicator of outcome in HIV patients.

Repeated physical examination is invaluable for the assessment of the pathologic process. Signs of peritoneal inflammation may well be delayed or absent even in the face of a surgical emergency.

Additionally, more than one disease may be present in the immunocompromised patient [14].

Physical examination may as well reveal the occurrence of organomegaly and lymphadenopathy, oral candidiasis, generalized lymphadenopathy, and Kaposi skin lesions, evidence associated with the stage of disease and degree of immunosuppression.

Full blood count and differential white cell count are rather unreliable, particularly in advanced HIV disease, since relative leukopaenia is usually noticed [15,16]. CD4 counts and viral loads could also be helpful since rates of morbidity and mortality are directly related to the CD4 count [13,17]. Yet, getting these results soon enough to help in establishing a management strategy is usually difficult. Thus a general rule may be remembered: The number of CD4 cells is roughly 10% of the lymphocyte count [18,19].

Laboratory investigations should be methodical and incorporate besides full blood count, serum urea and electrolytes, amylase, liver function tests, urinalysis and radiography of the abdomen as well as the chest. Plain radiographs of the abdomen may reveal extraluminal gas, indicating perforated bowel, or dilated loops of bowel, related to bowel obstruction. However, the diagnostic yield of plain abdominal radiographs remains low. Thus, abdominal computed tomography (CT) scan is used almost routinely [20]. Pneumatosis intestinalis, readily identified on CT scan, suggests bowel necrosis and impending perforation[21]. Intraperitoneal fluid collections characteristic of opportunistic infections may also be recognized only on CT scan. Fluid collections can be aspirated with ultrasound or CT scan guidance for microbiologic testing. If infected, they may be resolved with the aid of image-guided percutaneous drainage. Ultrasound is mainly useful for examination of suspected calculous disease, such as cholecystitis, cholangitis, pancreatitis, and nephrolithiasis.

## 3. Differential diagnosis

Before setting up a definite management plan, it should be reminded that *non-specific abdominal pain and fever are frequent among patients with AIDS who do not suffer from a surgical illness* [14,22]. The surgeon must consider that the possible causes of abdominal pain include a variety of conditions, some of which are frequent amongst the immunocompetent population, while others are directly HIV related (Tables 1,2,3, and 4), before a decision is made that the acute abdomen in the HIV patient is actually a "surgical abdomen".

| Appendicitis |
|---|
| Peptic ulcer disease |
| Diverticulitis |
| Cholecystitis |
| Hepatitis |
| Alcohol-related |
| Ischemic bowel |
| Abdominal aortic aneurysm |

Table 1. Non–HIV-related causes of abdominal pain.

| Opportunistic gastrointestinal (GI) infections<br>a) (Mycobacterium avium complex [MAC]<br>b) cytomegalovirus [CMV]<br>c) microsporidia |
|---|
| Cholecystitis (CMV) |
| Abscesses |
| Sexually transmitted disease-related |
| Proctitis |

Table 2. HIV-related causes of abdominal pain.

| Lymphomas (GI) |
|---|
| Kaposi's sarcoma (KS) |
| Cancer-related obstructions |
| Other cancers/metastatic disease |

Table 3. Immunosurveillance-related.

| Perforations secondary to procedures (upper/lower GI tract) |
|---|
| GI upset/GI reflux/gastritis |
| Kidney stones – indinavir |
| Pancreatitis |

Table 4. Medication-related/iatrogenic.

Finally there are non-specific causes of abdominal pain, i.e. no specific diagnosis is reached and the symptoms finally resolve [1,21,23].

Differentiating surgically treatable conditions from atypical HIV-related diseases, a number of which do not require surgery, may prove rather difficult. In fact, HIV-AIDS patients undergo emergency abdominal procedures more often than the age-matched non-AIDS population, since they present the anticipated rates of operation for commonly observed indications, e.g. appendicitis but also have additional indications specific for AIDS [24,25].

## 4. Therapy

When a decision is made that the abdominal symptoms require emergency surgery, appropriate resuscitation is initiated, such as fluid replacement, antibiotic administration, nasogastric decompression, transfusion of blood products, and (if not already started) consultation for antiviral therapy.

*Early* surgery should allow for rapid recovery, similar to immunocompetent surgical patients [1,26,27]. Even patients with restricted lifespan may find some profit in palliative surgery, which may offer relief from severe problems and improve the quality of life considerably.

The current experience with abdominal surgery points out that patients with HIV infection tolerate surgical procedures well and do not have an extremely high frequency of postoperative complications.

### 4.1 Most common indications for surgery

#### 4.1.1 Acute appendicitis

Acute appendicitis in the AIDS patient may occur due to the conventional obstruction of the appendiceal orifice by a fecalith, a lymphoid hyperplasia, Kaposi's sarcoma lesions, acute CMV infection, and mycobacterial infection [5,28,29,30,31,32]. Reports of cases among AIDS patients reveal accumulated cases of appendicitis in aged patients, which indicates that it is caused by complications of AIDS-related conditions [14]. The clinical presentation is with characteristic right lower quandrant pain, frequently associated with a low to normal white blood cell count [33]. Most patients have fever, but *non-specific abdominal pain and fever are frequent among patients with AIDS who do not suffer from a surgical illness.*

Patients with AIDS may have an opportunistic infection mimicking acute appendicitis. In that case, an operation may be carried out, leading to increased morbidity postoperatively [17,33]. For instance, typhlitis may well mimic appendicitis [34]. This infection originates from normal gut flora, possibly as a result of immunosuppression or cytotoxic drugs during chemotherapy. Medical management with broad-spectrum intravenous antibiotics is the treatment of choice [34]. Consequently, CT scan or even laparoscopy should be considered before surgical intervention [14,17].

Nevertheless, there seems to be an increased rate of perforation, gangrenous appendicitis, and early appendiceal abscess among patients with AIDS [14]. This observation may be the result of delay in patient presentation, as well as delay by the physician owing to a normal or low white blood cell count, which is in fact elevated over the chronically low white blood cell count, or to the erroneous assumption that the cause of the abdominal pain is not surgical [35].

#### 4.1.2 Bowel perforation

The previously high incidence of perforation of the gastrointestinal tract resulting from CMV infections and Kaposi sarcoma has been reduced with new retroviral drug therapy [1,2,36]. Currently, perforations are usually the result of lymphomas or disseminated mycobacterial disease [25,37]. Still, in case of acute bowel perforation, a high suspicion for underlying opportunistic infections is necessary [38]. Biopsies of the perforation site are required in order to ascertain the cause [39].

Management of the perforation site includes suture plication of gastroduodenal perforations, resection and anastomosis of small-bowel perforations, and colostomy for colonic perforations. Cytomegalovirus infection involves the arterioles of long segments of bowel; thus, perforations are ischemic lesions [38]. Consequently, healing of bowel anastomoses may be hindered, and performing a diverting stoma must be considered in selected patients. Antiviral chemotherapy should be initiated if not already established.

Acute bowel perforation in general carries a grave prognosis because it indicates advanced HIV disease [4,5,14].

#### 4.1.3 Gastrointestinal *obstruction*

Gastric outlet obstruction will take place due to lymphoma, small bowel obstruction secondary to mycobacterial disease, intussusception owing to Kaposi's sarcoma, and an

Ogilvie-like syndrome progressing to toxic megacolon as a result of CMV infection. Differential diagnosis must include more usual causes of obstruction. Yet, in the typical young patients with AIDS, especially when there is not a history of prior abdominal operation and the risk of obstruction caused by adhesions is eliminated, most cases will be related to AIDS.

Bowel obstruction and intussusception owing to Kaposi's sarcoma, lymphoma, and opportunistic infections may possibly be the result of multifocal disease or widespread dissemination. Thus, the prognosis is unfortunate[40,41,42]. Surgery will offer no more than palliation of the acute problem with slight advantage in prognosis [4,8,14,42]. Small-bowel resection can be carried out with primary anastomoses, whereas large bowel resection may call for fecal diversion [38].

### 4.1.4 Toxic megacolon

Toxic megacolon may be the result of CMV opportunistic infections, as already mentioned, or Clostridium difficile colitis. Clostridium difficile infection is predisposed by use of antibiotics and numerous hospitalizations or chemotherapeutic agents [43]. Megacolon is a sign of advanced disease and unfortunate prognosis because of the possibility of peritonitis [1,44]. Medical management including colonoscopic decompression of the dilated colon appears to have a favourable short-term outcome [44]. Nevertheless, emergent colectomies performed early, when peritoneal contamination is not extensive, may be successful in carefully selected patients who are able to sustain bowel resection [5].

### 4.1.5 Cholecystitis

Although occurrence of gallstone cholecystitis is the same in HIV patients and the general population, acute acalculous cholecystitis arises more often in HIV/AIDS patients [45]. Cholecystectomy is usually warranted. The outcome is favourable even in immunosuppressed patients and the mean survival period is more than 2 years [46].

### 4.1.6 Splenomegaly

Emergent splenectomy is usually necessary in the HIV-AIDS population on account of spontaneous rupture of an enlarged spleen (splenomegaly is common in patients with AIDS), traumatic rupture, or hemorrhagic rupture from splenic abscess [37,47,48].

## 5. Occupational risk of infection

A main surgical concern has been the possibility of accidental exposure and infection occupationally acquired while providing care for HIV-infected patients. Knowledge about the risk of transmission has reduced hesitation but should not decrease carefulness in the operating room.

The risk of occupational transmission of HIV disease is low, but not zero. Blood or bloody body fluids are the source of infection. The risk of HIV infection after percutaneous exposure is 0.3% [49,50]. Major percutaneous needle-stick injury with a hollow-bore needle is the major cause of occupational HIV infection. The possibility of transmission depends on the volume of the inoculum, the quantity of virus, the depth of penetration, and the type of needle; a hollow-bore needle, a device evidently contaminated with blood, a needle placed directly in a vein or artery, or a deep injury is associated with a higher risk than that of suture, solid needle [51].

The risk of transmission is higher if the patient suffers from terminal disease. Minor viral load is a sign of a lower titer exposure, but it does not eliminate the risk of transmission completely [51]. Although transmission by mucocutaneous exposure has been reported, it seems to be too low to calculate accurately (approximately 0.09%) [49,50]. Transmission after nonintact skin exposure has been documented. This risk is estimated to be less than the risk after mucous membrane exposure [52,53].

The risk after exposure to fluids or tissues other than blood has not been calculated but is most likely significantly lower than after blood exposure [54].

Transmission by usual contact or aerosols has not been documented.

Consequently, surgeons should feel secure in providing care for HIV-infected patients but all surgical team members must routinely practice standardized techniques to avoid blood-borne viral infection.

## 6. Role of laparoscopic surgery

Emergency laparoscopy for acute abdomen in patients infected with HIV has not been advocated widely. It appears that the rate of conversion to laparotomy is high (40%-60%) (55,56). Nenertheless a laparoscopic approach, when feasible, may be applicated as an initial step in the diagnosis and treatment of AIDS patients with acute abdominal complaints.

## 7. Conclusion

Acute abdomen in the HIV-AIDS patients involves abnormal presentation of common diseases as well as problems unique to this population, which are results of the immunosuppression. There is an increased probability of emergent abdominal operations in addition to a considerable possibility of non-surgical causes of abdominal pain, demanding a judicious differentiating assessment. Operative results are now favourable, reaching mortality and morbidity rates similar to patients without HIV infection. Care of these patients is best provided by surgeons with experience and interest in AIDS, together with infectious diseases physicians.

## 8. References

[1] Wilson SE, Robinson G, Williams RA, et al. Acquired immune deficiency syndrome (AIDS). Indications for abdominal surgery, pathology and outcome. *Ann Surg.* 1989;210:428-433.

[2] Robinson G, Wilson SE, Williams RA. Surgery in patients with acquired immunodeficiency syndrome. *Arch Surg.* 1987;122:170-175.

[3] Nuggent P, O"Connell T. The surgeon's role in treating acquired immunodeficiency syndrome. *Arch Surg.* 1986;121:1117-1120.

[4] Wexner SD, Smithy WB, Trillo C, Hopkins BS, Dailey TH. Emergency colectomy for cytomegalovirus ileocolitis in patients with the acquired immune deficiency syndrome. *Dis Colon Rectum.* 1988;31:755-761.

[5] Davidson T, Allen-Mersh TG, Miles AJ, et al. Emergency laparotomy in patients with AIDS. *Br J Surg.* 1991;78(8):924-6.
[6] Ming K Y, Saunder A, Scott D F. Abdominal surgery in HIV/AIDS patients: Indications, operative management, pathology and outcome. Aust N Z J Surg 1995; 65:320-6.;78:924-926.
[7] Buehrer J L, Weber D J, Meyer A A. Wound infection rates after invasive procedures in HIV-1 seropositive versus HIV-1 seronegative hemophiliacs. Ann Surg 1990; 211:492-8.
[8] Yii MK, Saunder A, Scott DF. Abdominal surgery in HIV/AIDS patients: indications, operative management, pathology and outcome. *Aust N Z J Surg.* 1995;65:320-326.
[9] Tran HS, Moncure M, Tarnoff M, et al. Predictors of operative outcome in patients with human immunodeficiency virus infection and acquired immunodeficiency syndrome. *Am J Surg.* 2000;180:228-233.
[10] Poles MA, Dieterich DT. HIV and Hepatitis Virus Infection. *Curr Infect Dis Rep.* 2000;2:177-184.
[11] Dassopoulos T, Ehrenpreis ED. Acute pancreatitis in human immunodeficiency virus-infected patients: a review. *Am J Med.* 1999;107:78-84.
[12] Kohan AD, Armenakas NA, Fracchia JA. Indinavir urolithiasis: an emerging cause of renal colic in patients with human immunodeficiency virus. *J Urol.* 1999;161:1765-1768.
[13] Albaran RG, Webber J, Steffes CP. CD4 cell counts as a prognostic factor of major abdominal surgery in patients infected with the human immunodeficiency virus. *Arch Surg.* 1998;133:626-631.
[14] Whitney TM, Macho JR, Russell TR, Bossart KJ, Heer FW, Schecter WP. Appendicitis in acquired immunodeficiency syndrome. *Am J Surg.* 1992;164:467-471.
[15] LaRaja R D, Rothenberg R E, Odom J W, Mueller S C. The incidence of intraabdominal surgery in acquired immunodeficiency syndrome: a statistical review of 904 patients. Surgery 1989; 105:175-9.
[16] Lowy A M, Barie P S. Laparotomy in patients infected with human immunodeficiency virus: indications and outcome. Br J Surg 1994; 81:942-5.
[17] Savioz D, Chilcott M, Ludwig C, et al. Preoperative counts of CD4 T-lymphocytes and early postoperative infective complications in HIV-positive patients. *Eur J Surg.* 1998;164:483-487.
[18] Blatt SP, Lucey CR, Butzin CA, Hendrix CW, Lucey DR. Total lymphocyte count as a predictor of absolute CD4+ count and CD4+ percentage in HIV-infected persons. *JAMA.* 1993;269:622-626.
[19] Shapiro NI, Karras DJ, Leech SH, Heilpern KL. Absolute lymphocyte count as a predictor of CD4 count. *Ann Emerg Med.* 1998;32:323-328.
[20] Ahn SH, Mayo-Smith WW, Murphy BL, Reinert SE, Cronan JJ. Acute nontraumatic abdominal pain in adult patients: abdominal radiography compared with CT evaluation. *Radiology.* 2002;225:159-164.

[21] Wiesner W, Mortele KJ, Glickman JN, Ji H, Ros PR. Pneumatosis intestinalis and portomesenteric venous gas in intestinal ischemia: correlation of CT findings with severity of ischemia and clinical outcome. *AJR Am J Roentgenol.* 2001;177:1319-1323.

[22] Darin J. Saltzman, Russell A. Williams, Dmitri V. Gelfand Samuel E. Wilson. The Surgeon and AIDS Twenty Years Later. *Arch Surg.* 2005;140:961-967.

[23] Slaven EM, Lopez F, Weintraub SL, Mena JC, Mallon WK. The AIDS patient with abdominal pain: a new challenge for the emergency physician. *Emerg Med Clin North Am.* 2003;21:987-1015.

[24] Ferguson CM. Surgical complication of human immunodeficiency virus infection. Am Surg 1988;54:4-9.

[25] Yoshida D, Caruso JM. Abdominal pain in the HIV infected patient. *J Emerg Med.* 2002;23:111-116.

[26] Diettrich N A, Cacioppo J C, Kaplan G, Cohen S M. A growing spectrum of surgical disease in patients with human immunodeficiency virus/acquired immunodeficiency syndrome: Experience with 120 major cases. Arch Surg 1991; 126:860-6.

[27] Hammund R, Achrafi H, Megegaux F, Caumes E. Abdominal surgical emergencies in human immunodeficiency virus (HIV) infected patients. Apropos of 34 cases. Ann Chir 1995; 49:922-7.

[28] Fry DE. Surgical problems in the immunosuppressed patient. In: Townsend CM, Beauchamp RD, Evers BM, Mattox KL, eds. *Sabiston Textbook of Surgery: The Biological Basis of Modern Surgical Practice.* 17th ed. Philadelphia, Pa: Elsevier Saunders; 2004:285-286.

[29] Blackman E, Vimadalal S, Nash G. Significance of gastrointestinal cytomegalovirus infection in homosexual males. *Am J Gastroenterol.* 1984;79:935-940.

[30] Visvanathan K, Jones PD, Truskett P. Abdominal mycobacterial infection mimicking acute appendicitis in an AIDS patient. *Aust N Z J Surg.* 1993;63:558-560.

[31] Dezfuli M, Oo MM, Jones BE, Barnes PF. Tuberculosis mimicking acute appendicitis in patients with human immunodeficiency virus infection. *Clin Infect Dis.* 1994;18:650-651.

[32] Baker MS, Wille M, Goldman H, Kim HK. Metastatic Kaposi's sarcoma presenting as acute appendicitis. *Mil Med.* 1986;151:45-47.

[33] Binderow SR, Shaked AA. Acute appendicitis in patients with AIDS/HIV infection. *Am J Surg.* 1991;162:9-12.

[34] Till M, Lee N, Soper WD, Murphy RL. Typhlitis in patients with HIV-1 infection. *Ann Intern Med.* 1992;116:998-1000.

[35] Bova R, Meagher A. Appendicitis in HIV-positive patients. *Aust N Z J Surg.* 1998;68:337-339.

[36] Burke G, Nichols L, Balogh K, et al. Perforation of the terminal ileum with cytomegalovirus vasculitis and Kaposi's sarcoma in a patient with acquired immunodeficiency syndrome. *Surgery.* 1987;102:540-545.

[37] Chambers AJ, Lord RS. Incidence of acquired immune deficiency syndrome (AIDS)-related disorders at laparotomy in patients with AIDS. *Br J Surg.* 2001;88:294-297.

[38] Williams RA, Wilson SE. Surgery in HIV-infected patients. In: R H, ed. *Infectious risks in surgery*. New York: Appleton and Lange; 1991:83-96.
[39] Culpepper-Morgan JA, Kotler DP, Scholes JV, Tierney AR. Evaluation of diagnostic criteria for mucosal cytomegalic inclusion disease in the acquired immune deficiency syndrome. *Am J Gastroenterol.* 1987;82:1264-1270.
[40] Horsburgh CR Jr. Mycobacterium avium complex infection in the acquired immunodeficiency syndrome. *N Engl J Med.* 1991;324:1332-1338.
[41] Levine AM. Lymphoma in acquired immunodeficiency syndrome. *Semin Oncol.* 1990;17:104-112.
[42] Cappell MS, Botros N. Predominantly gastrointestinal symptoms and signs in 11 consecutive AIDS patients with gastrointestinal lymphoma: a multicenter, multiyear study including 763 HIV-seropositive patients. *Am J Gastroenterol.* 1994;89:545-549.
[43] Monkemuller KE, Wilcox CM. Diagnosis and treatment of colonic disease in AIDS. *Gastrointest Endosc Clin N Am.* 1998;8:889-911.
[44] Beaugerie L, Ngo Y, Goujard F, et al. Etiology and management of toxic megacolon in patients with human immunodeficiency virus infection. *Gastroenterology.* 1994;107:858-863.
[45] French AL, Beaudet LM, Benator DA, Levy CS, Kass M, Orenstein JM. Cholecystectomy in patients with AIDS: clinicopathologic correlations in 107 cases. *Clin Infect Dis.* 1995;21:852-858.
[46] Flum DR, Wallack MK. Cholecystectomy and AIDS. *J Am Coll Surg.* 1997;184:669-760.
[47] O'Reilly RA. Splenomegaly in 2,505 patients at a large university medical center from 1913 to 1995. 1963 to 1995: 449 patients. *West J Med.* 1998;169:88-97.
[48] Aboolian A, Ricci M, Shapiro K, Connors A, LaRaja RD. Surgical treatment of HIV-related immune thrombocytopenia. *Int Surg.* 1999;84:81-85.
[49] Bell DM. Occupational risk of human immunodeficiency virus infection in healthcare workers: an overview. *Am J Med.* 1997;102:9-15.
[50] Ippolito G, Puro V, De Carli G. The risk of occupational human immunodeficiency virus infection in health care workers: The Italian Study Group on Occupational Risk of HIV infection. *Arch Intern Med.* 1993;153:1451-1458.
[51] Cardo DM, Culver DH, Ciesielski CA, et al. A case-control study of HIV seroconversion in health care workers after percutaneous exposure: Centers for Disease Control and Prevention Needlestick Surveillance Group. *N Engl J Med.* 1997;337:1485-1490.
[52] Centers for Disease Control. human immunodeficiency virus infections in health-care workers exposed to blood of infected patients. *MMWR Morb Mortal Wkly Rep.* 1987;36:285-289.
[53] Fahey BJ, Koziol DE, Banks SM, Henderson DK. Frequency of nonparenteral occupational exposures to blood and body fluids before and after universal precautions training. *Am J Med.* 1991;90:145-153.

[54] Henderson DK, Fahey BJ, Willy M, et al. Risk for occupational transmission of human immunodeficiency virus type 1 (HIV-1) associated with clinical exposures: a prospective evaluation. *Ann Intern Med.* 1990;113:740-746.

# 8

# Metabolic Alterations of HIV Infection

E.F. Silva
*Federal University of São Paulo – São Paulo, Brazil*

## 1. Introduction

Changes in lipid profile, like increased serum triglycerides (TG) and decreased cholesterol levels have been described in patients with HIV infection before the introduction of highly active antiretroviral therapy (HAART) (Constans et al., 1994; Grunfeld et al., 1991; Shor-Posner et al., 1993). However, with the widespread use of HAART it has been worsening. After the introduction of protease inhibitors (PIs) in 1996, patients developed a syndrome of fat redistribution with peripheral loss and central gain, generally associated with metabolic abnormalities and insulin resistance (lipodistrophy syndrome) (Carr et al., 1998). High levels of TG and total cholesterol (TC) concentrations are well known and often associated with abnormal body fat distribution and glucose metabolism disturbs (Carr et al., 1998). On persons treated with HAART, TG and TC elevations are associated with the use of protease inhibitors/nonnucleoside reverse transcriptase inhibitor (PIs/NNRTI) regimens (54 and 44% respectively), followed by PIs regimes (40 and 27% respectively) and NNRTI-containing combinations (32 and 23% respectively) (Friss Moller et al., 2003). All these symptoms are related to metabolic syndrome that could act to increase the cardiovascular risk in HIV-infected patients. Another aspect of these metabolic alterations is non-alcoholic fatty liver disease. Its prevalence is higher in HIV infected patients (30-40%) than in general population (14-31%) (Crum-Cianflone et al., 2009; Guaraldi et al., 2008). It is believed that there is a potential role of the antiretroviral therapy in the pathology of non-alcoholic fatty liver disease due to its negative effects on glucose control, lipid metabolism, body fat redistribution, insulin resistance and mitochondrial toxicity (Crum-Cianflone et al., 2009; Guaraldi et al., 2008).
HAART has change dramatically the natural history of HIV-infection, leading to a notable extension of life expectancy and decline in mortality (Palella et al., 1998). Thus, mortality rates in HIV-infected patients who have experienced a CD4 recovery (> 500 cells/mm$^3$) on long-term treatment resemble that of the general population (Lewden et al., 2007). However, prolonged metabolic imbalances could act on the long-term prognosis and outcome of HIV-infected persons. There is an increasing concern about the cardiovascular risk in this population despite the virological control (Graham, et al., 2000; Manfredi et al., 2000; Palella et al., 1998). Cardiovascular disease is emerging as one of the most important co morbidity and cause of death (Sackoff et al., 2006). Early identification and proper management of traditional cardiovascular risk factors, such as smoking, overweight or hypertension is imperative (Barbaro, 2006; Triant et al., 2007). As the prevalence of metabolic disorders is age-related their incidence will increase as HIV population becomes older (Triant et L., 2007). Thus, active prevention, together with prompt diagnosis and management of cardiovascular risk factors must be integrated on the routine of HIV care.

## 2. Dyslipidemia and antiretroviral therapy

The degree of dyslipidemia and lipid changes is different among the several classes of antiretroviral drugs and even among the individual drugs within each class. Furthermore, the magnitude of lipid changes varies widely among patients on the same antiretroviral regimen, reflecting the likely important role of host genomics. While the PI and NNRTI have well-described effects on lipids, there have been no reported significant changes in lipid profiles or cardiovascular risk associated with the new classes of antiretroviral such as, fusion inhibitors (enfuvirtide), CC chemokine receptor type 5 (CCR5) receptor inhibitors (maraviroc) or integrase inhibitors (raltegravir) as described in table 1. Nonnucleoside reverse transcriptase inhibitors are also associated with lipid abnormalities, but to a lesser extent than PIs. Nucleoside reverse transcriptase inhibitors have been associated with mitochondrial toxicity and insulin resistance, but the lipid changes associated with them are normally less significant than those caused by PI or NNRTIs (Malvestutto & Aberg, 2010, Hammond et al., 2004).

| **PI** | **Lipid Change** |
|---|---|
| Atazanavir | No change |
| Atazanavir/ritonavir | ↑ LDL-c. TG and no change HDL-c |
| Darunavir/ritonavir | ↑ TC, LDL-c, TG and no change HDL-c |
| Fosamprenavir/ritonavir | ↑ TC, LDL-c, TG and no change HDL-c |
| Indinavir | ↑ TC, LDL-c, TG and |
| Lopinavir/ritonavir | ↑ TC, LDL-c, TG and no change HDL-c |
| Nelfinavir | ↑ TC, LDL-c, TG and no change HDL-c |
| Ritonavir | ↑ TC, LDL-c, TG and ↓ HDL |
| Saquinavir/ritonavir | ↑ TC, LDL-c, TG and no change HDL-c |
| Tipranavir/ritonavir | ↑ TC, LDL-c, TG and not known in HDL-c |
| **ITRN** | |
| Stavudine | ↑ TG |
| **ITRNN** | |
| Efavirenz | ↑ TC, LDL-c, TG and HDL-c |
| Nevirapine | ↑ TC, LDL-c, TG and HDL-c |
| Etravirine | No change |
| **Integrase Inhibitor** | |
| Raltegravir | No change |
| **Fusion Inhibitor** | |
| Enfuvirtude | No change |
| **CC Chemokine receptor** | |
| Maraviroc | No change |

Table 1. Lipid changes with antiretroviral therapy.

## 3. Cardiovascular risk evaluation

Primary prevention must be indicated and periodic assessment could be done every 3-6 months in HIV-infected person on treatment and annually in patients not treated (Blanco et al., 2010). Factors to be evaluated include: age, smoking habit, diet, physical activity, alcohol consumption, personal and family history of coronary heart disease, hyperlipidemia, diabetes mellitus and hypertension (Adult Treatment Panel III, 2002). In women, the menopausal status is relevant. Baseline blood pressure, body mass index and waist circumference should be recorded together with lipid profile, glucose and renal function (Blanco et al., 2010). In addition, virologic control with HAART use may also decrease the risk of noninfectious co morbidities including cardiovascular disease.

To predict the cardiovascular risk, Framingham Risk Score could be use (Anderson et al., 1991). Using this score, which includes: age, gender, TC, HDL-c, systolic blood pressure and smoking, an individual could be stratified into three risk categories: low (<10%), medium (10-20%) and high risk (> 20%) in 10 year. The extent to which this model could be used from the general population to HIV-infected people is still under discussion. The Framingham Risk Score has not been specifically validated for HIV-infected subjects and factors related to the HIV/AIDS could not be adequately evaluated, but until more evidence is available, management strategies for cardiovascular risk proposed for the general population could be applied to HIV-infected subjects. In the D:A:D study (Data Collection on Adverse events of Anti-HIV Drugs), myocardial infarction rates seen in HIV-infected person treated and untreated were higher and lower respectively, than those predicted with Framingham Risk Score. Nevertheless, it predicted cardiovascular events at increased rates in parallel with time exposure to antiretroviral treatment (Friss-Moller et al., 2003). According to these findings, Framingham Risk Score may be useful for an initial estimation of cardiovascular risk in HIV-infected persons, although a more accurate model needs to be developed.

To contribute with the discussion about HIV and cardiovascular risk, it was recently showed by the Kaiser Permanent Members that HIV infection confers a high independent risk for coronary heart disease (Klein et al., 2011). They matched HIV-infected adults of Kaiser Permanent California health plan with HIV negative members (1:10 ratio) on age, sex, medical center and start year follow-up. The cohort was followed from first Kaiser Permanent enrollment in 1996 until the end of December 2008. Coronary heart disease rates among HIV-infected members stratified by antiretroviral use and the most recent and lowest CD4 cell counts recorded were compared with rates among HIV negative members- Adjusted rate ratios (RRs) for any CHD diagnosis and for MIs were obtained from Poisson regression models adjusting for age, sex, race, tobacco use, alcohol/drug abuse, obesity, diabetes, and use of lipid lowering and hypertension therapy. 20,775 HIV-infected and 215,158 HIV negative members contributed to 90,961 and 1,133,333 persons-years (py) respectively. HIV-infected and not infected individuals had respectively 399 (447/100,00 py) and 3,463 (311/100,00 py) coronary heart disease events and 248 and 1,825 myocardial infarction. In the HIV-infected group, the only significant HIV-related factor associated with an increased risk of coronary heart disease was the lowest CD4 ≤ 200 cells/mm$^3$ recorded (relative risk = 1.3 [95% CI: 10.-1.6, p = 0,022) (Klein et al., 2011). HIV-infected patients on antiretroviral therapy and with CD4 count > 500 cells/mm$^3$ (recent or lowest) had similar coronary heart disease risk compared with HIV negative group. These findings support early initiation of antiretroviral therapy and aggressive management of cardiovascular disease risk.

Nowadays, the recommendations suggest that HIV-infected people undergo evaluation and treatment on the basis of the Third National Cholesterol Education Program (ATP III) for dyslipidemia (Adult Treatment Panel III, 2002). Lipoprotein profiles should be done with at least 9 to 12 hours of fasting (Adult Treatment Panel III, 2002). Dyslipidemia is defined as TC ≥ 200 mg/dL, LDL-c ≥ 130 mg/dL, TG ≥ 150 mg/dL, HDL-c < 40 mg/dL and TC/HDL ≥ 6.5. Therapeutic indications are made regarding the time for initiating specific lifestyle modifications and prescription of lipid-lowering therapy in order to achieve LDL-c goals (Adult Treatment Panel III, 2002). As for the general population, distinct drugs are suggested regarding the lipid alterations: hypercholesterolemia and/or hypertriglyceridemia. An update from ATP III (Grundy et al., 2004) included diabetes in high risk category for cardiovascular risk, and there is an additional benefit adding LDL-lowering therapy in this population.

## 4. Lifestyle interventions

Counseling on healthy diet habits, regular exercise, alcohol consumption and quitting smoking should be the first step to decrease cardiovascular risk. Hyperglycemia due to diabetes mellitus must be managed aggressively, with consideration of treatment with insulin sensitizers, such as metformin and thiazolidenediones when appropriate (Kalra et al., 2011).

Smoking is one well-know modifiable risk factor for coronary heart disease and its cessation leads to a decrease in cardiovascular and malignances risk (Mohiuddin et al., 2007). The smoking prevalence in HIV-infected patients is generally high, around 45-70%, much more than observed in uninfected controls (Friss-Moller et al., 2003; Mamary et al., 2002; Saves et al., 2003). Smoking cessation should be a priority in managing cardiovascular risk in HIV-infected persons.

The prevalence of hypertension in HIV-infected patients is around 25% (Glass et al., 2006; Jung et al., 2004,). The current recommendations for general population should be followed for HIV-infected patients, considering drug-interactions between antiretroviral drugs and antihypertensive drugs, particularly calcium-channel blockers. The management of hypertension should include lifestyle modifications such as weight loss if needed, incorporating low total and saturated fat in the diet, reduction of dietary sodium to 2.5 g/day, aerobic exercise and decreasing alcohol consumption (Malvestutto & Aberg, 2010).

Diet and exercise could help improve dyslipidemia, high blood pressure and glucose metabolism (Barrios et al., 2002; Fitch et al., 2006). Comprehensive dietary interventions have been demonstrated to decrease LDL-c by 20% in short term interventions in which adherence is maximal (Jenkins et al., 2003; Skeaff et al., 2005). The majority of the cholesterol lowering effect may be achieved by substituting unsaturated fats for saturated fats and increasing intake of plant sterols to at least 1.5 g/day. Each strategy could decrease the levels of LDL-c around 10% (Clifton et al., 2009). Further cholesterol lowering is also possible through weight loss and increasing intake of soluble fiber and soy protein (Clifton et al., 2009). Replacing saturated and *trans* fats with unsaturated fats is therefore a key strategy for lowering serum LDL-c (Clifton et al., 2009). Weight loss in those who are overweight lowers serum TC, LDL-c and TG and increases HDL-c (Datillo & Kris-Etherton,

1992). Weight reduction should be strongly encouraged if obesity is present. There are several dietary components that may be protective against cardiovascular disease through known and unknown mechanisms and their consumption may be encouraged as part of a cholesterol lowering and cardiovascular protective diet such as fish oil, whole grains, fruit, vegetables and nuts. Low intake of alcohol may also be advised (Cheng et al., 2004; Clifton et al., 2009).

Clinicians should be alert for potential exacerbating conditions, such as hypothyroidism, renal and liver disease and hypogonadism. They should also consider the effects of glucocorticoids, beta-blockers, thiazide diuretics, thyroid preparations and hormonal agents (such as androgens, progestins, and estrogens) on both cholesterol and triglyceride levels (Dube et al., 2003).

## 5. Lipid lowering therapy for HIV-infected patients

The benefits of lipid-lowering therapy interventions have been extended to HIV-infected persons. Enthusiasm for drug therapy for dyslipidemia should be tempered with the understanding that interventions for advanced immunosuppression, opportunistic infections, malignancies, and HIV-associated wasting, should be done during the initial stages of treatment. There is currently no basis for a more aggressive dyslipidemia intervention among HIV-infected patients than what is currently recommended for the general population. Due to a significant possibility for drug interaction between some lipid-lowering agents and antiretroviral drugs, special attention should be given to the choice of lipid-lowering therapy (Dube et al., 2003). Some advises should be instituted before pharmacological interventions as explained in life style modification section, except when there is an urgent need to prompt treatment (individuals with high risk for cardiovascular disease or with previous coronary heart disease or diabetes mellitus) (Adult Treatment Panel III, 2002).

### 5.1 Statins

The 3-hydroxy-3-methylglutaryl coenzyme A (HMG-CoA) reductase enzyme catalyzes the first step of cholesterol synthesis in the mevalonate pathway. Statins lower LDL-c levels through the inhibition of this specific enzyme. The more potent statins have been shown to reduce LDL-c levels by up to 55%. In addition, they also decrease TG levels to a lesser extent (up to 20%), probably through the inhibition of its synthesis in the liver and increase of lipoprotein lipase enzyme activity in the adipocytes (Jones et al., 2003; Saiki et al., 2005). Furthermore, statins are known to modestly increase levels of HDL-c (up to 10%). The precise mechanism by which statins increase HDL-c levels is not known; however, it is thought to result from apolipoprotein A1 gene induction through the activation of peroxisome proliferator activated receptors (Yano et al., 2007). It is also postulated that statins have pleiotropic effects, (certain lipid-independent effects) that contribute to some degree to their antiatherothrombotic properties. Among the proposed mechanisms are modulation of inflammatory response, improvement of endothelial function and inhibition of coagulation factors (Ray & Cannon, 2005).

Lovastatin and simvastatin are highly metabolized through the cytrocrome P450 (CYP3A4), which is inhibited by most PIs. Thus, their concomitant use is contraindicated to avoid serious side effects of statins overexposure such as rhabdomyolysis. Pravastatin and fluvastatin appear to be safe for use in association with HAART (Dube et al., 2003). Pravastatin is eliminated mostly by glucoronidation, fluvastatin by CYP 2C9 isoform, and CYP 3A4 has no role in their metabolism (Willians & Feely, 2002). Table 2 has a summary of the lipid lowering therapy in HIV infected people.

Rosuvastatin and atorvastatin have higher efficacy than pravastatin in decreasing LDL-c. Due to partial metabolism of atorvastatin by CYP3A4, it must be used with caution when co administered with a PI, with hepatitis and myositis being potential toxicities. Rosuvastatin is the most potent statin to reduce LDL-c and TG, with serum levels being only slightly modified when co administered with a PI (Aslangui et al., 2010; Calza et al., 2008). It can also reduce TG and increase HDL-c. Moreover, pharmacokinetic studies have demonstrated that its metabolism is not dependent on the CYP 450 3A4 isoenzyme and its use could be considered in PI-treated individuals since the risk of drug-drug interactions are low (Martin et al., 2003). Only 10% of the administered dose is metabolized by CYP 2C9 isoenzyme into N-desmethyl rosuvastatin and its metabolite are 90% eliminated by the fecal route (Cheng, 2004; Martin et al., 2003; Willians & Feely, 2002). The usual recommended starting dose of rosuvastatin is 10 mg daily, but initiation at 5 mg daily may be considered for patients who have predisposing factors for myopathy or are taking cysclosporine. In subjects with severe renal impairment or taking fibrates, therapy with rosuvastatin should be used with great caution, daily dose should be initiated at 5 mg and not exceed 10 mg (Cheng, 2004).

Until recently, pravastin and rosuvastatin were thought to be safer than other statins because their metabolism do not utilize the CYP450 3A4 enzyme system influenced by many antiretroviral medications. However, recent studies have demonstrated increased plasma levels (expressed as area under the plasma concentration-time curve [AUC] and maximum concentration [Cmax] values) of these statins as a result of exposure to certain antiretroviral drugs (Busti et al., 2008; Calza et al., 2005; Mazza et al., 2008; Townsend et al., 2007).These increased levels may be the result of inhibition of the organic anion transporting polypeptide (OATP) 1B1 that facilitates statin uptake into the liver (Ray, 2009). The disposition of pravastatin and rosuvastatin may be more dependent than other statins on OATPB1B1. In agreement with this theory, a study showed that atazanavir/ritonavir was associated with an increased in rosuvastatin levels. This finding led the authors to conclude that the maximum rosuvastatin dose with atazanavir/ritonavir should be 10-20 mg, similar to current recommendation of a maximum rosuvastatin dose of 10 mg when used with lopinavir-ritonavir (Busti et al., 2008). Although increased statins levels may enhance the effectiveness of these drugs, this benefit may come at the expense of an increase in toxicity. To date there is no known interactions between rosuvastatin and NNRTIs (Ray, 2009). Rosuvastatin may be a particularly good option in the setting of NNRTI-based therapy, given its greater effectiveness and lack of proven interactions, although additional pharmacokinetic studies would be useful (Ray, 2009).

Statins should be initiated at the lowest dose established for each agent. Subsequent, adjustments of dosing can be done according to response, and potential side effects must be closely monitored during follow-up, especially elevations in creatine phosphokinase and abnormal liver parameters (Blanco et al., 2010). Statins may improve abnormal baseline transaminases levels in patients with steatohepatitis (Millazo et al., 2007). Although the mechanism is not well defined, the removal of the lipids from the liver by statins might explain their benefits on liver function.

| Goal | Lipid lowering therapy |
|---|---|
| Elevated LDL-c or non-HDL cholesterol with triglycerides level of 200-500 mg/dL | Statins:<br>- Pravastatin: 10-40 mg daily<br>- Atorvastatin: 10-40 mg/daily<br>- Fluvastatin: 20-40 mg/daily<br>- Rosuvastatin 5-20 mg<br>- Lovastatin - not recommended with PI<br>- Simvastatin - not recommended with PI<br>- Ezetimibe: 10 mg daily |
| Triglycerides level > 500 mg/dL | Fibrates and Fish Oil:<br>- Gemfibrozil: 1200 mg daily<br>- Fenofibrate: 200 mg daily<br>- Omega-3 polyunsaturated fatty acids/fish oil: 3-5g (alternative treatment) |

Adapted from Bader & & Kelly, 2008; Bennet et al., 2007; Calza et al., 2003; Soler et al., 2006; Stebbing et al., 2009.

Table 2. Lipid lowering therapy for HIV-infected people.

### 5.2 Fibrates

For patients with triglycerides > 500 mg/dL, fibrates may be the first choice, especially in order to prevent pancreatitis (Dube et al., 2003). When extreme elevations are present (>1000 mg/dL in persons with a history of pancreatitis), it is reasonable to institute both drug and nondrug therapies concomitantly (Dube et al., 2003). Fibrates are metabolized by CYP4A, and there is less issue of interactions with antiretroviral drugs. They exert their effects by activating PPAR- ɣ. These drugs reduce plasma TG between 30% to 50%, and raise the level of HDL-c by 2% to 20%. Their effect on LDL-c is variable, ranging from a small decrease around 10% to no change or even a slight increase (Barter & Rye, 2006).

Gemfibrozil is generally initially recommended due to its efficacy in reducing TG. When concomitant hypercholesterolemia is present, statins can be added to fibrates, but the risk of rabdomimyolysis should be closely monitored (Henry et al., 1998). Clinicians treating HIV-infected patients must be aware of the interaction between Lopinavir/ritonavir and Gemfibrozil. Lopinavir/ritonavir decreases the systemic exposure to gemfibrozil by reducing the absorption of this drug (Busse et al., 2009). Fenofibrate is recommended by current guidelines for hypertrigliceridemia in antiretroviral treated patients. (Dube et al., 2003). Fenofibrate, could decrease triglyceride levels in HIV-infected persons on antiretroviral therapy, but only moderately (Aberg et al., 2005).

### 5.3 Niacin

Niacin has also been used in HIV-infected persons to improve lipid profiles. In the AIDS Clinical Trials Group study A5148, hyperlipidemia was treated with long-acting niacin during 48 weeks. Treatment resulted in significant improvements in TG, TC, HDL-c, and LDL-c, but a transient worsening in insulin sensitivity was also observed (Dube et al., 2006). The use of niacin with antiretroviral drugs may reduce the effect of niacin (Martinez et al., 2008). Patients treated with niacin should have regular evaluation of fasting glucose levels, and a standard 75-g, 2-h oral glucose-tolerance test should be considered, particularly when lipodystrophy or traditional risk factors for type 2 diabetes mellitus are present (Dube, 2000; Schambelan et al., 2002).

### 5.4 Fish oils

The metabolic effects of N-3 polyunsaturated fatty acids (PUFAs) derived from marine sources (known as "fish oils") have been demonstrated to reduce fasting and postprandial triglycerides levels in individuals without HIV infection (Simons et al., 1985). Omega-3 is considered an alternative treatment in non-HIV infected populations. It has been reported that 3-5 g per day of omega-3 fatty acids can reduce triglycerides by 30-50%, thereby potentially minimizing the risk of coronary heart disease and pancreatitis (O'Keefe & Harris, 2000). Treatment with fish oil is well tolerated, although potential effects on platelets must be checked, especially in persons taking drugs that may favor bleeding (Gerber et al., 2009).

### 5.5 Ezetimibe

Ezetimibe is the first lipid-lowering drug that inhibits intestinal uptake of dietary and biliary cholesterol at the brush border of the intestine, resulting in a reduction of hepatic cholesterol stores and an increase in clearance of cholesterol form in the blood (Kosoglou et al., 2005). It doesn't affect the absorption of fat-soluble nutrients and is an attractive option for HIV-infected patients because it lacks CYP P450 metabolism and therefore is not expected to interact with antiretroviral drugs (Kosoglou et al., 2005; Negredo et al., 2006]. The major metabolic pathway for Ezetimibe is the glucuronidation of 4-hydroxyphenyl group by uridine 5'-diphosphate-glucuronosyltransferase isoenzymes to form ezetimibe-glucuronide in the intestine and liver (Kosoglou et al., 2005). It reduces cholesterol absorption in the duodenum by approximately 50%, thereby attaining reductions in LDL-c of 20% (Gagne et al., 2002). This benefit is significantly greater when it is associated with any of the statins, achieving reductions in LDL-c of up to 50% (Bennett et al., 2007; Gagne et al., 2002, Pearson et al., 2005,). This synergistic effect of the two drugs in combination results from the inhibition of duodenal cholesterol absorption by ezetimibe, together with the reduction of hepatic cholesterol production by statins (Kosoglou et al., 2005). The recommended dose is 10 mg/day, and can be administered in the morning or evening with or without food (Kosoglou et al., 2005).

Ezetimibe has a favorable drug-drug interaction profile. It does not have significant effects on plasma levels of statins (atorvastatin, fluvastatin, lovastatin, pitavastatin, pravastatin, rosuvastatin, simvastatin), fibric acid derivatives (gemfibrozil, fenofibrate), digoxin, glipizide, warfarin and triphasic oral contraceptives (ethinylestradiol and levonorgestrel). Concomitant administration of food, antiacids, cimetidine or statins had no significant effect on ezetimibe bioavailability (Kosoglou et al., 2005). For this reason, it could be recommended as a second line therapy for dyslipidemia associated with antiretroviral drug use if hypercholesterolemia is refractory to statins or if patient does not tolerate statins. Its high tolerability and the lack of interactions with the CYP 3A4 indicate that ezetimibe will not increase the risk of toxicity or pharmacokinetic interactions with the use of antiretroviral medications. In HIV-infected patients ezetimibe results in a significant decrease in LDL-c, without significant changes in TG (Berg-Wolf et al., 2008; Chow et al., 2009). Creatine phosphokinase levels should be monitored due to potential risk of rhabdomyolisis.

Reductions in lipid levels with lipid-lowering therapy are greater in non-HIV infected patients than in HIV positive subjects (Martinez et al., 2008; Silverberg et al., 2009). Many studies that evaluated the effect of statins for the treatment of antiretroviral-associated dyslipidemia have shown only partial responses to such therapy, with total and LDL-c values being reduced by about 25% (Calza et al., 2003; Silverberg et al., 2009). The effectiveness and toxicity of statins among HIV-infected individuals may differ from those of the general population for several reasons. The patterns of dyslipidemia commonly seen among HIV-infected individuals are different from those observed in the general population (Riddler et al., 2003) and may be less responsive to treatment (Silverberg et al., 2009). Second, drug interactions between statins and antiretroviral drugs may impact the metabolism, effectiveness and toxicity associated with various forms of statins (Aberg et al., 2006; Gerber et al., 2005; Kiser et al., 2008, Ray, 2009). Response to any lipid lowering therapy must be evaluated after 3-6 months by repeating a fasting lipid profile.

## 6. Conclusion

Metabolic alterations and traditional cardiovascular risk factors are common in HIV-infected patients. Due to the success of antiretroviral therapy in the last years in reducing AIDS events and mortality, the population is aging and naturally the risk of cardiovascular disease increases. Early detection and management of cardiovascular risk factors is necessary to prevent coronary heart disease. All HIV-infected patients should have their fasting plasma lipid profile prior to starting antiretroviral treatment and then at every three or four months regularly. Efforts should be done including incorporating healthy diet habits, regular exercise, decrease alcohol consumption and smoking cessation prior to start of pharmacological interventions, to avoid excess medication and undesirable side effects. Virologic control and immune recovery should be the first priority in the management of HIV-infected patients due to their associations with high mortality.

## 7. References

Aberg, J.; Zackin, R.; Brobst, S.; Evans, S., Alston, B.; Henry, W.K. & Fichtenbaum, C.J. (2005). A randomized trial of the efficacy and safety of fenofibrate versus pravastatin in HIV-infected subjects with lipid abnormalities: AIDS Clinical Trial Group Study 5087. *AIDS* Research and Human Retroviruses, Vol.21, No.9 (September 2005) pp. 757-767, ISSN 0889-2229.

Aberg, J.A.; Rosenkranz, S.L.; Fichtenbaum, C.J.; Alston, B.L.; Brobst, S.W.; Segal, Y.; Gerber, J.G. and the AIDS Clinical Trials Group A5108 Team (2006). Pharmacokinetic interaction between nelfinavir and pravastatin in HIV-seronegative volunteers: ACTG Study A5108. *AIDS*, Vol.20, No. 5, (March 2006) pp. 725–729, ISSN 0269-9370.

Anderson, K.M.; Odell, P.M; Wilson, P.W. & Kannel W.B. (1991). Cardiovascular disease risk profiles. *Am Heart J*, Vol. 121 No. 1pt2, (January 1991), pp. 293-298, ISSN 0002-8703.

Aslangul, E; Assoumou, L; Bittar, R, Valantin, MA; Kalmykova, O; Peytavin, G, Fiévet, MH, Boccara, F, Bonnefont-Rousselot, D, Melchior, JC, Giral, P. & Costagliola D. (2010). Rosuvastatin versus pravastatin in dyslipidemic HIV-1-infected patients receiving protease inhibitors: a randomized trial. *AIDS*, Vol.24, No.1 (January 2010), pp. 77-83, ISSN 0269-9370

Bader, M.S. & Kelly, D.V. (2008). Diagnosis and Management of Common Chronic Metabolic Complications in HIV-infected patients. *Postgrad Med*, Vol.120, No. 4, (November 2008), pp. 1-11, ISSN 0022-3859.

Barbaro, G. (2006). Highly active antiretroviral therapy-associated metabolic syndrome: pathogenesis and cardiovascular risk. *Am J Ther*, Vol. 13, No. 3, (May-Jun 2006), pp. 48-60, ISSN 1075-2765.

Barrios, A.; Blanco, F.; García-Benayas, T.; Gómez-Viera, J.M., de la Cruz, J.J.; Soriano, V. & González-Lahoz, J. (2002). Effect of dietary intervention on highly active antiretroviral therapy-related dyslipemia. *AIDS*, Vol.18, No. 16(15), (October 2002), pp. 2079-81, ISSN 0269-9370

Barter, P.J. & Rye, K.A. (2006). Cardioprotective properties of fibrates: which fibrate, which patients, what mechanism? *Circulation*, Vol.113, No. 12 (March 2006); pp. 1553-5, ISSN 0009-7322.

Bennett, M.T.; Johns, K.W. & Bondy, G.P. (2007). Ezetimibe is effective when added to maximally tolerated lipid lowering therapy in patients with HIV. *Lipids Health Dis*, Vol.6, No. 15, (June 2007), pp. 6-15, ISSN 1476-511X.

Berg-Wolf, M.V.; Klibanov, O.M.; Gaughan, J.P. & Tedaldi, E.M. (2008). Ezetimibe Combined with Low-Dose Statin Effectively Lowers LDL in Protease Inhibitor Treated Patients. *AIDS Patient Care STDS*, Vol.22, No.6, (May 2008), pp. 483-488, ISSN 1087-2914.

Blanco, F.; San Román, J.; Vispo, E.; López, M.; Salto, A.; Abad, V. & Soriano, V. (2010). Management of metabolic complications and cardiovascular risk in HIV-infected patients. *AIDS Rev*, Vol.12, No.4, (October-December 2010), pp. 31-41.

Busse, K.H.; Hadigan, C.; Chairez, C.; Alfaro, R.M.; Formentini, E.; Kovacs, J.A. & Penzak, S.R. (2009). Gemfibrozil concentrations are significantly decreased in the presence of lopinavir-ritonavir. *J Acquir Immune Defic Syndr*, Vol.52, No.2, (October 2009), pp. 235-239, ISSN 1525-4135.

Busti, A.J.; Bain, A.M.; Hall, R.G.; 2nd, Bedimo, R.G.; Leff, R.D.; Meek, C. & Mehvar. R. (2008). Effects of atazanavir/ritonavir or fosamprenavir/ritonavir on the pharmacokinetics of rosuvastatin. *J Cardiovasc Pharmacol*, Vol.51, No.6, (June 2008), pp. 605–610, ISSN 0160-2446.

Calza, L., Manfredi, R. & Chiodo, F. (2003). Statins and fibrates for the treatment of hyperlipidaemia in HIV-infected patients receiving HAART. *AIDS*, Vol.17, No.6, (April 2003), pp. 851-859, ISSN 0269-9370.

Calza. L.; Colangeli, V.; Manfredi, R.; Legnani, G.; Tampellini. L.; Pocaterra.;D. & Chiodo, F. (2005). Rosuvastatin for the treatment of hyperlipidaemia in HIV-infected patients receiving protease inhibitors: A pilot study. *AIDS*, Vol.19, No. 10, (July 2005), pp. 1103–1105, ISSN 0269-9370.

Calza, L.; Manfredi, R.; Pocaterra, D. & Chiodo, F. (2008). Risk of premature atherosclerosis and ischemic heart disease associated with HIV infection and antiretroviral therapy. *J Infect*, Vol.57, No.1 (July 2008), pp. 16-32, ISSN 0163-4453.

Calza, L.; Manfredi, R.; Colangeli, V.; Pocaterra, D.; Pavoni, M. & Chiodo, F. (2008). Rosuvastatin, pravastatin, and atorvastatin for the treatment of hypercholesterolaemia in HIV-infected patients receiving protease inhibitors. *Curr HIV Res*, Vol.6, No.6, (November 2008), pp. 572-578, ISSN 1570-162X.

Carr, A.; Samaras, K.; Burton, S.; Law, M.; Freund, J.; Chisholm, D.J. & Cooper, D.A. (1998). A syndrome of peripheral lipodystrophy, hyperlipidaemia and insulin resistance in patients receiving HIV protease inhibitors. *AIDS*, Vol.12, No. 7, (May 1998), pp.F51-F58, ISSN 0269-9370.

Cheng. C; Graziane, C. & Diamond, J.J. (2004). Cholesterol-Lowering Effect of the Food for Heart Nutrition Education Program. *J Am Diet Assoc*, Vol. 104, No. 12, (Decembre 2004), pp. 1868-1872, ISSN 1878-3570.

Cheng, J.W. (2004). Rosuvastatin in the management of hyperlipidemia. Clin Ther, Vol,26, No.9, (September 2004), pp. 1368-1387, ISSN 0149-2918.

Chow, D.; Chen, H.; Glesby, M.J.; Busti, A.; Souza, S.; Andersen, J.; Kohrs, S.; Wu, J. & Koletar S.L. (2009). Short-term ezetimibe is well tolerated and effective in combination with statin therapy to treat elevated LDL cholesterol in HIV-infected patients. *AIDS*, Vol. 23, No. 16, (October 2009), pp. 2133-2141, ISSN 0269-9370.

Clifton,P.,Colquhoun, D. & Hewat, C. (2009). Dietary Intervention to lower serum cholesterol. *Australian Family Physician*, Vol.38, No. 6, (June 2009), pp.424-428, ISSN 0300-8495

Constans, J.; Pellegrin, J.L.; Peuchant, E.; Dumon, M.F.; Pellegrin, I.; Sergeant C, Simonoff M, Brossard G, Barbeau P. & Fleury H. (1994). Plasma lipids in HIV-infected patients: a prospective study in 95 patients. *Eur J Clin Invest*, Vol.24, No.6, (June 1994), pp. 416-420, ISSN 0014-2972.

Crum-Cianflone, N.; Dilay, A.; Collins, G.; Asher, D.; Campin, R.; Medina, S;. Goodman, Z.; Parker, R.; Lifson, A.; Capozza, T.; Bavaro, M.; Hale, B.; Hames, C. (2009). Nonalcholic fatty liver disease among HIV-infected persons. *J Acquir Immune Defic Syndr*, Vol. 50, No. 5, (April 2009), pp. 464–473, ISSN 1525-4135.

Dattilo, A.M. & Kris-Etherton, P.M. (1992). Effects of weight reduction on blood lipids and lipoproteins: a meta-analysis. *Am J Clin Nutr*, Vol. 56, No. 2, (August 1992), pp. 320–328, ISSN 0002-9165.

Dubé, M.P. (2000). Disorders of glucose metabolism in patients infected with human immunodeficiency virus. *Clin Infect Dis*, Vol. 31, No.6, (December 2000), pp. 1467–1475, ISSN 1058-4838.

Dubé, M.P.; Stein, J.H.; Aberg, J.A.; Fichtenbaum, J.G.; Gerber, K.; Sprecher, D. & Glesby M.J. (2003). Guidelines for the Evaluation and Management of Dyslipidemia in Human Immunodeficiency Vírus (HIV) – Infected Adults Receiving Antiretroviral Therapy: Recommendations of the HIV Medicine Association of the Infectious Disease of America and the Adult AIDS Clinical Trials Group. *Clin Infect Dis*, Vol.37, No. 5, (September 2003), pp. 613-627, ISSN 1058-4838.

Dubé, M.P.; Wu, J.W.; Aberg, J.A.; Deeg, M.A.; Alston-Smith, B.L.; McGovern, M.E.; Lee, D.; Shriver, S.L.; Martinez, A.I.; Greenwald, M. & Stein, J.H. AIDS Clinical Trials Group A5148 Study Team. (2006). Safety and efficacy of extended-release niacin for the treatment of dyslipidaemia in patients with HIV infection: AIDS Clinical Trials Group Study A5148. *Antivir Ther*, Vol.11. No.8, (April 2006), pp. 1081-1089, ISSN 1359-6535.

Fitch, K.V.; Anderson, E.J.; Hubbard, J.L.; Carpenter, S.J.; Waddell, W.R.; Caliendo, A.M. & Grinspoon, S.K. (2006). Effects of a lifestyle modification program in HIV-infected patients with the metabolic syndrome. *AIDS*, Vol.20, No.14, (September 2006), pp. 1843-1850, ISNN 0269-9370.

Friis-Møller, N.; Weber, R.; Reiss, P.; Thiébaut, R.; Kirk, O.; d'Arminio Monforte, A.; Pradier, C.; Morfeldt, L.; Mateu, S.; Law, M.; El-Sadr, W.; De Wit, S.; Sabin, C.A.; Phillips, A.N. & Lundgren, J.D.; DAD study group. (2003). Cardiovascular disease risk factors in HIV patients-association with antiretroviral therapy. Results from the DAD study. *AIDS*, Vol.17, No.8, (May 2003), pp. 1179-1193, ISSN 0269-9370.

Gagné, C.; Bays, H.E.; Weiss, S.R.; Mata, P.; Quinto, K.; Melino, M.; Cho, M.; Musliner, T.A. & Gumbiner, B. (2002). Ezetimibe Study Group. Efficacy and safety of ezetimibe added to ongoing statin therapy for treatment of patients with primary hypercholesterolemia. *Am J Cardiol*, Vol.90, No. 10, (November 2002), pp. 1084-1091, ISSN 0002-9149.

Gerber, J.G.; Kitch, D.W.; Fichtenbaum, C.J.; Zackin, R.A.; Charles, S.; Hogg, E.; Acosta, E.P.; Connick, E.; Wohl, D.; Kojic, E.M.; Benson, C.A. & Aberg, J.A. (2009). Fish oil and fenofibrate for the treatment of hypertriglyceridemia in HIV-infected subjects on antiretroviral therapy: results of ACTG A5186. *J Acquir Immune Defic Syndr*, Vol.47, No.4, (April 2008), pp. 459-466, ISSN 1525-4135.

Glass, T.R.; Ungsedhapand, C.; Wolbers, M.; Weber, R.; Vernazza, P.L.; Rickenbach, M.; Furrer, H.; Bernasconi, E.; Cavassini, M.; Hirsche,l B.; Battegay.; M. & Bucher, H.C.; Swiss HIV Cohort Study. (2006). Prevalence of risk factors for cardiovascular disease in HIV-infected patients over time: the Swiss HIV Cohort Study. *HIV Med*, Vol.7, No.6, (September 2006), pp.404-410, ISSN 1464-2662.

Guaraldi, G.; Squillace, N.; Stentarelli.; C, Orlando, G.; D'Amico, R;. Ligabue, G.; Fiocchi, F;. Zona, S;. Loria, P;. Esposito, R;. Palella, F. (2008).Nonalcoholic fatty liver disease in HIV-infected patients referred to a metabolic clinic: prevalence, characteristics, and predictors. *Clin Infect Dis*, Vol.47, No.2 (July 2008), pp. 250-257, ISSN 1058-4838.

Graham, N.M. (2000). Metabolic disorders among HIV-infected patients treated with protease inhibitors: A review. *J Acquir Immune Defic Syndr*, Vol. 25, Suppl 1, (October 2000), pp.S4-11, ISNN 1525-4135.

Grundy, S.M.; Cleeman, J.I.; Merz ,C.N.; Brewer, H.B Jr.; Clark, L.T.; Hunninghake, D.B.; Pasternak, R.C.; Smith, S.C. Jr. & Stone, N.J. Coordinating Committee of the National Cholesterol Education Program. (2004). Implications of recent clinical trials for the National Cholesterol Education Program Adult Treatment Panel III Guidelines. *J Am Coll Cardiol*, Vol.44, No.3, (August 2004), pp.720-732, ISNN 0735-1097.

Grunfeld, C.; Kotler, D.P.; Shigenaga, J.K.; Doerrler, W.; Tierney, A.; Wang, J.; Pierson, R.N. Jr. & Feingold, K.R. (1991). Circulating interferon-alpha levels and hypertriglyceridemia in the acquired immunodeficiency syndrome. *Am J Med*, Vol.90, No.2, (February 1991), pp.154-162, ISSN 0002-9343.

Hammond, E.; Nolan, D.; James, I.; Metcalf, C. & Mallal S. (2004). Reduction of mitochondrial DNA content and respiratory chain activity occurs in adipocytes within 6-12 months of commencing nucleoside reverse transcriptase inhibitor therapy. *AIDS*, Vol.26, No.18, (Mars 2004), pp. 815-817, ISSN 0269-9370.

Henry, K.; Melroe, H.; Huebesch, J.; Hermundson, J. & Simpson, J. (1998). Atorvastatin and gemfibrozil for protease-inhibitor-related lipid abnormalities. *Lancet,* Vol.26, No. 352(9133), (September 1998), pp.1031-1032, ISSN 0140-6736.

Jenkins, D.J.; Kendall, C.W.; Marchie, A.; Faulkner, D.A.; Wong, J.M.; de Souza, R.; Emam, A.; Parker, T.L.; Vidgen, E.; Lapsley, K.G.; Trautwein, E.A;, Josse, R.G.; Leiter, L.A. & Connelly, P.W. (2003). Effects of a dietary portfolio of cholesterol-lowering foods vs lovastatin on serum lipids and C-reactive protein. *JAMA,* Vol.290, No.4, (July 2003); pp. 502-510, ISNN 0003-9926.

Jones, P.H.; Davidson, M.H.; Stein, E.A.; Bays, H.E.; McKenney, J.M.; Miller, E.; Cain, V.A. & Blasetto, J.W. (2003). Comparison of the efficacy and safety of rosuvastatin versus atorvastatin, simvastatin, and pravastatin across doses (STELLAR* Trial). *Am J Cardiol,* Vol.92, No.2, (July 2003), pp.152-160, ISNN 0002-9149.

Jung, O.; Bickel, M.; Ditting, T.; Rickerts, V.; Welk, T.; Helm, E.B.; Staszewski, S. & Geiger, H. (2004). Hypertension in HIV-1-infected patients and its impact on renal and cardiovascular integrity. *Nephrol Dial Transplant,* Vol.19, No.9, (September 2004), pp. 2250-2258, ISNN 0931- 0509.

Kalra, S.; Kalra, B.; Agrawal, N. & Unnikrishnan, A. (2001). Understanding diabetes in patients with HIV/AIDS. *Diabetol Metab Syndr,* Vol.3, No.1, (January 2011), pp.2.

Klein, D.; Leyden, W.; Xu, L.; Chao, C.; Horberg, M.; Towner, W.; Hurley, L.; Quesenberry, C. & Silverberg, M. (2011). Contribution of Immunodeficiency to CHD: Cohort Study of HIV+ and HIV- Kaiser Permanente Members. *Proceedings of 18th Conference on Retrovirus and Opportunistic Infections,* ISBN 0-9793191-8-8, Boston, USA feb 27- 2 mars 2011.

Kiser, J.J.; Gerber J.G.; Predhomme, J.A.; Wolfe, P.; Flynn, D.M. & Hoody, D.W. (2008). Drug/Drug interaction between lopinavir/ritonavir and rosuvastatin in healthy volunteers. *J Acquir Immune Defic Syndr,* Vol.47, No.5, pp. 570–578, ISSN 1525-4135.

Kosoglou, T.; Statkevich, P.; Johnson-Levonas, A.O.; Paolini, J.F.; Bergman, A.J. & Alton, K.B. (2005). Ezetimibe: a review of its metabolism, pharmacokinetics and drug interactions. *Clin Pharmacokinet,* Vol.44, No.5, (May 2005), pp. 467-494, ISSN 0312-5963.

Lewden, C.; Chene, G.;.Morlat, P.; Raffi, F.; Dupon, M.; Dellamonica, P.; Pellegrin, J.L.; Katlama, C.; Dabis, F. & Leport, C. Agence Nationale de Recherches sur le Sida et les Hepatites Virales (ANRS) CO8 APROCO-COPILOTE Study Group; Agence Nationale de Recherches sur le Sida et les Hepatites Virales (ANRS) CO3 AQUITAINE Study Group. (2007). HIV-infected adults with a CD4 cell count greater than 500 cells/mm3 on long-term combination antiretroviral therapy reach same mortality rates as the general population. *J Acquir Immune Defic Syndr,* Vol.46, No.1 (September 2007), pp. 72-77, ISSN 1525-4135.

Malvestutto, C.D. & Aberg, J.A. (2010). Coronary heart disease in people infected with HIV. *Cleve Clin J Med,* Vol.77, No.8, (August 2010), pp. 547-556, ISSN 0891-1150.

Mamary, E.M.; Bahrs, D. & Martinez, S. (2002). Cigarette smoking and the desire to quit among individuals living with HIV. *AIDS Patient Care STDS,* Vol.16, No.1, (January 2002), pp. 39-42, ISSN 1087-2914.

Manfredi, R. (2000). Management of dyslipidemia in patients with HIV disease. *Clin Microbiol Infect*, Vol.6, No. 11, (November 2000), pp.579-584, ISSN 1469-0691

Martínez, E.; Leyes, P. & Ros, E. (2008). Effectiveness of lipid-lowering therapy in HIV patients. *Curr Opin HIV AIDS*, Vol.3, No.3, (May 2008), pp.240-246, ISSN 1746-6318.

Mazza, F.; Stefanutti, C.; Di Giacomo, S.; Vivenzio, A. ; Fraone, N. ; Mazzarella, B. & Bucci A. (2008). Effects of low-dose atorvastatin and rosuvastatin on plasma lipid profiles: A long-term, randomized, open-label study in patients with primary hypercholesterolemia. *Am J Cardiovasc Drugs*, Vol.8, No. 4 (July 2008), pp. 265–270, ISSN 1175-3277.

Martin, P.D.; Warwick, M.J.; Dane, A.L.; Hill, S.J.; Giles, P.B.; Phillips, P.J. & Lenz E. (2003). Metabolism, excretion, and pharmacokinetics of rosuvastatin in healthy adult male volunteers. *Clin Ther*, Vol.25, No.11, (November 2003), pp. 2822-2835, ISSN 0149-2918.

Milazzo, L.; Menzaghi, B.; Corvasce, S.; Bonfanti, P.; Rusconi, S.; Ridolfo, A.L. & Antinori, S. (2007). Safety of statin therapy in HIV/hepatitis C virus-coinfected patients. *J Acquir Immune Defic Syndr*, Vol.46, No.2, (October 2007), pp. 258-260, ISSN 1525-4135.

Mohiuddin, S.M.; Mooss, A.N.; Hunter, C.B.; Grollmes, T.L.; Cloutier, D.A. & Hilleman, D.E. (2007). Intensive smoking cessation intervention reduces mortality in high-risk smokers with cardiovascular disease. *Chest*, Vol.131, No.2, (February 2007), pp. 446-452, ISSN 0012-3692.

Negredo, E.; Molto.; J, Puig J.; Cinquegrana, D.; Bonjoch, A.; Pérez-Alvarez, N.; López-Blázquez, R.; Blanco, A.; Clotet, B. & Rey-Joly, C. (2006). Ezetimibe, a promising lipid-lowering agent for the treatment of dyslipidaemia in HIV-infected patients with poor response to statins. *AIDS*, Vol. 20, No. 17, (November 2006), pp. 2159-2164, ISSN 0269-9370.

O'Keefe, J.H. &Harris, W.S. (2000). From Inuit to implementation: omega-3 fatty acids come of age. *Mayo Clin Proc*, Vol. 75, No.6, (June 2000), pp.607-614, ISSN1942-5546.

Palella, F.J.; Delaney, K.M.; Moorman, A.C.; Loveless, M.O.; Fuhrer, J.; Satten G.A.; Aschman, D.J. & Holmberg, S.D. (1998). Declining Morbidity and Mortality among Patients with Advanced Human Immunodeficiency Virus Infection. *N Engl J Med*, Vol. 338, No. (March 1998), pp. 853-860, ISSN 1533-4406.

Pearson, T.A.; Denke, M.A.; McBride, P.E.; Battisti, W.P.; Brady, W.E. & Palmisano, J. (2005). A community-based, randomized trial of ezetimibe added to statin therapy to attain NCEP ATP III goals for LDL cholesterol in hypercholesterolemic patients: the ezetimibe add-on to statin for effectiveness (EASE) trial. *Mayo Clin Proc*, Vol. 80, No.5, (May 2005), pp. 587-595, ISSN 0025-6196.

Ray, G.M. (2009). Antiretroviral and statin drug-drug interactions. *Cardiol Rev*, Vol.17, No. 1 (January-February 2009), pp. 44–47, ISSN 1061-5377.

Ray, K.K. & Cannon, C.P. (2005). The potential relevance of the multiple lipid-independent (pleiotropic) effects of statins in the management of acute coronary syndromes. J *Am Coll Cardiol*, Vol. 46, No. 8, (October 2005), pp.1425-1433, ISSN 0735-1097.

Riddler, S.A.; Smit, E.; Cole, S.R.; Li, R.; Chmiel, J.S.; Dobs, A.; Palella, F.; Visscher, B.; Evans, R. & Kingsley, L.A. (2003). Impact of HIV infection and HAART on serum lipids in men. *JAMA*, Vol. 289, No. 22, (June 2003), pp.2978–2982, ISSN 00987484.

Sackoff, J.E.; Hanna, D.B.; Pfeiffer, M.R. & Torian, L.V. (2006). Causes of death among persons with AIDS in the era of highly active antiretroviral therapy: New York City. *Ann Intern Med*, Vol.145, No.6, (September 2006), pp. 397-406, ISSN 0003-4819.

Saiki, A.; Murano, T.; Watanabe, F.; Oyama, T.; Miyashita, Y. & Shirai, K. (2005). Pitavastatin enhanced lipoprotein lipase expression in 3T3-L1 preadipocytes. *J Atheroscler Thromb*, Vol. 12, No. 3 (January 2005), pp. 163-168, ISSN 1880-3873.

Savès, M.; Chêne, G.; Ducimetière, P.; Leport, C.; Le Moal, G.; Amouyel, P.; Arveiler, D.; Ruidavets, J.B.; Reynes, J.; Bingham, A. & Raffi, F; French WHO MONICA Project and the APROCO (ANRS EP11) Study Group. (2003). Risk factors for coronary heart disease in patients treated for human immunodeficiency virus infection compared with the general population. *Clin Infect Dis*, Vol.37, No.2 (July 2003), pp. 292-298, ISSN 1058-4838.

Schambelan, M.; Benson, C.A.; Carr A.; Currier, J.S.; Dubé, M.P.; Gerber, J.G.; Grinspoon, S.K.; Grunfeld, C.; Kotler, D.P.; Mulligan, K.; Powderly, W.G. & Saag, M.S. (2002). Management of metabolic complications associated with antiretroviral therapy for HIV-1 infection: recommendations of an International AIDS Society-USA Panel. *J Acquir Immune Defic Syndr*, Vol. 31, No. 3, (November 2002), pp. 257–275, ISSN 1525-4135.

Silverberg, M.J.; Leyden, W.; Hurley L.; Go, A.S.; Quesenberry, C.P.;Jr, Klein, D. & Horberg, M.A. (2009). Response to newly prescribed lipid-lowering therapy in patients with and without HIV infection. *Ann Intern Med*, Vol. 150, No. 5 (March 2009), pp. 301–313, ISSN 0003-4819.

Shor-Posner, G.; Basit, A.; Lu, Y.; Cabrejos, C.; Chang, J.; Fletcher, M.; Mantero-Atienza, E. & Baum, M.K. (1993). Hypocholesterolaemia is associated with immune dysfunction in early human immunodeficiency virus-1 infection. *Am J Med*, Vol. 94, No. 5, (May 1993), pp. 515-519, ISSN 0098-8588.

Simons, L.A.; Hickie, J.B. & Balasubramaniam, S. (1985). On the effects of dietary n-3 fatty acids (Maxepa) on plasma lipids and lipoproteins in patients with hyperlipidaemia. *Atherosclerosis*, Vol. 54, No. 1, (January 1985), pp. 75-88, ISSN 0021-9150.

Skeaff, C.M.; Thoma, C.; Mann, J.; Chisholm, A.; Williams, S. & Richmond, K. (2005). Isocaloric substitution of plant sterol-enriched fat spread for carbohydrate-rich foods in a low-fat, fibre-rich diet decreases plasma low-density lipoprotein cholesterol and increases high-density lipoprotein concentrations. *Nutr Metab Cardiovasc Dis*, Vol 15, No. 5 (March 2005), pp.337–344, ISSN 0939-4753.

Soler, A.; Deig, E.; Guil, J.; Rodríguez-Martín, M.; Guelar, A. & Pedrol, E. (2006). Effectiveness and tolerance of atorvastatin for antiretroviral therapy-secondary dyslipemia. *Med Clin (Barc)*, Vol. 127, No. 7, (July 2006), pp. 250-252, ISSN 0025-7753.

Stebbing, J.; Asghar, A.K.; Holmes, P.; Bower, M.; Isenman, H.L. & Nelson, M. (2009). Use of ezetimibe during HIV infection. *J Antimicrob Chemother*, Vol. 63, No. 1, (January 2009), pp. 218-220, ISSN 0305-7453.

Third Report of the National Cholesterol Education Program (NCEP). Expert Panel on Detection, Evaluation and Treatment of High Blood Cholesterol in Adults (Adult Treatment Panel III) final report. (2002). *Circulation*, Vol. 106, No. 25 (December 2002), pp. 3143-3421, ISSN 0009-7322.

Townsend, M.L.; Hollowell, S.B.; Bhalodia, J.; Wilson, K.H.; Kaye, K.S. & Johnson, M.D. (2007). A comparison of the effectiveness of lipid-lowering therapy between HIV- and non-HIV-infected subjects with hyperlipidaemia. *Int J STD AIDS*, Vol. 18, No. 12, (December 2007), pp. 851–855, ISSN 0956-4624.

Triant, V.A.; Lee, H.; Hadigan, C. & Grinspoon, S.K. (2007). Increased acute myocardial infarction rates and cardiovascular risk factors among patients with human immunodeficiency virus disease. *J Clin Endocrinol Metab*, Vol. 92, No. 7, (July 2007), pp. 2506-2012, ISSN 0021-972X.

Williams. B. & Feely, J. (2002). Pharmacokinetic-pharmacodynamic drug in interactions with HMG-CoA reductase inhibitors. *Clin Pharmacokinetic*, Vol. 41, No. 5, (May 2002), pp. 434-470, ISSN 0312-5963.

Yano, M.; Matsumura, T.; Senokuchi, T.; Ishii, N.; Murata, Y.; Taketa, K.; Motoshima, H.; Taguchi, T.; Sonoda, K.; Kukidome, D.; Takuwa, Y.; Kawada, T.; Brownlee, M.; Nishikawa T. & Araki, E. (2007). Statins activate peroxisome proliferator-activated receptor gamma through extracellular signal-regulated kinase 1/2 and p38 mitogen-activated protein kinase-dependent cyclooxygenase-2 expression in macrophages. *Circ Res*, Vol.100, No. 10, (May 2007), pp. 1442-1451, ISSN 0009-7330.

9

# HIV Associated Neuropathies

Katrin Hahn[1] and Ingo Husstedt[2]
[1]*Universitätsklinikum Charité Campus Mitte, Klinik für Neurologie, Berlin*
[2]*Universitätsklinikum Münster, Klinik und Poliklinik für Neurologie, Münster*
*Germany*

## 1. Introduction

Over the past decade there have been significant demographic changes in the HIV epidemic. The overall population of people living with HIV/AIDS is aging. The effect of HAART, aging and resulting comorbidities, such as hypertension, and diabetes add new complexity to HIV and related conditions such as HIV neuropathies.

HIV -associated polyneuropathy is still the most common neurological complication of HIV infection and is one of the main risk factors for development of a neuropathy worldwide. Many types of peripheral neuropathies are seen in HIV infection depending on the stage of infection. The inflammatory demyelinating neuropathies both acute (Guillain-Barré syndrome [GBS] and chronic (chronic inflammatory demyelinating neuropathy [CIDP] occur mainly at the time of seroconversion or early in the course of the disease while syndromes associated with opportunistic infections like CMV (i.e. polyradiculoneuropathy) occur in the late phase of HIV infection and are related to the loss of immune function. The most common neuropathy in HIV-infected patients is the sensory HIV associated neuropathy which includes distal symmetrical polyneuropathy (DSP) and antiretroviral toxic neuropathy (ATN). Those patients may experience painful symptoms such as burning or hyperalgesia in the feet and treatment is very often focussed on management of neuropathic pain. However one should be aware that the high prevalence of HIV-DSP in the HIV population makes the coexistence of more than one neuropathic condition likely either because of comorbidities or aging. These complexities have led to neuropathic syndromes that do not meet diagnostic criteria because of overlapping syndromes. We review the clinical manifestations, epidemiology, clinical diagnostics, and pathophysiology as well as management strategies for HIV-associated polyneuropathies.

## 2. Diagnostic evaluation

One way to classify HIV-neuropathies is according to the stage of HIV disease in which they occur. Therefore it is mandatory to have an actual CD4 cell count. Some types of neuropathies such as inflammatory demyelinating neuropathies often occur during seroconversion, before strong immunosuppression [1-4] while others such as progressive polyradiculopathies associated with CMV infection are common in late stages of AIDS.

Over the past decade there have also been significant demographic changes in the HIV population, which has consequently brought attention to common so called "age related neuropathies" now also occurring in the HIV population. Figure 1 summarizes laboratory parameters that are recommended as a baseline diagnostic in patients representing with the clinical symptoms of neuropathy.

erythrocyte sedimentation rate or C-reactive protein, complete blood count, comprehensive metabolic panel (blood glucose or glucose tolerance testing (GTT), renal function, liver function), thyroid function tests, serum B12 (serum methylmalonic acid with or without homocysteine for low normal vitamin B12 levels), serum immunofixation electrophoresis, hepatitis B and C panel, Treponema pallidum screening test, immune status, HIV viral load, antinuclear antigen profile.
In case of a co infection with hepatitis C: cryoglobulins.

Fig. 1. Basic laboratory parameters in HIV-infected patients presenting with distal symmetric neuropathy.

Cerebrospinal fluid (CSF) analysis is usually acquired when an inflammatory or an opportunistic/neoplastic neuropathy is suspected. You have to be aware that it may reveal confusing results in cases of GBS or CIDP, which occur mainly in patients with high CD4 counts. This is because asymptomatic HIV patients may show an elevated protein and a mild lymphocytic pleocytosis [1, 2]. CSF analysis is however very important in patients with CD4 counts below 200/µl in whom there is a strong suspicion of an underlying infectious or malignant etiology.

### 2.1 Functional and morphological assessment of nerve fibers

Neurophysiological examination has do be done in every patient presenting with neuropathic symptoms in order to classify the neuropathy as either axonal or demyelinating and to assess a subclinical large fiber involvement in patients presenting with typical small fiber symptoms such as burning, aching or stubbing pain mainly localized in the feet. Somatosensory evoked potential may be useful if a myelopathy is suspected.

HIV-infected patients represent very often with a pure small fiber neuropathy with burning feet, which may be difficult to objectify because of a paucity of clinical signs and unremarkable electrodiagnostic studies. Advances have been made in identifying those patients during the last decade. Skin biopsy from the distal leg and assessment of epidermal nerve fiber density (ENFD) using antibodies to protein-gene product 9.5 is nowadays a validated tool [5, 6]. ENFD declines with age [7], which has to be taken into account with the increased aging of HIV-infected individuals. Beyond skin biopsy, functional measurements are applicable such as quantitative sensory testing or contact heat-evoked potentials (CHEP`s) the later evaluating late potentials of A-delta and C fibers at the scalp following cutaneous stimulation. It has been shown that by using CHEP`s the sensitivity to detect patients with predominant small fiber involvement is higher compared to convential electrodiagnostic techniques [8].

### 2.2 Nerve biopsy

Nerve and muscle biopsies are only required in selected cases especially in patients representing with rapid progressing neuropathies. Reasons to perform a biopsy are patients were vasculitis, amyloidosis or storage diseases are suspected. Neuropathic pain on the biopsy site remains in 10 to 20 % of the patients.

## 3. Subtypes of HIV-associated neuropathies

HIV-associated neuropathies can be classified according to clinical, neurophysiological or histomorphological criteria. Figure 2 summarizes the HIV-associated subtypes.

**HIV-associated neuropathies**

HIV- associated sensory neuropathy (HIV-SN)

- distal symmetric polyneuropathy (DSP)
- antiretroviral toxic neuropathy (ATN)

Inflammatory Demyelinating Polyneuropathies

- acute inflammatory demyelininating polyneuropathy (AIDP)
- chronic inflammatory demyelininating polyneuropathy (CIDP)

Mononeuropathy multiplex

Autonomic neuropathy

Diffuse infiltrative lymphocytosis syndrome

Neuropathies due to opportunistic infections

Fig. 2. HIV-associated neuropathies.

## 4. HIV-associated sensory neuropathy (HIV-SN)

HIV-SN is by far the most common neurological complication in HIV infection [9, 10]. HIV-SN summarizes 2 subtypes that are clinically undistinguishable: distal symmetric polyneuropathy (DSP) which occurs mainly during advanced stages of HIV infection and antiretroviral toxic neuropathy (ATN) as a result of neurotoxic antiretroviral treatment.

### 4.1 Epidemiology

The prevalence of HIV-SN has been found to increase further. In various cohorts, its prevalence reaches up to 50% [11, 12]. Early epidemiological studies conducted during the pre HAART-era describe an annual incidence of 36% for HIV-SN compared to 21% in the HAART-era [11, 13]. The increasing life expectancy of HIV-infected individuals and the high cumulative dosage of neurotoxic antiretroviral substances, in particular ddC, ddl and d4T, represent the causes for the increasing prevalence [14]. Markers of advanced HIV disease such as low CD4 cell count (especially a CD4 nadir below 50 cells/µl), a high HIV viral load (> 10.000 cop./ ml) as well as a diabetes and demographic factors such as age are associated with increased risk of HIV-SN [15, 16]. There seems to be evidence that the prevalence of the mitochondrial Haplotyp T as well as the E4 isoform for Apolipoprotein E act as an independent risk factor for ATN and HIV-DSP [17, 18]. Moreover it is argued that APOE epsilon4 may play a role in nerve regeneration [18, 19].

Newer analyses demonstrate that HIV-SN also occurs increasingly with protease inhibitors as Indinavir, Saquinavir and Ritonavir [20]. However, these patients demonstrate additional factors that are combined with an increased prevalence of polyneuropathies, such as increased age and glycometabolic disturbances. Since protease inhibitors are often applied as first-line therapies, the progressing HIV infection likewise induces an increase of polyneuropathy, which is caused by the HIV virus itself [20].

### 4.2 Clinical manifestation

The clinical presentation of HIV-DSP and ATN is undistinguishable and similar to other forms of DSP. Symptoms are usually length-dependent, symmetric, mainly sensory and often painful. Patients may describe burning, tightness or hyperalgesia in the feet and hands in a classic "stocking-and-glove" like pattern. Negative sensory symptoms such as numbness or hypalgesia often occur while strength is relatively preserved. Deep tendon reflexes are reduced at the ankles compared to the knees. Hyperactive reflexes may occur in cases of coexisting central nervous system disease such as myelopathy as well as HIV dementia. Significant motor involvement raises severe doubt about the diagnosis HIV-SN, although slight to moderate weakness and atrophy of the intrinsic muscles of the feet may be a feature of advanced HIV-SN.

### 4.3 Diagnostic evaluation

Nerve conduction studies (NCS`s) show predominantly an axonal sensory pattern with reduction of the sensory nerve action potential (SNAP) and mild reduction of the conduction velocities. As it is stated above, 20% of the patients represent exclusively with small fiber symptoms and therefore show unremarkable NCS`s [21]. One may consider conducting skin biopsy in those patients, which has been shown an objective and sensitive tool [6, 22]. Decreased ENFD was significantly associated with high plasma HIV viral levels and low CD4 counts as well as higher levels of neuropathic pain [6].

### 4.4 Pathogenesis

Although HIV-DSP and HIV-ATN represent identically in clinical and neurophysiological examination they have different pathogenesis.

#### 4.4.1 HIV-DSP

The pathogenesis of HIV-DSP is incompletely understood, but is likely immune mediated.
The most characteristic pathological feature is the distal degeneration of long axons [4] accompanied by macrophage infiltration [4, 23] and either the absence or modest loss of neurons in the sensory dorsal root ganglia (DRG) [24-26]. Furthermore, there is degeneration within the centrally directed extension of sensory DRG neurons [26]. These findings have led to the hypothesis that the primary pathology could be at the level of the sensory neurons in the DRG, leading secondarily to a dying back process with axonal degeneration. The diminution and degeneration of epidermal nerve fibers as seen in skin biopsies proves this hypothesis [6]. People with HIV infection have also significantly reduced rates of both collateral and regenerative sprouting in skin biopsy experimental injury models [27].
The presence of HIV-infected perivascular macrophages has been shown in the DRG of patients with and without DSP. These studies demonstrated the presence of HIV proviral DNA, mRNA, p24 antigen in these cells [28-31]. Another consistent neuropathological abnormality in the DRG appears to be the presence of activated macrophages, which express MHC antigens and pro-inflammatory cytokines [4, 29, 31]. HIV-DSP correlates with the

degree of macrophage activation [32]. Taken together, this has led to the hypothesis that activated macrophages play an important role in the pathogenesis of peripheral neuropathy. Two possible neuropathogenetic mechanisms have been proposed; the direct effect of HIV or HIV proteins such as gp120 on DRGs [33-35] and the indirect neurotoxicity of products secreted by activated macrophages [32]. The later assumption is underlined by our observation that supernatants from HIV-infected macrophages induce neuritic retraction in DRG culture, suggesting that activated macrophages may secrete neurotoxic mediators [36].

#### 4.4.2 ATN

The increased survival time in the AIDS stage leads to a significantly higher cumulative dosage of antiretroviral agents. The toxicity of HAART is produced by a dysfunction in the mitochondria itself and mitochondrial DNA. There is evidence that the primary target in ATN is not the DRG itself but the axon [37]. Dalakas et al. described structural abnormalities in axonal mitochondria as well as mitochondria of Schwann cells in patients with ATN [38]. Mitochondrial DNA in subcutaneous fat was significantly reduced in patients currently taking Nucleoside reverse transcriptase inhibitors (NRTIs) but did however not correlate to the incidence of ATN [39].

Ddl, ddC and d4T show toxic effects on the mitochondrial DNA in tissue cultures as well. PC12 cells exposed to ddl and ddC triggered structural modifications to the mitochondria and an increase in lactate production [40]. These effects are correlated with the concentration of these substances. The initial changes to the mitochondrial ultrastructure occurred after only a few days. The toxic potential for the induction of these changes can be arranged in the following sequence: ddC > d4T > ddI [41]. The higher toxicity of ddl, ddC and d4T in comparison to other antiretroviral agents results from the diverse inhibition of mitochondrial enzymes as γ-polymerase. However there seems to be γ-polymerase independent pathways of mitochondrial damage [42].

### 4.5 Therapy

#### 4.5.1 Causal

There is no approved causal treatment for HIV-associated DSP. There is however some evidence that HAART may improve symptoms [43]. Early epidemiological studies conducted during the pre HAART-era describe an annual incidence of 36% for HIV-SN compared to 21% in the HAART-era [11, 13] which also indicate some positive influence of HAART.

If the patient is taking neurotoxic medications they should be stopped or changed if it is possible. One has to check for potentially neurotoxic co medications that are often used for HIV-related conditions such as chloramphenicol, dapsone, ethambutol, etopside, isoniazid, metronidazole, pyridoxine, thalidomide, and vincristine [44].

Clinical trials of potentially neuroregenerative therapies such as nerve growth factor [45], prosaptide [46] and timcodar [47], agents that were neurotrophic in vitro and in animal models have failed.

#### 4.5.2 Pain management

Neuropathic pain can be quite disabling for the patients and treatment is often challenging because of concomitant diseases and relevant interactions of neuropsychopharmacologically active drugs with HAART.

Recommendations are based on studies performed specifically in HIV-SN, but also extrapolated from studies performed in various conditions such as painful diabetic neuropathy as well as postherpetic neuralgia. Six main classes of agents are used: anticonvulsants (calcium- and sodium-dependent), antidepressants, opioids, topical treatments, nonspecific analgesics and alternatives therapies.

A recently published review and meta-analysis describes randomized controlled trials (RCT`s) evidence of analgesic efficacy superior to placebo in the context of HIV-SN pain only for smoked cannabis, recombinant nerve growth factor (rhNGF) and high dose (8%) topical capsaicin [48]. Several other agents have been examined in RCTs and found to be not effective such as acetyl-L carnitine (1g/day), amitriptyline (100mg/day), topical capsaicin 0.075%, gabapentin (2.4g/day), mexilitine (600mg/day), peptide –T (6mg/day), pregabalin (600mg/day), lamotrigine (600mg/day) and prosaptide (16mg/day) [48, (Simpson, Schifitto et al. 2010)]. Prospective RCT´s show however an effectiveness for gabapentin (up to 3.6g/d) [49] in HIV-DSP as well as lamotrigene in ATN [50].

Gabapentin and pregabalin do not induce the cytochrome P-450 system and are therefore preferred agents. Older antiepileptics such as carbamazepine should be avoided as a result of multiple and pronounced interactions [51, 52]. There are also promising data for duloxetine in reducing pain. However RCT´s were performed in patients with painful diabetic neuropathy [53, 54]. Duloxetine is characterized by nearly no interactions with HAART and is therefore an interesting alternative. Even though the older, tricyclic antidepressants have not be convincing in one RCT [55] they are very well suited for neuropathic pain therapy in our clinical experience. However it has to be taken into consideration that amitriptyline levels are increased by protease inhibitors, which may provoke side effects.

## 5. Inflammatory demyelinating polyneuropathies

Acute inflammatory demyelinating polyneuropathy (AIDP or Guillain-Barré- syndrome [GBS]) or chronic inflammatory demyelinating polyneuropathy (CIDP) may occur early in the course of HIV disease as a part of the acute antiretroviral syndrome or in a stage where the CD4 cell count is above 250/µl [1, 2, 56].

### 5.1 HIV-AIDP

In our clinical experience HIV-AIDP is a rare disease. It has not been seen in prospective studies of HIV infection [57]. A Zimbabvian study of 32 consecutive patients with AIDP found that 55% suffered from HIV, while the seroprevalence of HIV infection during the time the study took place was estimated at 4.3%, clearly indicating a relationship [2].

Cornblath et al. [1] described three patients with HIV-AIDP early in HIV infection, prior to AIDS. Subsequent reports also indicated that HIV-AIDP occurs at time of seroconversion [58, 59]. HIV-AIDP is considered to precede AIDS but has been described in HIV-infected patients with a CD4 cell count below 200 but above 50/µl [56, 60]. The last remark is important as one has always to consider an opportunistic polyradiculitis in patients presenting with symptoms consistent with HIV-AIDP but CD4 cells below 50/µl. Those patients should be treated presumptively for CMV infection until the CMV polymerase chain reaction (PCR) in CSF is negative.

The clinical manifestation is similar to those seen in HIV-negative patients with AIDP. First symptoms are distal pain, numbness, paraesthesia, or weakness in the limbs rapidly progressing into a relatively symmetric weakness of the limbs with or without involvement of respiratory muscles or cranial nerve-innervated muscles [61]. Diagnostic evaluation for HIV-AIDP typically includes cerebrospinal fluid analysis (CSF) which might be misleading on the first glance because about 50% of the patients show mild lymphocytic pleocytosis (up to 50/µl) and elevated protein [62]. CSF analysis is especially important in patients with CD4 cell counts far below 200/µl in whom the suspicion of an underlying opportunistic or malignant etiology is high.

Treatment recommendations are derived from experiences in HIV-negative patients and include either plasmapheresis (5-7 times) or intravenous immunoglobulin (IVIg) (2g/kg/body weight) [61]. The prognosis is in general good with an almost complete remission in more than 50% of the patients [10, 56]. It seems that the relapse rate of HIV-AIDP or the development of a secondary chronic disease (CIDP) seems to occur more often [56].

### 5.2 HIV-CIDP

HIV-CIDP is a rare disease but in our clinical experience more common than HIV- AIDP.

Patients may present with similar clinical features like their HIV-negative counterparts but one may observe overlaps with other subtypes of HIV-associated neuropathies such as HIV-DSP or ATN which can make the diagnose challenging.

Typical clinical features include an acute or subacute onset of symptoms progressing for at least 8 weeks, a relapsing/remitting course, sometimes an asymmetrical pattern, a lack of length-dependent sensory deficits, or the presence of marked large fiber sensory deficits [63]. Sensory symptoms usually consist of numbness and tingling, but painful paresthesias may be present. Many patients have impaired balance due to proprioceptive deficits [63]. Weakness usually involves both proximal and distal muscles, but can be purely distal. Patients may reveal concomitant cranial nerve deficits [63]. As stated previously, there seems to be a higher risk for HIV-infected patients to progress from AIDP into CIDP. Those patients warrant careful consideration and follow-up as they are at risk for relapses that will require sustained treatment.

CSF analysis is usually performed, but as already mentioned shows mild lymphocytic pleocytosis (up to 50/µl) and elevated protein in up to 50% of the patients [62]. Diagnostic evaluation includes NCS´s showing features of demyelination such as slowing of conduction velocity, prolonged distal latencies, and F-waves as well as conduction blocks and temporal dispersion [64]. Electromyography may reveal mild pathological spontaneous activity [1, 64]. A magnetic resonance image (MRI) with and without gadolinium of the corresponding spinal segments is not obligatory but is strongly recommended in patients with a CD4 cell count below 200/µl to exclude infiltrative processes in the nerve roots. A sural nerve biopsy is rarely necessary but may be helpful in patients representing with atypical clinical signs.

There are no RCT´s in HIV-CIDP investigating treatment options. Therefore we follow the treatment recommendation for the non HIV-CIDP counterparts, where RCT´s have demonstrated the efficacy of corticosteroids [65], plasma exchange [66, 67], and IVIg [68, 69]. In our view IVIgs (loading dose 2g/kg/body weight) are the best choice to start with. Corticosteroids (1mg/kg/body weight for 2-4 weeks and than tapering down or switching into an alternate-day therapy) might be another option, but one has to consider potential side effects such as immunosuppression, increased risk of osteonecrosis of the femoral head, osteoporosis and metabolic derangement. They are only a choice if the patient receives a stable HAART. Plasma exchange is typically used if patients are severely weak or if they relapse on prednisone or IVIg [63]. Many patients require a sustained therapy but there is no general paradigm.

## 6. Mononeuropathy and mononeuropathy multiplex

We do see mononeuropathies with HIV-infection and they are often described in the literature [10, 22, 70]. There are however no data about the incidence. They are occurring mainly as focal cranial neuropathies such as unilateral or bilateral facial palsy [71-73]. They are described in the context of seroconversion [71] but can occur also during later stages of HIV disease. If a patient is relevantly immunosuppressed one has to consider varicella zoster virus (VZV) as well as neoplastic etiologies [72].

It is unclear whether HIV-associated mononeuropathies should prompt one to start HAART. Since we are lacking data to answer that question it cannot be recommended yet. The prognosis is in general good.

Mononeuropathy multiplex (MM) is a rare disease in HIV. Patients represent often with rapidly progressive multifocal deficits and pain. The underlying etiology differs according to the stage of HIV-disease. Mononeuropathy multiplex in patients with a high CD4 count is probably immune-mediated. In contrast in patients with advanced AIDS it represents mainly an opportunistic infection like CMV-MM and shows a more severe course compared to the immune-mediate variant. Because of the high rate of co-infection with hepatitis C and secondary cryoglobulinemia it should be always considered a potential differential diagnosis.

Nerve conduction studies reveal axonal damage [74] and electromyography relevant pathological spontaneous activity in the clinically involved muscles. A CSF analysis is obligatory in patients with AIDS to search for the underlying pathology (PCR for CMV). Sural (or an alternative clinically involved nerve) biopsy if often required to show inflammatory CD8 infiltrates.

If a CMV associated mononeuropathy multiplex is suspected you may choose to treat empirically with ganciclovir and attempt HAART. The prognosis is however poor.

In patients with a high CD4 count and a suspected immune-mediated form patients may benefit from IVIg (2g/kg/body weight) or corticosteroids (100mg/d for 2 weeks, than tapering down). There are however no evidence based guidelines.

## 7. Autonomic neuropathy

It is not clear whether an autonomic HIV-associated neuropathy should be described as an isolated entity because according to our knowledge it is not known, that patients present with purely autonomic symptoms [10]. Autonomic symptoms however are often in other HIV-neuropathies, for instance HIV-SN. Studies investigating autonomic functions in HIV-infected patients describe different in part contrary results [75-79], which urges the need for larger RCT´s.

## 8. Diffuse infiltrative lymphocytosis syndrome (DILS)

DILS is a very rare systemic disease involving several organs including the peripheral nervous system. To our knowledge it occurs exclusively in HIV-infected patients [80, 81] during the middle or advanced stages of HIV disease while the CD4 cells are below 500/µl. The most common manifestations are bilateral parotid enlargement, pulmonary insufficiency, and lymphadenopathy [81]. Neurological manifestations of DILS include peripheral neuropathy, which can be the presenting symptom [82]. It has been described as a painful, symmetric neuropathy with acute or subacute onset. Other neurological manifestations are facial nerve palsy (uni- or bilateral) as well as myositis [83]. Recently a lumbosacral radiculoplexus neuropathy has been described as a clinical presentation of DILS [84].

The typical syndrome includes CD8-lymphomatosis (>1200/µl) and secondary infiltration of the visceral organ and peripheral nerves [81, 82, 85-87]. Sural nerve biopsy reveals epi- and endoneural infiltration by CD8 cells and vascular mural necrosis [82, 85]. Increased expression of HIV p24 has been demonstrated in macrophages infiltrating the nerves [80, 82, 88].

DILS is a rare disease so there are no RCT´s for treatment regimens. It is described, that patients show improvement with corticosteroids and zidovudine [82]. It is therefore recommends to initiate or continue HAART and start with corticosteroids (1 mg/kg body weight for 4 weeks than tapering slowly down to 10-20 mg) [70].

## 9. Radiculopathies

Progressive polyradiculopathy is seen in patients with advanced AIDS [89]. They are mainly CMV-associated but can be also caused by Treponema pallidum, VZV, EBV, HSV, mycobacterium tuberculosis or cryptococcus neoformans [62, 90-92]. Patients present with a rapidly evolving cauda equina syndrome, including weakness and numbness in the lower extremities and sphincter dysfunction [90].

Mandatory diagnostic evaluation includes an MRI of the lumbosakral spine, which may show meningeal enhancement [93] as well as CSF analysis. A spinal tap is essential to confirm the underlying opportunistic infection in the CSF (PCR) as well as malignancy (cytology). CSF can be surprisingly unremarkable which would still not exclude the diagnosis [94] because of the severe immunosuppression. Nerve conduction studies reveal severe axonal damage in the lower extremities combined with extensive pathological spontaneous activity in the electromyography. If a CMV infection is suspected it would speed up the diagnose to search for evidence of CMV infection in other organs (retinitis, pneumonitis, hepatitis) [10, 22].

Treatment follows the underlying etiology [95]. In cases of CMV - polyradikulitis ganciclovir is effective or alternative foscarnet, and cidofovir [89, 96, 97].

## 10. References


[1] Cornblath, D.R., et al., *Inflammatory demyelinating peripheral neuropathies associated with human T-cell lymphotropic virus type III infection.* Ann Neurol, 1987. 21(1): p. 32-40.

[2] Thornton, C.A., A.S. Latif, and J.C. Emmanuel, *Guillain-Barre syndrome associated with human immunodeficiency virus infection in Zimbabwe.* Neurology, 1991. 41(6): p. 812-5.

[3] Dalakas, M.C. and G.H. Pezeshkpour, *Neuromuscular diseases associated with human immunodeficiency virus infection.* Ann Neurol, 1988. 23 Suppl: p. S38-48.

[4] Pardo, C.A., J.C. McArthur, and J.W. Griffin, *HIV neuropathy: insights in the pathology of HIV peripheral nerve disease.* J Peripher Nerv Syst, 2001. 6(1): p. 21-7.

[5] McCarthy, B.G., et al., *Cutaneous innervation in sensory neuropathies: evaluation by skin biopsy.* Neurology, 1995. 45(10): p. 1848-1855.

[6] Polydefkis, M., et al., *Reduced intraepidermal nerve fiber density in HIV-associated sensory neuropathy.* Neurology, 2002. 58(1): p. 115-119.

[7] Bakkers, M., et al., *Intraepidermal nerve fiber density and its application in sarcoidosis.* Neurology, 2009. 73(14): p. 1142-8.

[8] Katsarava, Z., et al., *Pain related potentials by electrical stimulation of skin for detection of small-fiber neuropathy in HIV.* J Neurol, 2006. 253(12): p. 1581-4.

[9] Brinley, F.J., Jr., C.A. Pardo, and A. Verma, *Human immunodeficiency virus and the peripheral nervous system workshop.* Arch.Neurol., 2001. 58(10): p. 1561-1566.

[10] Verma, A., *Epidemiology and clinical features of HIV-1 associated neuropathies.* J Peripher Nerv Syst, 2001. 6(1): p. 8-13.

[11] Schifitto, G., et al., *Incidence of and risk factors for HIV-associated distal sensory polyneuropathy.* Neurology, 2002. 58(12): p. 1764-1768.

[12] Morgello, S., et al., *HIV-associated distal sensory polyneuropathy in the era of highly active antiretroviral therapy: the Manhattan HIV Brain Bank.* Arch.Neurol., 2004. 61(4): p. 546-551.

[13] Schifitto, G., et al., *Markers of immune activation and viral load in HIV-associated sensory neuropathy.* Neurology, 2005. 64(5): p. 842-8.

[14] Cherry, C.L., et al., *Antiretroviral use and other risks for HIV-associated neuropathies in an international cohort.* Neurology, 2006. 66(6): p. 867-73.

[15] Lichtenstein, K.A., et al., *Modification of the incidence of drug-associated symmetrical peripheral neuropathy by host and disease factors in the HIV outpatient study cohort.* Clin Infect Dis, 2005. 40(1): p. 148-57.

[16] McArthur, J.C., B.J. Brew, and A. Nath, *Neurological complications of HIV infection.* Lancet Neurol, 2005. 4(9): p. 543-55.

[17] Hulgan, T., et al., *Mitochondrial haplogroups and peripheral neuropathy during antiretroviral therapy: an adult AIDS clinical trials group study.* Aids, 2005. 19(13): p. 1341-9.

[18] Bedlack, R.S., et al., *APOE genotype is a risk factor for neuropathy severity in diabetic patients.* Neurology, 2003. 60(6): p. 1022-4.

[19] Bedlack, R.S., W.J. Strittmatter, and J.C. Morgenlander, *Apolipoprotein E and neuromuscular disease: a critical review of the literature.* Arch Neurol, 2000. 57(11): p. 1561-5.

[20] Pettersen, J.A., et al., *Sensory neuropathy in human immunodeficiency virus/acquired immunodeficiency syndrome patients: protease inhibitor-mediated neurotoxicity.* Ann Neurol, 2006. 59(5): p. 816-24.

[21] Tagliati, M., et al., *Peripheral nerve function in HIV infection: clinical, electrophysiologic, and laboratory findings.* Arch Neurol, 1999. 56(1): p. 84-9.

[22] Keswani, S.C., et al., *HIV-associated sensory neuropathies.* AIDS, 2002. 16(16): p. 2105-2117.

[23] Bradley, W.G., et al., *Morphometric analysis of the peripheral neuropathy of AIDS.* Muscle Nerve, 1998. 21(9): p. 1188-1195.

[24] Esiri, M.M., C.S. Morris, and P.R. Millard, *Sensory and sympathetic ganglia in HIV-1 infection: immunocytochemical demonstration of HIV-1 viral antigens, increased MHC class II antigen expression and mild reactive inflammation.* J Neurol Sci, 1993. 114(2): p. 178-87.

[25] Griffin, J.W., et al., *Peripheral nerve disorders in HIV infection. Similarities and contrasts with CNS disorders.* Res Publ Assoc Res Nerv Ment Dis, 1994. 72: p. 159-82.

[26] Rance, N.E., et al., *Gracile tract degeneration in patients with sensory neuropathy and AIDS.* Neurology, 1988. 38(2): p. 265-71.

[27] Hahn, K., et al., *Impaired reinnervation in HIV infection following experimental denervation.* Neurology, 2007. 68(16): p. 1251-6.

[28] Brannagan, T.H., 3rd, et al., *Human immunodeficiency virus infection of dorsal root ganglion neurons detected by polymerase chain reaction in situ hybridization.* Ann Neurol, 1997. 42(3): p. 368-72.

[29] Nagano, I., et al., *Parvalbumin and calbindin D-28 k immunoreactivity in dorsal root ganglia in acquired immunodeficiency syndrome.* Neuropathol Appl Neurobiol, 1996. 22(4): p. 293-301.

[30] Rizzuto, N., et al., *Role of HIV in the pathogenesis of distal symmetrical peripheral neuropathy.* Acta Neuropathol, 1995. 90(3): p. 244-50.

[31] Yoshioka, M., et al., *Expression of HIV-1 and interleukin-6 in lumbosacral dorsal root ganglia of patients with AIDS.* Neurology, 1994. 44(6): p. 1120-30.

[32] Jones, G., et al., *Peripheral nerve-derived HIV-1 is predominantly CCR5-dependent and causes neuronal degeneration and neuroinflammation.* Virology, 2005. 334(2): p. 178-193.

[33] Apostolski, S., et al., *Complement dependent cytotoxicity of sensory ganglion neurons mediated by the gp120 glycoprotein of HIV-1.* Immunol Invest, 1994. 23(1): p. 47-52.

[34] Keswani, S.C., et al., *Schwann cell chemokine receptors mediate HIV-1 gp120 toxicity to sensory neurons.* Ann.Neurol., 2003. 54(3): p. 287-296.

[35] Apostolski, S., et al., *The gp120 glycoprotein of human immunodeficiency virus type 1 binds to sensory ganglion neurons.* Ann Neurol, 1993. 34(6): p. 855-63.

[36] Hahn, K., et al., *Differential effects of HIV infected macrophages on dorsal root ganglia neurons and axons.* Exp Neurol, 2008. 210(1): p. 30-40.

[37] Melli, G.a.H.A., *In Vitro Models of HIV-associated Neuropathies Differ in Pathogenic Site of Action.* 12th conference on retroviruses and opportunistic infections . 2005.

[38] Dalakas, M.C., C. Semino-Mora, and M. Leon-Monzon, *Mitochondrial alterations with mitochondrial DNA depletion in the nerves of AIDS patients with peripheral neuropathy induced by 2'3'-dideoxycytidine (ddC).* Lab Invest, 2001. 81(11): p. 1537-44.

[39] Cherry, C.L., et al., *Exposure to dideoxynucleosides is reflected in lowered mitochondrial DNA in subcutaneous fat.* J Acquir Immune Defic Syndr, 2002. 30(3): p. 271-7.

[40] Keilbaugh, S.A., W.H. Prusoff, and M.V. Simpson, *The PC12 cell as a model for studies of the mechanism of induction of peripheral neuropathy by anti-HIV-1 dideoxynucleoside analogs.* Biochem Pharmacol, 1991. 42(1): p. R5-8.

[41] Medina, D.J., et al., *Comparison of mitochondrial morphology, mitochondrial DNA content, and cell viability in cultured cells treated with three anti-human immunodeficiency virus dideoxynucleosides.* Antimicrob Agents Chemother, 1994. 38(8): p. 1824-8.

[42] Keswani, S.C., et al., *FK506 is neuroprotective in a model of antiretroviral toxic neuropathy.* Ann.Neurol., 2003. 53(1): p. 57-64.

[43] Martin, C., et al., *Antiretroviral therapy may improve sensory function in HIV-infected patients: a pilot study.* Neurology, 2000. 54(11): p. 2120-7.

[44] Estanislao, L.G.A.D.R.A.S.D., *HIV myelopathy, peripheral neuropathy and myopathy.*, in *Clicial Neurovirology*, A.B.J. Nath, Editor. 2003, Informa healthcare: New York. p. 283.

[45] Schifitto, G., et al., *Long-term treatment with recombinant nerve growth factor for HIV-associated sensory neuropathy.* Neurology, 2001. 57(7): p. 1313-1316.

[46] Evans, S.R., et al., *A randomized trial evaluating Prosaptide for HIV-associated sensory neuropathies: use of an electronic diary to record neuropathic pain.* PLoS ONE, 2007. 2(6): p. e551.

[47] Hahn, K., et al., *Collateral sprouting of human epidermal nerve fibers following intracutaneous axotomy.* J.Peripher.Nerv.Syst., 2006. 11(2): p. 142-147.

[48] Phillips, T.J., et al., *Pharmacological treatment of painful HIV-associated sensory neuropathy: a systematic review and meta-analysis of randomised controlled trials.* PLoS ONE, 2010. 5(12): p. e14433.

[49] Hahn, K., et al., *A placebo-controlled trial of gabapentin for painful HIV-associated sensory neuropathies.* J Neurol, 2004. 251(10): p. 1260-6.

[50] Simpson, D.M., et al., *Lamotrigine for HIV-associated painful sensory neuropathies: a placebo-controlled trial.* Neurology, 2003. 60(9): p. 1508-14.

[51] d'Arminio Monforte, A., et al., *Insights into the reasons for discontinuation of the first highly active antiretroviral therapy (HAART) regimen in a cohort of antiretroviral naive patients. I.CO.N.A. Study Group. Italian Cohort of Antiretroviral-Naive Patients.* Aids, 2000. 14(5): p. 499-507.

[52] Husstedt, I.W., et al., *[Highly active antiretroviral therapy of neuro-AIDS. Side effects on the nervous system and interactions].* Nervenarzt, 2009. 80(10): p. 1133-4, 1136-8, 1140-2.

[53] Wernicke, J.F., et al., *A randomized controlled trial of duloxetine in diabetic peripheral neuropathic pain.* Neurology, 2006. 67(8): p. 1411-20.

[54] Goldstein, D.J., et al., *Duloxetine vs. placebo in patients with painful diabetic neuropathy.* Pain, 2005. 116(1-2): p. 109-18.

[55] Kieburtz, K., et al., *A randomized trial of amitriptyline and mexiletine for painful neuropathy in HIV infection. AIDS Clinical Trial Group 242 Protocol Team.* Neurology, 1998. 51(6): p. 1682-8.

[56] Brannagan, T.H., 3rd and Y. Zhou, *HIV-associated Guillain-Barre syndrome.* J Neurol Sci, 2003. 208(1-2): p. 39-42.

[57] Fuller, G.N., J.M. Jacobs, and R.J. Guiloff, *Nature and incidence of peripheral nerve syndromes in HIV infection.* J Neurol Neurosurg Psychiatry, 1993. 56(4): p. 372-81.

[58] Piette, A.M., et al., *Acute neuropathy coincident with seroconversion for anti-LAV/HTLV-III.* Lancet, 1986. 1(8485): p. 852.

[59] Vendrell, J., et al., *Guillain-Barre syndrome associated with seroconversion for anti-HTLV-III.* Neurology, 1987. 37(3): p. 544.

[60] Parry, O., et al., *Peripheral neuropathy in individuals with HIV infection in Zimbabwe.* Acta Neurol Scand, 1997. 96(4): p. 218-22.

[61] van Doorn, P.A., L. Ruts, and B.C. Jacobs, *Clinical features, pathogenesis, and treatment of Guillain-Barre syndrome.* Lancet Neurol, 2008. 7(10): p. 939-50.

[62] Hahn, K. and I.W. Husstedt, *[HIV-associated neuropathies].* Nervenarzt, 2010. 81(4): p. 409-17.

[63] Saperstein, D.S., *Chronic acquired demyelinating polyneuropathies.* Semin Neurol, 2008. 28(2): p. 168-84.

[64] Fuglsang-Frederiksen, A. and K. Pugdahl, *Current status on electrodiagnostic standards and guidelines in neuromuscular disorders.* Clin Neurophysiol, 2011. 122(3): p. 440-55.

[65] Dyck, P.J., et al., *Prednisone improves chronic inflammatory demyelinating polyradiculoneuropathy more than no treatment.* Ann Neurol, 1982. 11(2): p. 136-41.

[66] Dyck, P.J., et al., *Plasma exchange in chronic inflammatory demyelinating polyradiculoneuropathy.* N Engl J Med, 1986. 314(8): p. 461-5.

[67] Hahn, A.F., et al., *Plasma-exchange therapy in chronic inflammatory demyelinating polyneuropathy. A double-blind, sham-controlled, cross-over study.* Brain, 1996. 119 ( Pt 4): p. 1055-66.

[68] Hahn, A.F., et al., *Intravenous immunoglobulin treatment in chronic inflammatory demyelinating polyneuropathy. A double-blind, placebo-controlled, cross-over study.* Brain, 1996. 119 ( Pt 4): p. 1067-77.

[69] Mendell, J.R., et al., *Randomized controlled trial of IVIg in untreated chronic inflammatory demyelinating polyradiculoneuropathy.* Neurology, 2001. 56(4): p. 445-9.

[70] Wulff, E.A., A.K. Wang, and D.M. Simpson, *HIV-associated peripheral neuropathy: epidemiology, pathophysiology and treatment.* Drugs, 2000. 59(6): p. 1251-1260.

[71] Serrano, P., et al., *Bilateral Bell palsy and acute HIV type 1 infection: report of 2 cases and review.* Clin Infect Dis, 2007. 44(6): p. e57-61.

[72] Belec, L., et al., *Peripheral facial paralysis and HIV infection: report of four African cases and review of the literature.* J Neurol, 1989. 236(7): p. 411-4.

[73] Schielke, E., H.W. Pfister, and K.M. Einhaupl, *Peripheral facial nerve palsy associated with HIV infection.* Lancet, 1989. 1(8637): p. 553-4.

[74] Lange, D.J., *AAEM minimonograph #41: neuromuscular diseases associated with HIV-1 infection.* Muscle Nerve, 1994. 17(1): p. 16-30.

[75] Sakhuja, A., et al., *Heart rate variability and autonomic function tests in HIV positive individuals in India.* Clin Auton Res, 2007. 17(3): p. 193-6.

[76] Craddock, C., et al., *Cardiorespiratory arrest and autonomic neuropathy in AIDS.* Lancet, 1987. 2(8549): p. 16-8.

[77] Lohmoller, G., A. Matuschke, and F.D. Goebel, *[False-positive test of autonomic neuropathy in HIV infection and AIDS? Case control study of heart rate variability in 62 HIV positive patients].* Med Klin (Munich), 1989. 84(5): p. 242-5.

[78] Compostella, C., L. Compostella, and R. D'Elia, *The symptoms of autonomic dysfunction in HIV-positive Africans.* Clin Auton Res, 2008. 18(1): p. 6-12.

[79] Chittiprol, S., et al., *Progressive dysregulation of autonomic and HPA axis functions in HIV-1 clade C infection in South India.* Psychoneuroendocrinology, 2008. 33(1): p. 30-40.

[80] Berger, J.R. and D.M. Simpson, *The pathogenesis of diffuse infiltrative lymphocytosis syndrome: an AIDS-related peripheral neuropathy.* Neurology, 1998. 50(4): p. 855-7.

[81] Itescu, S., L.J. Brancato, and R. Winchester, *A sicca syndrome in HIV infection: association with HLA-DR5 and CD8 lymphocytosis.* Lancet, 1989. 2(8661): p. 466-8.

[82] Moulignier, A., et al., *Peripheral neuropathy in human immunodeficiency virus-infected patients with the diffuse infiltrative lymphocytosis syndrome.* Ann Neurol, 1997. 41(4): p. 438-45.

[83] Attarian, S., et al., *Myositis in infiltrative lymphocytosis syndrome: clinicopathological observations and treatment.* Neuromuscul Disord, 2004. 14(11): p. 740-3.

[84] Chahin, N., et al., *HIV lumbosacral radiculoplexus neuropathy mimicking lymphoma: diffuse infiltrative lymphocytosis syndrome (DILS) restricted to nerve?* Muscle Nerve, 2010. 41(2): p. 276-82.

[85] Gherardi, R.K., et al., *Neuropathy in diffuse infiltrative lymphocytosis syndrome: an HIV neuropathy, not a lymphoma.* Neurology, 1998. 50(4): p. 1041-4.

[86] Franco-Paredes, C., et al., *Diagnosis of diffuse CD8+ lymphocytosis syndrome in HIV-infected patients.* AIDS Read, 2002. 12(9): p. 408-13.

[87] Kazi, S., et al., *The diffuse infiltrative lymphocytosis syndrome. Clinical and immunogenetic features in 35 patients.* Aids, 1996. 10(4): p. 385-91.

[88] Price, R.W., *Neuropathy complicating diffuse infiltrative lymphocytosis.* Lancet, 1998. 352(9128): p. 592-4.

[89] Miller, R.G., J.R. Storey, and C.M. Greco, *Ganciclovir in the treatment of progressive AIDS-related polyradiculopathy.* Neurology, 1990. 40(4): p. 569-74.

[90] Robinson-Papp, J. and D.M. Simpson, *Neuromuscular diseases associated with HIV-1 infection.* Muscle Nerve, 2009. 40(6): p. 1043-53.

[91] Leger, J.M., et al., *Lymphoma-induced polyradiculopathy in AIDS: two cases.* J Neurol, 1992. 239(3): p. 132-4.

[92] Lanska, M.J., D.J. Lanska, and J.W. Schmidley, *Syphilitic polyradiculopathy in an HIV-positive man.* Neurology, 1988. 38(8): p. 1297-301.

[93] Bazan, C., 3rd, et al., *Gadolinium-enhanced MRI in a case of cytomegalovirus polyradiculopathy.* Neurology, 1991. 41(9): p. 1522-3.

[94] Miller, R.F., et al., *Acute lumbosacral polyradiculopathy due to cytomegalovirus in advanced HIV disease: CSF findings in 17 patients.* J Neurol Neurosurg Psychiatry, 1996. 61(5): p. 456-60.

[95] *[Peripheral nerve diseases and myopathies associated with HIV infection].* Nervenarzt, 2000. 71(6): p. 442-50.

[96] Fuller, G.N., et al., *Ganciclovir for lumbosacral polyradiculopathy in AIDS.* Lancet, 1990. 335(8680): p. 48-9.

[97] Anders, H.J., et al., *Ganciclovir and foscarnet efficacy in AIDS-related CMV polyradiculopathy.* J Infect, 1998. 36(1): p. 29-33.

[98] Simpson, D. M., G. Schifitto, et al. (2010). "*Pregabalin for painful HIV neuropathy: a randomized, double-blind, placebo-controlled trial.*" Neurology 74(5): 413-20.

# 10

# Bone Metabolism and HIV Infection

Stefano Coaccioli
*Dept of Internal Medicine and Rheumatology, Perugia University Medical School, "Santa Maria" General Hospital, Terni, Italy*

## 1. Introduction

Osteoporosis (OP) is the most widely spread metabolic osteopathy in the Western world, and is defined as a generalised state of the skeletal structure, characterised by a low bone mass and microarchitectural alterations, with an increase in bone fragility and risk of fracture (1). OP is now considered as an evolutive disorder affecting both the mineral and organic components leading to a progressive reduction in bone density, due to an imbalance in the regulation of hormones, which normally regulates the skeletal tissues (2). There are numerous classifications of OP in existence based on its pathogenesis , age of onset, association with other pathologies and pharmacological treatment or skeletal districts involved. Alongside primary OP is the heterogeneous group of secondary OP, which is either the consequence of the core disease or of the use of drugs. HIV infection has been shown to play an important role in the development of OP (3) and high prevalence of both osteopenia (OPe) and OP have been reported in subjects with chronic HIV infection (4). Loss of body weight, low body mass index (BMI) and diminished functional capacity are among some of the risk factors which, to a large extent, contribute to the loss of bone tissues in subjects suffering from chronic HIV infection (2-8).Furthermore, the drugs used to treat HIV+ patients can also interfere with bone metabolism and contribute to loss of bone mass (16). A reduction in bone mineral density (BMD) was observed in both HIV+ patients with hypogonadism and in those without (9-11). OP seems to be most frequently observed in subjects undergoing intense antiretroviral therapy, however, the mechanism by which antiretroviral treatments interfere with bone metabolism has not yet been clearly demonstrated.

The success of highly active antiretroviral therapy (HAART) has dramatically increased the life expectancy of HIV+ patients in the developed world, however, their use has been associated with a range of side effects and complications. As people with HIV now live longer, bone disease is among the metabolic complications presenting physicians with new challenges in the management of the HIV+ patients (12). Although, OP is the most common bone disease described in HIV, but osteomalacia, usually in association with Fanconi's syndrome or in patients treated with tenofovir, is also reported (15).

The reduction in bone mass and the disruption of bone architecture increases the risk of bone fracture leading to disability, morbidity and mortality especially in the older population. One in two women and one in five men over the age of 50 years will suffer a fracture due to OP during their lifetime (13). There are concerns that as the HIV+ population ages, increased rates of bone loss may give rise to an 'epidemic' of fragility fractures (17).

Evidence is needed to inform judicious use of bone protective agents so that this situation can be avoided.

## 2. Does HIV cause low bone mineral density?

Validated risk factors for reduced BMD and fragility fracture are well established for the general population (19). They include,old age, low BMI, previous fragility fracture, low BMD at the femoral neck, parental history of hip fracture; glucocorticoid exposure; rheumatoid arthritis; current smoking; alcohol consumption of more than 3 units per day; hypogonadism, including post-menopausal status in women; prolonged immobility; malabsorption and liver cirrhosis (20). In addition, other well reported associations exist, including vitamin D deficiency, opiate (21) and other substance dependence (22) and the use of selective serotonin uptake inhibitor (SSRI) antidepressants (23). Some of the risk factors for OP described in the general population are also prevalent in people with HIV infection. The HIV+ population also has high rates of vitamin D insufficiency, high prevalence of smoking, alcohol abuse and injection drug use, opiate use and depression requiring SSRI treatment that are also risk factors for OP (25). Patients presenting late in their illness with AIDS usually have a low BMI. Immune reconstitution inflammatory syndrome (IRIS), which arises when HAART-associated immune reconstitution leads to an unmasking or worsening of features of infections such as tuberculosis, may require prolonged courses of glucocorticoid therapy (26), as may treatment of malignancies. Chronic diarrhoea resulting in malabsorption and nutritional deficiency can occur secondary to opportunistic infections or HIV directly. Androgen deficiency was common in the pre-HAART era in men presenting with AIDS-associated wasting (27) and is still seen in HIV-infected men on HAART presenting with weight loss (28). Low testosterone levels have also been reported in association with intravenous drug use (29). Of note, menstrual abnormalities are not more prevalent in HIV-infected women compared with non-infected women (30). There are growing numbers of studies reporting an increased prevalence of vitamin D deficiency in HIV-positive individuals compared to HIV-negative controls. Other studies have also demonstrated reduced 25-hydroxyvitamin D serum levels in HIV+ individuals taking HAART compared to age- and sex-matched HAART-naïve HIV+ individuals, with non-nucleoside reverse transcriptase inhibitor (NNRTI) use and, moreover, cumulative exposure to efavirenz (but not nevirapine) being specifically implicated. Considering the high prevalence of the above risk factors in the HIV-infected population, it could be argued that the increased prevalence of decreased BMD in HIV-positive individuals is not surprising. It is very challenging, however, to separate HIV-specific factors from the confounding effect of traditional risk factors which are over-represented in the HIV-positive population.

**HIV-specific risk factors.** As well as establishing the contribution of known OP risk factors within the HIV-positive population, cross-sectional and longitudinal studies have also related changes in BMD to HIV-specific factors, for example duration of HIV infection, HIV viral load and CD4 cell count, to determine whether these represent independent risk factors for reduced BMD in the HIV-positive population and consequently whether HIV infection is a risk factor for reduced BMD in its own right. The extent of the rise in CD4 cell count was directly proportional to the BMD increase at the lumbar spine in one longitudinal study of patients on HAART (31). Similar findings were seen in another longitudinal study, although without adjustment for simultaneous rise in BMI (28). The BMD increase in these two studies was also independently associated with having an undetectable HIV viral load.

In support of these findings a high HIV viral load at the time of assessment by Dual Energy X-Ray Absorptiometry (DXA) correlated positively with reduced BMD in one cross-sectional study (32), although neither high HIV viral load nor low CD4 count were associated with reduced BMD in other studies (33). A low nadir CD4 cell count has been shown to be an independent risk factor for both reduced BMD and increased fracture incidence after adjustment for BMI (34). Time from date of diagnosis and prolonged exposure to unsuppressed HIV was also found to be an independent risk factor for loss of BMD in three studies (33).

## 3. HIV-1 infection has direct influence on bone turnover

The mechanical competence of bone is maintained by the process of bone remodelling, which consists of the removal of old bone by osteoclasts and its subsequent replacement with new bone by osteoblasts. In young adult skeleton, the amounts of bone resorbed and formed are similar, thus maintaining bone mass. Bone loss may occur in OP as a result of increased resorption, decreased formation or a combination of the two. In age-related bone loss in women, both mechanisms play a role, whereas in men, reduced bone formation is the predominant changes (49).The cellular mechanisms underlying bone loss in HIV+ individuals are not well defined, although in one study, reduced bone formation and turnover were reported in iliac crest biopsies (49,50). The association between chronic inflammatory conditions and OP is well documented and receptor activator of NFkB ligand (RANKL), the key mediator of osteoclast activity, is produced by activated T cells (46). Even in the asymptomatic phase of HIV infection, levels of inflammatory cytokines such as interleukin-1 (IL-1), IL-6 and tumor necrosis factor alpha (TNFa) are increased, and these cytokines also stimulate bone resorption (51). TNFa has also been shown to mediate apoptosis of human osteoblasts in response to HIV gp120 (52). Studies recently reported that levels of RANKL were higher in HIV-infected men and correlated with reduced BMD. Osteoblast and osteoclast function is influenced by a number of factors during HIV-1 infection, including pro-inflammatory cytokines such as TNF-a, expression of receptor of activated NF-kB ligand (RANKL) and osteoprotegerin (OPG), vitamin D and calcium metabolism and hormone levels (36). Although there is not convincing evidence that osteoblasts or osteoclasts are directly infected, their function may be modulated by a variety of HIV proteins. The HIV envelope glycoprotein, gp 120, can induce TNF-a dependent apoptosis of osteoblast cell lines or primary cells (37); however many HIV-mediated effects occur without affecting cell viability. Inflammatory conditions modify bone metabolism, including a variety of factors released by T-cells and macrophages such as TNF-a, IFN-c, IL-4, macrophage inflammation protein-1 (MIP-1) and RANKL. Markers of bone resorption in advanced HIV infection correlate with TNF-a levels (38). During HIV infection the cytokine profile favors TNF-a expression and increased viral replication, whilst there is a shift towards a TH2 cytokine balance, with decreased production of IFN-c (34). In turn enhanced TNF-a levels increases expression of RANKL with resulting stimulation of osteoclast activity (39). A number of studies suggest HIV proteins can shift the OPG/RANKL ratio in favour of RANKL-mediated osteoclastic activation (40). HIV Vpr (viral protein R), a factor needed for viral replication being required for the nuclear import of the HIV-1 pre-integration complex, up-regulates RANKL, potentiating glucocorticoid-induced stimulation of RANKL (41). gp120 also stimulates RANKL (42). ARV naïve HIV-positive individuals have increased serum RANKL levels and reduced OPG/RANKL ratios, which correlate negatively with the

HIV viral load and the Z-score obtained by densitometry (43). RANKL is not only produced by osteoblasts but also by activated T-cells, which represent a likely source of enhanced RANKL expression in light of their increased numbers during HIV infection. Although the natural inhibitor of RANKL, OPG, is also enhanced in the serum of ARV naïve individuals, increased binding of OPG to another factor up regulated by HIV, TNF-related apoptosis-inducing ligand (TRAIL), in preference to RANKL, limits its availability to inhibit osteoclast activation by RANKL (44). RANK (receptor of activated NF-kB) signalling via tumour necrosis factor receptor-associated factor 6 (TRAF-6) facilitates nuclear factor kappa B (NF-kB) activation and phosphorylates (activates) c-Jun NH2- terminal kinase (JNK) 1 and Akt facilitating osteoclastogenesis. gp120 may also stimulate RANKL via activation of extracellular signal-regulated kinase (ERK) signaling. Nevertheless the specific RANK signaling events activated by HIV-1 are still being delineated. RANKL appears to limit the susceptibility of mitochondria to oxidative stress induced dysfunction in response to nucleoside reverse transcriptase inhibitors (NRTIs) by mechanisms that do not involve alterations in levels of mitochondrial superoxide dismutase (SOD) (45). These observations, in macrophage cell lines, if replicated in osteoclasts, may suggest a potential mechanism for enhanced osteoclastogenesis in response to RANKL could therefore be maintenance of mitochondrial metabolism despite increasing cell stress and therefore maintenance of osteoclast viability and prevention of apoptotic death (46). HIV proteins gp120 and the gag structural protein p55 suppress osteoblast activity in cell lines with up-regulation of the transcription factor RUNX-2 and decreased release of RANKL. p55 also suppresses osteoblast differentiation from mesenchymal stem cells (47).

## 4. Does HAART increase the risk of osteoporosis?

Protease inhibitors (PIs) and nucleoside reverse transcriptase inhibitors (NRTIs) have been the agents most widely investigated as causes for reduced BMD in HIV+ populations. However, consistent evidence for their effects is lacking and it is increasingly recognized that these may be drug rather than class-specific (48). Potential mechanisms by which antiretroviral might negatively affect BMD have been identified in vitro. Some PIs have been shown to inhibit osteogenesis and increase osteoclastogenesis, whereas others may decrease bone loss (53). Metabolic and morphologic changes have been described in patients with HIV infection receiving antiretroviral therapy (ART), including alterations in body fat distribution, dyslipidemia, lactic acidosis, glucose metabolism abnormalities, and bone metabolism abnormalities. The etiologies of these disorders are being investigated and are likely to be multifactorial. It is clear, however, that ART plays a significant role in these alterations.

## 5. Pathophysiology of osteoporosis in HIV patients

In the light of these facts, we set out to determine the incidence of OPe and OP, within a population of subjects suffering from chronic HIV infection, by calculating the biochemical parameters using the ultrasonic densitometer. The Quantitative Ultrasound Densitometry (QUS) was chosen for the fact that this exam enabled us to predict the risk of fractures, also for the vertebrae, comparable to the DEXA method (56-58), in addition to its low cost and feasibility. This study consisted of 26 HIV+ patients (mean age 47.9 ± 12.8), with a average duration of infection equal to 6.7 ± 4.8 years and seropositive duration ranging from 6

months to 16 years. This group of patients did not exhibit any associated diseases, while the BMI was equal to 24.82±1.45. No other type of pharmacological treatment was introduced other than the one for HIV infection. In this group of patients, 6 exhibited illnesses associated with HIV, such as: *pneumocystis carinii* infection, hepatocellular carcinoma, tuberculosis, cerebral neoplasia and HIV-related encephalitis. From our samples, 4 belonged to class C under the CDC classification (Centers for Disease Control - USA; 23) (59).
The aim of our study was to determine has been to observe whether the presence of seropositivity for HIV could constitute to the development of OPe and/or overt OP. Meanwhile, our group of patients fell within the age bracket well below the limit for both post-menopausal and senile OP, with a superimposable average age for either sex. The different aspects evident at the bone level during the course of HIV infection stress that , in the various forms of genesis the IPs (Protease inhibitors (PIs) seem to play a causal predominant role. Other attributable factors are in play, like the possible interference of hormonal factors (behavioural and/or nutritional) directly correlated with the state of infection, but also the dysmetabolic effects of the antiretroviral drugs depending on the mechanism and the time involved. The protocols of the HAART therapy on the hand lead with a decisive improvement in the life expectancy and quality of life of HIV+ patients, but expose to toxic effects, which generally become more frequent and severe as the treatment is prolonged, and may take effect within diverse metabolic areas. As far as the skeletal structure is concerned, such effects can seriously impair the status of bone metabolism with pathological pictures of variable graveness, ranging from OPe to osteonecrosis (with a higher risk of developing pathological fractures). It is of extreme importance to have one or more of the instruments to safely and easily individualise the alterations of bone resistance readily available for diagnostic procedures aimed at various aspects of the disease and the adverse reactions of the antiretroviral therapy, before they advance into significant clinical events. In fact, a prompt diagnosis can allow for the implementation of more efficient therapeutic and prophylactic measures. Bone resistance must be considered, in a modern sense, as a fundamental characteristic of the bones themselves, which contribute to quantitative (bone density) and qualitative factors (structural properties, biomechanical properties, bone turnover). Our study also included an ultrasonometric bone assessment and biochemical assessment - in terms of neoformation marker and bone resorption markers. Motivations which have led us to use the ultrasonic densitometer to calculate the variations of bone resistance in the population in question were based on the grounds of employing a procedure which was safe and non invasive. This decision was also based on the possibility of obtaining accurate information on all the factors influencing bone resistance (biomechanical competence and elements associated to bone quality). In the course of our study, the ultrasonic densitometer also proved to be a highly sensitive diagnostic safeguard, allowing us to individualise an elevated incidence of cases of OPe/OP in HIV+ subjects. Analysis of the ultrasonometric parameters according to sex does not show significant variations, except for the broadband ultrasound attenuation (BUA), which seems to be significantly lower in females with respect to males. Significant variations can also be observed in relation to the duration of HIV infection, with ultrasonometric values highlighting its inclination towards OPe/OP with an increase in the number of years of infection-disease. Significant, indeed, is the reduction in the values of BMD relative to the duration of infection; proving the hypothesis that HIV inhibits osteoblastic activities and triggers osteoclastic activities, resulting in a negative skeletal balance, with an annual reduction in BMD values equal to approximately 1%. As for the dosage of sieric osteocalcin,

particularly the bone neoformation index, the data obtained does not allow for the complete explanation of the significance of the diagnosis, however, it does highlight the elevated sieric concentration in women after about 10-12 years of seropositivity, conferming the ultrasonometric results showing the presence of the aggressive processes of bone mineralisation. The assessment of other bone turnover markers does not reveal any significant variations - in terms of resorption marker - in subjects belonging to diverse classes under the CDC classification, with the exception of d-PYR in the group with the most serious conditions: this marker showed an unexpected lower mean level compared to the groups with patients in less aggressive situations. Although the results obtained from our study does not enable us to reach a definitive conclusion regarding the origin of the pictures of alterated bone mineralisation during the course of HIV infection, it does emphasise the considerable incidence, and destined to increase, thanks to the ever improving life expectancy as a result of more efficient antiretroviral therapies which are better tolerated by the patients. This problem presents a particularly serious connotation in younger subjects where the consequence of a chronic reduction in bone quality and quantity could result in irreversible disability. Bear in mind that it is, therefore, advisable to predispose accurate protocols when monitoring the skeletal development in these patients, based on the use of biochemical and instrumental research. Each patient should be followed with an individual programme, appropriately prepared based on age and personal characteristics, along with regular physical activities aimed at strengthening the skeletal muscles. It should also include a healthy diet, with particular reference to daily intakes of calcium and Vitamin D (60).

## 6. References


[1] NIH Consensus Development Panel on Osteoporosis, Prevention, Diagnosis and Therapy. JAMA 2001; 285:785-95.

[2] Peck WA. Consensus Development Conference: Diagnosis, prophylaxis, and treatment of osteoporosis. Am J Med 1993; 94:646-50.

[3] Ofotokun I, Weitzmann MN. HIV and bone metabolism, Discov Med. 2011 May; 11(60):385-93.

[4] Arora S, Agrawal M, Sun L, Duffoo F, Zaidi M, Iqbal J. HIVand bone loss. Curr Osteoporos Rep. 2010 Dec;8(4):219-26.

[5] Tebas P. Osteopenia, Osteoporosis, and Other Bone Problems in HIV-Infected individuals. The PRN Notebook 2001;6(3)

[6] Grinspoon SK, Bilezikian JP. HIV Disease and the endocrine system. N Engl J Med 1992; 327:1369-65.

[7] Aukurst C, Haug CJ, Ueland T, Lien E, Müller F, Espevik T, Bollerslev J, Frøland SS. Decreased bone formative and enhanced resorptive markers in human immunodeficiency virus infection: indication of normalization of the bone-remodeling process during highly active antiretroviral therapy. J Clin Endocrinol Metab 1999; 84:145-50.

[8] Stephens EA, Das R, Madge S, Barter J, Johnson MA. Symptomatic osteoporosis in two young HIV-positive African women. AIDS 1999; 13:2605-6.

[9] Paton NIJ, Macallan DC, Griffin GE, Pazianas M. Bone mineral density in patients with human immunodeficiency virus infection. Calcif Tissue Int 1997; 61:30-2.

[10] Mondy K, Yarasheski K, Powderly WG, Whyte M, Claxton S, DeMaarco D, Hoffman M, Tebas P. Longitudinal evolution of bone mineral density and bone markers in

human immunodeficiency virus-infected individuals. Clin Infect Dis 2003; 36:482-90.

[11] Fairfield WP, Finelstein JS, Klibanski A, Grinspoon SK. Osteopenia in eugonadal men with acquired immune deficiency syndrome. J Clin Endocrinol Metab 2001; 86:2020-6.

[12] Bhasin S, Storer TW, Javanbakht M, Berman N, Yarasheski KE, Phillips J, Dike M, Sinha-Hikim I, Shen R, Hays RD, Beall G. Testosteron replacement and resistance exercise in HIV-infected men with weight loss. JAMA 2000; 283:763-70.

[13] Grinspoon S, Corcoran C, Parlman K, Costello M, Rosenthal D, Anderson E, Stanley T, Schoenfeld D, Burrows B, Hayden D, Basgoz N, Klinbanski A. Effects of testosterone and progressive resistance training in eugonadal men with AIDS wasting, A randomized, controlled trial. Ann Intern Med 2000; 133:348-55.

[14] Morse CG, Kovacs J. Metabolic and skeletal complications of HIV infection: the price of success.JAMA, 296, 844–854. 2006.

[15] Johnell O, Kanis JA. An estimate of the worldwide prevalence and disability associated with osteoporotic fractures. Osteoporos Int, 17, 1726–1733. 2006

[16] Health Protection Agency (HPA) (2008) HIV in the United Kingdom. London.

[17] Brown TT, Qaqish RB. Antiretroviral therapy and the prevalence of osteopenia and osteoporosis: a meta-analytic review. AIDS, 20, 2165–2174,2006

[18] Triant VA, Brown TT, Lee H, Grinspoon SK Fracture prevalence among human immunodeficiency virus (HIV)-infected versus non-HIV-infected patients in a large U.S healthcare system. J Clin Endocrinol Metab, 93, 3499–3504.

[19] Singh K, Moyle GJ (2006) Bone mineral abnormalities in persons with HIV infection: signal or noise?AIDS Read, 16, 407–10–413–8.

[20] Amorosa V, Tebas P. HIV/AIDS bone disease and HIV infection. Clin Infect Dis, 42, 108–114. (2006)

[21] Rivas P, Go´ golas M, Garcia-Delgado R, Diaz-Curie M, Goyenechea A, Fernandez-Guerrero M (2008). Evolution of bone mineral density in AIDS patients on treatment with zidovudine/ lamivudiine plus abacavir or lopinavir/ritonavir. HIV Med, 9, 89–95.

[22] Bolland MJ, Grey AB, Gamble GD, Reid IR. Low body weight mediates the relationship between HIV infection and low bone mass density: a meta-analysis. J Clin Endocrinol Metab. 2007;92(12):4522-8.

[23] Pollock E, Klotsas AE, Compston J, Gkrania-Klotsas E. Bone health in HIV infection. Br Med Bull. 2009;92:123-33.

[24] Cazanave C, Dupon M, Lavignolle-Aurillac V, Barthe N, Lawson- Ayayi S, Mehsen N, et al; Groupe d'Epidémiologie Clinique du SIDA en Aquitaine. Reduced bone mineral density in HIV-infected patients: prevalence and associated factors. AIDS. 2008;22(3):395-402.

[25] Madeddu G, Spanu A, Solinas P, Calia GM, Lovigu C, Chessa F, et al. Bone mass loss and vitamin D metabolism impairment in HIV patients receiving highly active antiretroviral therapy. Q J Nucl Med Mol Imaging. 2004;48(1):39-48.

[26] Mondy K, Yarasheski K, Powderly WG, Whyte M, Claxton S, et al. Longitudinal evolution of bone mineral density and bone markers in human immunodeficiency virus-infected individuals. Clin Infect Dis. 2003;36(4):482-90.

[27] Aukrust P, Huag C, Ueland T, Lien E, Müller F, Espevik T, et al. Decreased bone formative and enhanced resorptive markers in human immunodeficiency virus infection: indication of normalization of the bone-remodeling process during highly active antiretroviral therapy. J Clin Endocrinol Metab. 1999;84(1):145-50.

[28] Yin MT, Shane E. Low bone-mineral in patients with HIV: pathogenesis and clinical significance. Curr Opin Endocrinol Diabetes. 13:497-502.

[29] Serrano S, Marinoso ML, Soriano JC, Rubiés-Prat J, Aubia J, Coll J, et al. Bone remodeling in human immunodeficiency virus-1-infected patients: histomophometric study. Bone. 1995;16:185-91.

[30] Grijsen ML, Vrouenraets SM, Steingrover R, Lips P, Reiss P, Wit FW, Prins JM. High prevalence of reduced bone mineral density in primary HIV-1-infected men. AIDS. 2010 Sep 10;24(14):2233-8.

[31] Stone B, Dockrell D, Bowman C, McCloskey E HIV and bone disease. Arch Biochem Biophys. 2010 Nov 1;503(1): 66-77

[32] NIH Consensus Development Panel. Osteoporosis prevention, diagnosis, and therapy. Journal of the American Medical Association. 2001;285(6):785–795

[33] Brown TT, Ruppe MD, Kassner R, Kumar P, Kehoe T, Dobs AS, et al. Reduced bone mineral density in human immunodeficiency virus-infected patients and its association with increased central adiposity and postload hyperglycemia. J Clin Endocrinol Metab. 2004;89(3):1200-6.

[34] Tsekes G, Chrysos G, Douskas G, Paraskeva D, Mangafas N, Giannakopoulos D, et al. Body composition changes in protease inhibitor-naive HIV-infected patients treated with two nucleoside reverse transcriptase inhibitors. HIV Med. 2002;3(2):85-90.

[35] Pan G, Yang Z, Ballinger SW, McDonald JM. Pathogenesis of osteopenia/osteoporosis induced by highly active anti-retroviral therapy for AIDS. Ann N Y Acad Sci. 2006;1068:297-308.

[36] Wang MW, Wei S, Faccio R, Takeshita S, Tebas P, Powderly WG, et al. The HIV protease inhibitor ritonavir blocks osteoclastogenesis and function by impairing RANKL-induced signaling. J Clin Invest. 2004;114:206-13.

[37] Amorosa V, Tebas P. Bone disease and HIV infection. Clin Infect Dis. 2006:42:108-14.

[38] Vescini F, Borderi M, Buffa A, Sinicropi G, Tampellini L, Chiodo F, et al. Bone mass in HIV-infected patients: focus on the role of therapy and sex. J Acquir Immune Defic Syndr. 2003;33(3):405-7.

[39] Serrano S, Marinoso ML, Soriano JC, Rubies-Prat J, Aubia J, Coll J et al. (1995) Bone remodeling in human immunodeficiency virus-1-infected patients. A histomorphometric study. Bone, 16, 185–191.

[40] Raisz LG (2005) Pathogenesis of osteoporosis: concepts, conflicts and prospects. J Clin Invest, 115, 3318–3325.

[41] Gibellini D, De Crignis E, Ponti C, Cimatti L, Borderi M, Tschon M et al. (2008) HIV-1 triggers apoptosis in primary osteoblasts and HOBIT cells through TNFalpha activation. J Med Virol, 80, 1507–1514.

[42] Gibellini D, Borderi M, De Crignis E, Cicola R, Vescini F, Caudarella R et al. (2007). RANKL/OPG/TRAIL plasma levels and bone mass loss evaluation in antiretroviral naïve HIV-1-positive men. J Med Virol, 79, 1446–1454.

[43] Chirch LM, Feiner J, Go R, Mynarcik D, McNurlan M, Gelato M et al. (2006). Osteopenia in patients with HIV infection is not associated with elevated sTNFR2 levels. Clin Infect Dis, 43, 1084–1085.

[44] Villamor E (2006) A potential role for vitamin D on HIV infection?Nutr Rev, 64, 226–233.

[45] Pan G, Yang Z, Ballinger SW, McDonald JM (2006). Pathogenesis of osteopenia/osteoporosis induced by highly active anti-retroviral therapy for AIDS. Ann N Y AcadSci, 1068, 297–308.

[46] Malizia AP, Vioreanu MH, Doran PP, Powderly WG (2007) HIV1 protease inhibitors selectively induce inflammatory chemokine expression in primary human osteoblasts. Antiviral Res, 74, 72–76.

[47] Tran H, Robinson S, Mikhailenko I, Strickland DK (2003) Modulation of the LDL receptor and LRP levels by HIV protease inhibitors. J Lipid Res, 44, 1859–1869.

[48] Carr A, Miller J, Eisman JA, Cooper DA (2001) Osteopenia in HIV-infected men: association with asymptomatic lactic acidemia and lower weight pre-antiretroviral therapy. AIDS, 15, 703–709.

[49] Gyllensten K, Josephson F, Lidman K, Saaf M (2006) Severe vitamin D deficiency diagnosed after introduction of antiretroviral therapy including efavirenz in a patient living at latitude AIDS, 20, 1906–1907

[50] Mondy K, Yarasheski K, Powderly WG, et al. Longitudinal evolution of bone mineral density and bone markers in human immunodeficiency virus infected individuals. Clin Infect Dis 2003;36:482–90.

[51] Nolan D, Upton R, McKinnon E, et al. Stable or increasing bone mineral density in HIV-infected patients treated with nelfinavir or indinavir. AIDS 2001;15:1275–80.

[52] Dolan SE, Kanter JR, Grinspoon S. Longitudinal analysis of bone density in human immunodeficiency virus-infected women. J Clin Endocrinol Metab 2006;91:2938–45.

[53] Kopicko JJ, Momodu I, Adedokun A, et al. Characteristics of HIV-infected men with low serum testosterone levels. Int J STD AIDS 1999;10:817–20.

[54] Rietschel P, Corcoran C, Stanley T. Prevalence of hypogonadism among men with weight loss related to human immunodeficiency virus infections who were receiving highly active antiretroviral therapy. ClinInfect Dis 2000;31:1240–4.

[55] Haug CJ, Aukrust P, Lien E, et al. Disseminated Mycobacterium avium complex infection in AIDS: immunopathogenic significance of an activated tumor necrosis factor system and depressed serum levels of 1,25 dihydroxyvitamin D. J Infect Dis 1996;173:259–62.

[56] Fakruddin M, Yin M, Laurence J. Pathophysiologic correlates of RANKL deregulation in HIV infection and its therapy [abstract]. In: Program and abstracts of the 12th Conference on Retroviruses and Opportunistic Infections (Boston). Alexandria, VA: Foundation for Retrovirology and Human Health, 2005.

[57] McKelvie ML, Palmer SB. The interaction of Ultrasound with cancellous bone. Phys Med Biol 1991; 36:1331-40.

[58] Luis O, Moreels X, Osteaux M. Reproducibility of the phalanx osteosonografy and relation forearm peripheral quantitative computed tomography. European Journal of Radiology 1998; 28:270-5.

[59] Feltrin GP, Nardin M, Marangon A, Khadin Y, Calderone M, De Conti G, Quantitative ultrasound at the hand phalanges: comparison with quantitative computed tomography of the lumbar spine in postmenopausal women. Eur Radiol 2000; 10:826-31.

[60] Coaccioli S., Del Giorno R., Crapa G. et al.: Study of bone metabolism in patients with chronic HIV infection. Clin Ter 2009; 160(6):451-6.

# 11

# Oral Manifestations of Paediatric HIV Infection

Omolola Orenuga[1], Mutiat Obileye[2],
Christiana Sowole[3] and Gbemisola Agbelusi[1]
[1]*Faculty of Dentistry, College of Medicine, University of Lagos, Lagos*
[2]*Dental Clinics, Lagos State University Teaching Hospital, Ikeja*
[3]*Dental Public Health, Chatham*
[1,2]*Nigeria*
[3]*United Kingdom*

## 1. Introduction

Immune defects in children have been shown to have profound effects on oral tissues. (Joint United Nations Program on HIV/AIDS [UNAIDS], 2002, 2005).

Oral lesions are among the earliest and most common clinical sign of infection with the Human Immunodeficiency Virus (HIV), are important indicators and can predict progression of HIV infection. A number of studies have shown that oral lesions are common in HIV infected patients. Knowledge and awareness of the signs and symptoms, of oral lesions that may be indicative of the patients' HIV status will assist in instituting the appropriate careful steps of management at an early stage for better prognosis. (Chadwick & Yogev, 1995; Eldridge & Gallagher, 2000; Fowler et al., 2000; Gray & McIntyre, 1999; Ramos-Gomez, 1997; Sullivan, 2003; Working Group on Mother To Child Transmission of HIV, 1995). A thorough understanding of these lesions has implications for all health care professionals.

HIV progression is faster and more severe in children, due to the immaturity of the immune system. Most children born with HIV infection are symptomatic at birth, however time between birth and initial symptoms and signs varies considerably. The median age of paediatric patients at the time of an AIDS diagnosis is 12 months with oral manifestations often the first sign of infection in approximately half of all infected children. (Magalhaes et al, 2001; Ramos-Gomez, 1997, Ramos-Gomez et al., 2000; Rosemberg & Faucias 1994).

Most children will develop one or more oral manifestation of HIV infection during the course of the disease, similar to that seen in adults. (Leao et al., 2009; UNAIDS 2002, 2004). AIDS has emerged as the seventh leading cause of death among infants and children in the United States of America (USA), and a leading cause of death among minority groups and in low income countries (LINCs). (Centres for Disease Control and Prevention [CDC] 1993; Ramos-Gomez et al., 2000; UNAIDS, 2009)

Majority of paediatric HIV infections are the result of Mother To Child Transmission (MTCT). The increasing proportion of infected children achieving adulthood highlights the need for multidisciplinary approach to management and thus facilitates transition to adult care while maintaining strategies specific for mother to child acquired infections. (Giaquinto et al, 2010; Massarente et al 2011; Swendeman et al, 2009).

Evidence of HIV disease progression in both adult and paediatric patients is marked by oral manifestations and general periodontal status, and oral symptoms and signs may have prognostic value that is independent of CD4 status or other commonly used markers. (Greenspan & Greenspan, 1999; Ramos-Gomez et al., 2000). Oral lesions commonly associated with paediatric HIV infection include oral candidiasis, herpes simplex virus infection, linear gingival erythema and recurrent aphthous ulcers. Oral candidiasis is the commonest oral manifestation in children and may be associated with burning sensation in the mouth, problems with nutrition and changes in taste. (Orne-Glieman et al., 2008) Oral candidiasis has also been associated with HIV disease progression and immune system deterioration as evidenced by low CD4 counts in both adults and children with the infection. However, parotid gland enlargement is indicative of a better prognosis, with slower disease progression or long term survival. (Katz et al., 1993; Magalhaes et al., 2001; Ramos-Gomez et al., 1999)

Recognition of these early oral signs during routine examinations and in surgical procedures is important for diagnosis and treatment, which allows for early intervention, clinical staging of the infection leading to better prognosis, reduced morbidity and improved quality of life in this population. The early diagnosis of these lesions will help in assessing disease progression especially in LINCs where limited resources hamper disease specific interventions.

## 2. Literature review

### 2.1 Epidemiology

HIV is a global pandemic, which continues to escalate throughout developing countries compared to a notable stabilization in new cases and fatalities in some developed countries. The number of people living with HIV worldwide continued to grow in 2008, reaching an estimated 33. 4 million. The total number of people living with the virus in 2008 was more than 20% higher than the number in 2000, and the prevalence reported to be roughly threefold higher than in 1990. (UNAIDS, 2009). The continuing rise in the population of people living with HIV reflects the combined effects of continued high rates of new HIV infections and the beneficial impact of antiretroviral therapy. As of December 2008, approximately 4 million people in low- and middle-income countries were receiving antiretroviral therapy. An estimated 430,000 new HIV infections occurred among children under the age of 15 in 2008. Most of these new infections are believed to stem from transmission in-utero, during delivery or post-partum as a result of breastfeeding. The number of children newly infected with HIV in 2008 was roughly 18% lower than in 2001. To date, UNAIDS estimates that 40 million are living with HIV/AIDS, with more than 95% in developing countries, including 28. 5% in sub-Saharan Africa, and out which at least 2. 1 million are children under the age of 15years. (Barnett & Whiteside, 2006; Greene, 2007; Nigeria, 1992; UNAIDS, 2002, 2004, 2005, 2006, 2009).

Studies on oral manifestations of HIV infection have reported that these lesions are common, with a wide variation in the prevalence of lesions; 41% to 99. 5% prevalence reported in studies carried out on populations of intravenous drug abusers and other risk groups. (Arendorf et al., 1998; Barone et al., 1990; Ceballos-Salobrena et al., 1996; Onunu & Obuekwe, 2002; Sauer et al.,1995; Schimdt-Westhausen et al 1997., Ukpebor & Braimoh, 2006; Wright, 2003). The wide variations in the prevalence of oral lesions in the literature have been attributed to a number of factors, and include sample randomization, sample size, clinical stage at presentation, risk group, education, race, socioeconomic status and access to health care. Most studies have reported a high prevalence of at least one oral lesion in children with HIV infection, with oral candidiasis being the most prevalent oral condition. (Barasch et al., 2000; Glick, 2005; Katz et al., 1993; Lamster et al., 1994; Ramos-Gomez et al., 1996; Yengopal et al., 2011).

### 2.2 Pathogenesis

The acquired immunodeficiency syndrome (AIDS) was first observed in 1981 in young male homosexuals in the United States of America (USA); though there are evidences that sporadic cases may have been in existence before then. (Olumide, 2002; Scully, 1997) The causative organism was identified and named as the Human Immunodeficiency Virus (HIV). It is a member of the lentevirus subfamily. Two strains HIV-1 and HIV-2 the primary aetiological viruses for AIDS were described in 1983 and 1986 respectively. However, HIV infection in children was first described in 1983. (Oleske et al., 1983). HIV disease in infants and children, as in adults, is a progressive disease with a clinical spectrum ranging from asymptomatic infection to profound and eventual fatal immunosuppression. AIDS is the point on this spectrum where significant immunodeficiency causes emergence of conditions that meet the criteria for the Centres for Disease Control (CDC) definition of AIDS diagnosis. (Ammann, 1999). The hallmark of immunodeficiency caused by HIV infection is the depletion of cells of the immune system: CD4+ T lymphocytes, macrophages, monocytes and dendritic cells that express the CD4 receptors. The gradual decrease in the number of cells of the immune system and the functional decline of these cells lead to the breakdown of the immune system, exposing infected individuals to a wide variety of viral, bacterial, fungal and parasitic infections as well as the development of malignancies that result in full blown AIDS. These conditions when occurring in the mouth constitute the oral manifestations of HIV/AIDS and may be indicators of HIV infection. (Agbelusi & Wright 2005; Zijenah & Katzenstein, 2002).

#### 2.2.1 Transmission

The epidemic in children has risen globally due to the worldwide increase in HIV prevalence in women of childbearing age. Majority of paediatric HIV/AIDS cases are as a result of transmission from mother to child. Though the source and route of transmission is multifactorial, mother to child transmission (MTCT) is the commonest mode of transmission of HIV in children. In the absence of any intervention, the risk of MTCT is 15–30% in non-breastfeeding populations and 20–45% among populations who practice prolonged breastfeeding. It is estimated that 50% of HIV-infected infants will die before the age of two. (De Cock et al., 2000; Newell et al., 2004).

Effective prevention of mother-to-child transmission involves simultaneous support for several strategies that work synergistically to reduce the odds that an infant will become infected as a result of exposure to the mother's virus. Through the reduction in overall HIV among reproductive-age women and men, the reduction of unwanted pregnancies among HIV-positive women, the provision of antiretroviral drugs to reduce the chance of infection during pregnancy and delivery and appropriate treatment, care and support to mothers living with HIV (including infant feeding), programmes are able to reduce the chance that infants will become infected. In ideal conditions, the provision of antiretroviral prophylaxis and replacement feeding can reduce transmission from an estimated 30% to 35% with no intervention to around 1% to 2%. Most countries have not yet reached all pregnant women with these services, let alone significantly reduced HIV prevalence among reproductive-age individuals or unwanted pregnancies among HIV-positive women. (Ammann 2006; UNAIDS 2009).

### 2.3 Clinical aspect of HIV disease in children

#### 2.3.1 Orofacial manifestations

The development of HIV infection in children has different characteristics to those noted in adults, due mainly to the earlier acquisition of the virus, combined with the immaturity of the immunologic system and other body structures. The clinical features of pediatric HIV infection includes the appearance of various oral lesions, some of which are considered AIDS diagnosis markers, such as recurrent oral candidiasis and chronic enlargement of the parotid. The most frequently associated oral lesions are: candidiasis, herpes simplex infection, linear gingival erythema (LGE), parotid enlargement and recurrent aphthous stomatitis. Other viral and bacterial infections, including periodontal infections are less commonly associated, while hairy leukoplakia and Kaposi's sarcoma are rarely seen in HIV-infected children. (Greenspan D, 1998; Soares et al., 2004). The oral manifestations of HIV disease in adults and children were classified before the advent of anti-retroviral drugs (ART). Patients who do not receive ART are likely still to have the common oral features of HIV disease: candidiasis (typically pseudomembranous candidiasis), hairy leukoplakia, Kaposi's sarcoma, non-Hodgkin's lymphoma and, perhaps periodontal disease. (Frezzini et al., 2006). Dry mouth as a result of decreased salivary flow rate may not only increase the risk of dental caries but further impact negatively on quality of life because of difficulty in chewing, swallowing and tasting food. According to the World Oral Health Report 2003 priority is given to effective prevention of oral manifestations of HIV/AIDS through additional actions. These actions are integral components of WHO and joint United Nations global programs for control of HIV/AIDS. These collaborative programs include but are not limited to the identification of the most indicative oral manifestations of HIV/AIDS, training of other health professional and dissemination of information on disease prevention and recognition. (Petersen, 2003; 2004; UNAIDS 2004; WHO, 2003).

#### 2.3.2 Overview of treatment

Anti retroviral drugs (ARDs) used in the management of HIV-infection now principally comprise four classes of retroviral agents:

Nucleoside analog reverse transcriptase inhibitors (NRTIs);

Non-nucleoside analog reverse transcriptase inhibitors (NNRTIs);

Protease inhibitors (Pis) and Entry inhibitors.

However, effective anti-retroviral therapies are rarely available to HIV-infected people in LINCs and the developing world, particularly areas of Africa. Moreover, only a handful of ARDs in the current WHO guidelines have solid formulations in doses appropriate for pediatric use and pediatric fixed-dose drug combinations are scarce.

## 3. Oral manifestations in paediatric HIV infection

### 3.1 Classification of oral lesions in HIV infection

Oral lesions seen in HIV disease have been classified by the EC Clearing house on oral problems related to HIV infection and WHO collaborating centre on Oral manifestations of

the immunodeficiency virus into three main groups. (Coogan et al 2005; Greenspan JS & D, 1995; Leao et al., 2009). These are:
Group 1: Lesions strongly associated with HIV infection
Group 2: Lesions less commonly associated with HIV infection
Group 3: Lesions seen in HIV infection
These lesions have also been grouped according to their aetiology as:

- Neoplastic conditions
- Bacterial infections
- Fungal infections
- Viral infections
- Autoimmune disorders
- Neurological disturbances
- Other conditions.

The spectrum of oral diseases in HIV infected children differs significantly from that of adults. These differences have been attributed to differences in the viral induced immunopathologic changes in these two different age groups as well as to being the result of decreased exposure at a young age to certain viruses, which reduces the risk for diseases such as oral hairy leukoplakia, oral warts, Kaposi's sarcoma and lymphoma. Despite this limited range of diseases, most children will develop one or more oral manifestation of HIV infection during the course of the disease, similar to that seen in adults Orofacial manifestations of paediatric HIV infection have been divided into four groups. (Flaitz &Hicks, 2003; Fonseca et al., 2000).

### 3.1.1 Oral lesions commonly associated with paediatric HIV infection

- Candidiasis-
  Pseudomembranous
  Erythematous
  Angular cheilitis
- Herpes simplex viral infection
- Linear gingival erythema
- Major salivary gland enlargement
- Recurrent aphthous ulcers-

Minor, major, and herpetiform

### 3.1.2 Oral lesions less commonly associated with paediatric HIV infection

- Bacterial infections
- Periodontal diseases
- Necrotizing ulcerative gingivitis (NUG)
- Necrotizing ulcerative periodontitis (NUP)
- Necrotizing stomatitis (NS)
- Viral infections (cytomegalovirus, human papilloma virus, varicella zoster virus, molluscum contagiosum)
- Xerostomia

### 3.1.3 Oral lesions strongly associated with HIV infection but rare in children

- Kaposi's sarcoma

- Non-Hodgkin's lymphoma
- Oral hairy leukoplakia
- Tuberculosis-related ulcers

### 3.1.4 Oral conditions with increased severity in paediatric HIV infection

- Gingivitis and periodontitis (increased gingival and plaque indices)
- Over-retained primary teeth
- Delayed eruption of primary and permanent teeth
- Primary dentition caries

## 4. Oral lesions commonly associated with paediatric HIV infection

### 4.1 Oral candidiasis

This is the most common oral soft tissue manifestation of paediatric HIV infection. (Barasch et al., 2000; Fonseca et al 2000; Kline 1996; Ramos-Gomez et al., 1999). Candidiasis is often the first clinically observable manifestation of HIV infection, with up to 72% of these children developing the disease. (Flaitz & Hicks 2003).

Candidiasis has been reported as the commonest oral lesion in several studies and has been used as a clinical marker of the disease as the frequency of oral candidiasis usually correlates with a falling CD4+ T lymphocyte count and a rising HIV viral load Pseudomembranous candidiasis remains the commonest variant, followed by erythymatous candidiasis and angular cheilitis. Studies indicate that oral candidiasis is prevalent in HIV/AIDS and has been reported in up to 72% of all pediatric HIV infection. (Flaitz & Hicks 2003; Kline 1996; Naidoo & Chikte 2004; Obileye 2006; Olaniyi & Sunday 2005; Ramos-Gomez et al 1999; Sowole et al., 2009). However, oral pseudo-membranous candidiasis is not uncommon in healthy infants in the first six months of life. However, in immuno-competent children, Candida lesions are often mild, readily amenable to treatment, or regress spontaneously and are rarely seen beyond infancy in the absence of predisposing factors. In addition, concurrent oral infection is the most common clinical presentation of oesophageal candidiasis, a very debilitating and symptomatic AIDS-defining condition in children. (Chiou et al., 2000) Candida albicans was the primary aetiological agent but recently other species including C. tropicalis, C. krusei, C. glabrata, C. parasilosis, C. pseudotropicalis, C. gulliermondi, have been identified. C. dubliniensis, a newly emerging pathogen. isolated almost exclusively in HIV infected and oncology patients has been identified. (Brown et al 2000).

Clinical features of candidiasis are variable depending on the form of the disease. The different forms associated with HIV
infection are:

#### 4.1.1 Pseudomembraneous candidiasis or thrush

This presents as non-adherent multifocal, creamy white to yellow papules or plaques overlying the oral mucosa. Removal of this material often leaves an erythematous mucosal surface, which occasionally bleeds. It typically occurs on the buccal mucosa, mucobuccal folds, dorsolateral tongue and the oropharynx, but may occur throughout the oropharyngeal region. (Flaitz & Hicks 1999, 2003; Ramos-Gomez et al 1999). (Figures 1, 2 & 3).

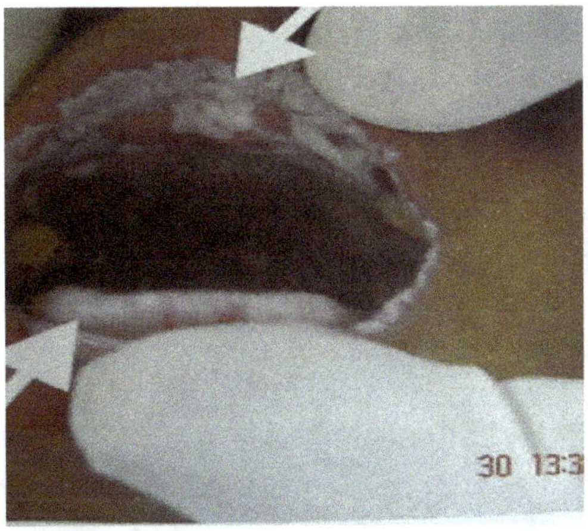


Fig. 1. Pseudomembranous candidiasis.

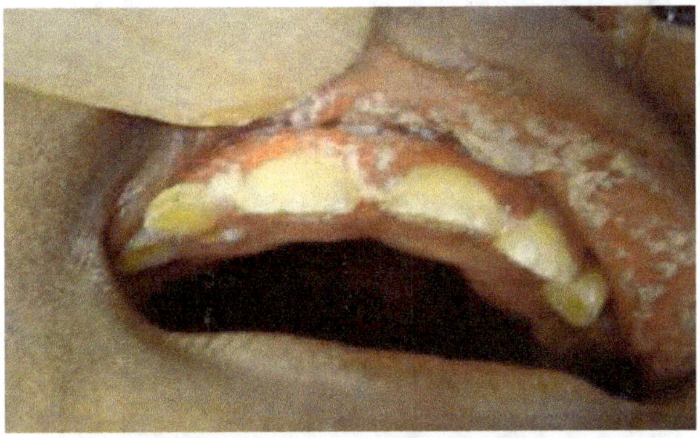

Fig. 2. Pseudomembranous candidiasis.

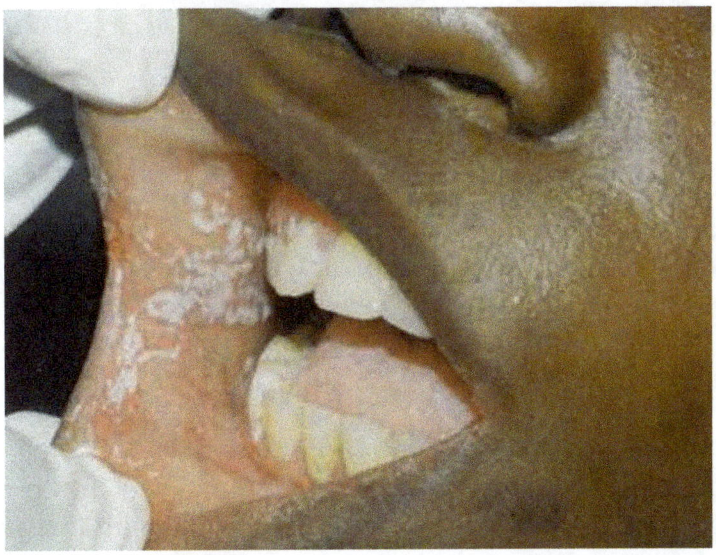

Fig. 3. Pseudomembranous candidiasis.

### 4.1.2 Erythematous (atrophic) candidiasis

This varies from diffuse to patchy redness throughout the oral mucosa. Multiple flat red patches of varying intensity occur. It sometimes presents as pinpoint to macular erythema,

which mimics a bleeding diathesis or submucosal trauma. They are most commonly located on the palate and the dorsum of the tongue. Non adherent filmy white to creamy plaques may be seen concurrently with this lesion. When the tongue is involved, there is selective loss of filiform papillae, resulting in a red, smooth to beaded mucosal surface.
Median Rhomboid Glossitis is a specific type of erythematous candidiasis that presents as red, smooth, depapillated, persistent oral patch in the middle of the dorsum of the tongue. Tenderness or a burning sensation may be experienced. (Flaitz & Hicks 2003; Ramos-Gomez et al 1999). (Figures 4, 5 & 6)

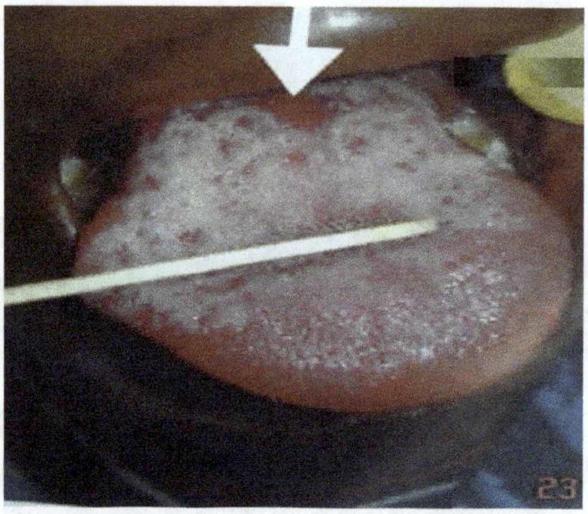

Fig. 4. Erythematous candidiasis.

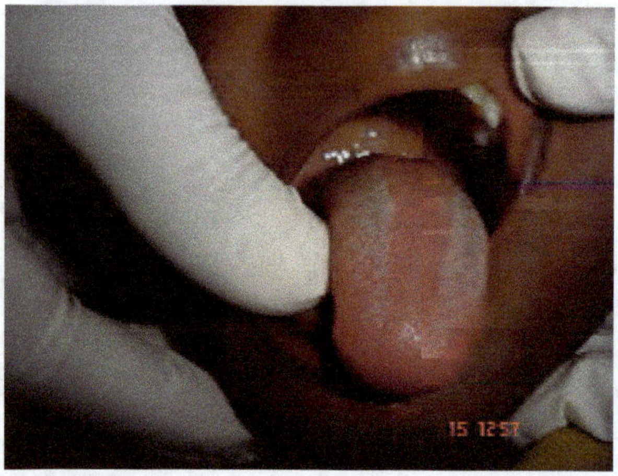

Fig. 5. Erythematous candidiasis.

#### 4.1.3 Angular cheilitis

This presents as linear red or ulcerated fissures radiating from the corners of the mouth. They are typically bilateral, and multiple red papules may be found when the adjacent peri-oral skin is involved. (Figure 7) It commonly occurs in conjunction with either of the other intraoral forms. (Flaitz & Hicks, 2003; Ramos-Gomez et al 1999)

**Diagnosis**

Definitive diagnosis of oral candidiasis is made from exfoliative cytological smears using PAS stain or potassium hydroxide or Gomori's methenamine silver stain. Detection of

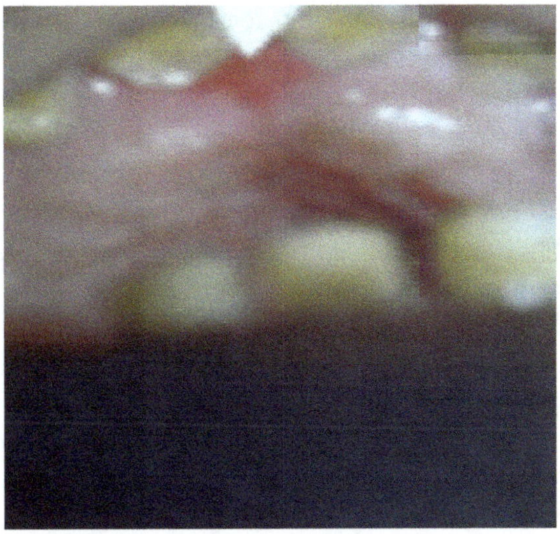

Fig. 6. Erythematous candidiasis (interdental papilla).

fungal hyphae and/or pseudohyphae is necessary for microscopic diagnosis. Biopsy of the oral lesion can also be carried out. Fungal cultures are not usually necessary but are helpful in species identification when lesions are refractory to antifungal therapy. (Flaitz & Hicks 1999, 2003).

**Treatment**

Candidiasis should be treated promptly and thoroughly with topical antifungal agents such as nystatin or clotrimazole. prognosis depends on disease severity, oesophageal involvement, recurrence rate, drug compliance, the child's age and previous history and response to antifungal therapy. (Abrams 2000; Flaitz & Hicks 1999). Both oral and esophageal candidiasis have a high propensity to recur unless antifungal therapy is continued. Therapy is indicated to prevent the symptoms of pain, burning sensation, soreness and dysphagia that may occur. (Ramos-Gomez et al.,1999)

Topical Antifungal Agents

These include Nystatin, Ketoconazole, Clotrimazole, Amphotericin B and Miconazole.

- Nystatin suspension (100,000U/ml) 100,000-500,000 U 6 hourly for 14days
  Oral pastille (200,000U) 6 hourly for 14 days
- Clotrimazole troche (10mg) 10mg 4-5 times daily for 14days
- Amphotericin B oral suspension (100mg/ml) 100mg 6 hourly for 14days
- Miconazole oral gel (25mg/ml) 2. 5-5ml 6 hourly for 14 days

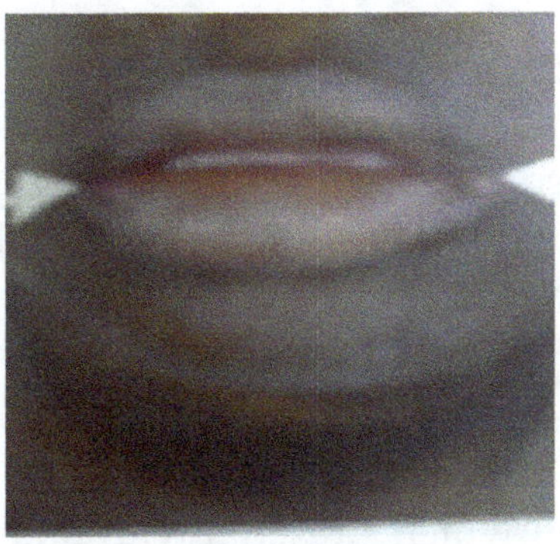

Fig. 7. Angular cheilitis.

The long term use of these preparations may lead to increased incidence of caries because of their high dextrose or sucrose content. Topical fluoride should thus be prescribed. Alternatively, antifungal preparations designed for vagina use such as pessaries which contain less dextrose and sucrose may be used. (Greenspan 1994).

Topical creams and ointments containing Nystatin, ketoconazole or Clotrimazole are used in the treatment of angular cheilitis and peri-oral skin or lip involvement. These are applied 3 times daily. Angular cheilitis frequently occurs as a mixed infection with staphylococcus aureus, therefore an antibacterial ointment such as mupirocin may be indicated. A combination of a low potency steroid ointment and an antifungal is valuable when deep fissures and cracks on the lips are present. (the middle of the dorsum of the tongue. Tenderness or a burning sensation may be experienced. (Abrams 2000; Flaitz & Hicks 1999, 2003; Greenspan 1993, 1994). Generally, antifungal therapy should be continued 1 to 2 weeks after clinical resolution of the lesions.

Systemic Antifungal Agents

These include Ketoconazole, Fluconazole and Itraconazole.

- Ketoconazole tablets (200mg/tablets) 5-10mg/kg in 1 or 2 doses for 14days
- Fluconazole suspension (50 or 200mg/5ml) 3-6mg/kg once daily to a maximum of 100mg for 14 days
- Fluconazole tablets (50 or 150mg/tab) - as above-
- Itraconazole caps (100mg/cap) 2-5mg/kg once daily for 14days
- Itraconazole oral liquid (10mg/ml) - as above-

In cases of drug resistant candidiasis, microbiologic culturing may be important but Fluconazole and Itraconazole have been found to be more effective empirically for treating lesions resistant to other polyenes and azoles and are associated with longer disease free periods. Suppressive maintenance antifungal therapy is indicated when frequent episodes are encountered. (Flaitz & Hicks 1999, 2000)Disinfection and/or replacement of contaminated oral pacifiers, toothbrushes and orthodontic appliances should be done as these contribute to disease recurrence in children. Restoration of carious teeth and continuous caries prevention is important, as it has been shown microscopically that deep dental caries may act as a reservoir for Candida species in HIV infected individuals.
(Jacob et al 1998)

**Recommended Prophylaxis Regimen (Flaitz & Hicks 1999)**

| | |
|---|---|
| Nystatin oral suspension | 100,000 to 400,000 units twice daily |
| Clotrimazole | 10mg twice daily |
| Fluconazole | 6mg/kg, once daily or weekly |
| Chlorhexidine mouth rinse | twice daily |

### 4.2 Herpes simplex virus infection

This is the most common viral muco-cutaneous disease affecting HIV-positive children. The majority of oral lesions are caused by herpes simplex virus type1 (HSV-1). Prevalence ranges from 2% - 24% in Paediatric HIV studies. HIV positive children who have two or more herpetic infection episodes within 1year are classified as having moderately symptomatic HIV disease. (Caldwell et al., 1994). There are 2 clinical forms:

#### 4.2.1 Primary herpetic gingivostomatitis

This is a systemic viral infection which presents with sudden onset of fever, swollen and tender cervical lymph nodes, irritability and malaise. Classically, there is widespread mucosal erythema, vesicles and painful coalescing ulcers. The gingiva, palate, dorsum of tongue, lip and the peri-oral skin are the commonest sites (Figures 8 &9). Excessive drooling of saliva and pharyngitis often accompanies this infection. Resolution usually occurs within 14days but the disease may linger for several more weeks in immuno-compromised children. (William1993).

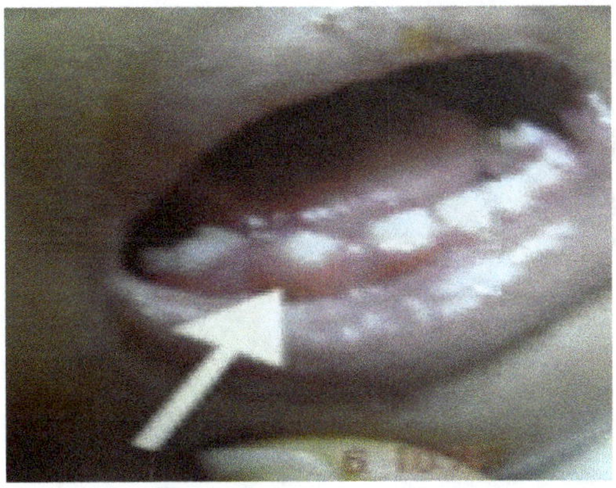

Fig. 8. Primary herpetic gingivostomatitis.

### 4.2.2 Recurrent herpes simplex virus infection

This occurs when the Herpes simplex virus is reactivated within the trigeminal ganglion by factors such as excessive exposure to sunlight, physical injury, febrile systemic illness, immunosuppression, emotional stress and hormonal alterations. It is characterized by sudden onset of focal erythema, clustered vesicles and painful coalescing ulcers. The ulcers usually involve the vermilion border of the lip, peri-oral skin, and nasal mucosa and may form crusts extraorally. Intraorally, the gingivae and palatal mucosa are usually involved. Lesions typically heal within 7 - 10days.

In immuno-suppressed children, lesions may be multifocal in distribution and occur on non-keratinized mucosa. The infection may run a chronic course, lasting 4 - 6weeks and producing large crater form lesions with irregular serpentine to scalloped margins. Extraoral vesicular to crusted lesions that bleed on manipulation are characteristic. Deep persistent lesions may result in significant scarring. Cytomegalovirus co-infection has been observed in these persistent ulcers. (Flaitz et al., 1996).

Some HIV and other immuno-compromised children develop an unusual disease pattern on the dorsum of the tongue called the geometric herpetic glossitis. This variant appears as multiple painful ulcerated fissures that radiate from the middle of the dorsum of the tongue. Herpetic lesions recur frequently in severe immunosuppression.

Diagnosis of herpes simplex viral infection is usually clinical but can be confirmed in atypical lesions by exfoliative cytology, incisional biopsy or tissue culture with viral isolation or presence of viral giant cell. Immuno-cytochemical and fluorescent monoclonal antibody typing can be performed on direct smears, biopsy samples, or infected cells grown in tissue culture for more accurate diagnosis. (Flaitz & Hicks 1999).

### 4.2.3 Treatment

Most herpetic lesions in HIV infected children are reported to be self-limiting. Antiviral therapy is recommended in moderately to severely immuno-compromised children and in cases with frequent recurrences. Oral acyclovir is most frequently used. Lesions resistant to acyclovir have been effectively managed with Foscarnet (Trisodium phosphonoformate hexahydrate).

Acyclovir 200 - 400mg tabs 6 hourly for 10-14days
Foscarnet 24 - 40mg/kg 8 hourly (very severe cases only) for 14-21days.

Suppressive maintenance therapy may be indicated for children who develop multiple episodes. (Ramos-Gomez et al., 1999)

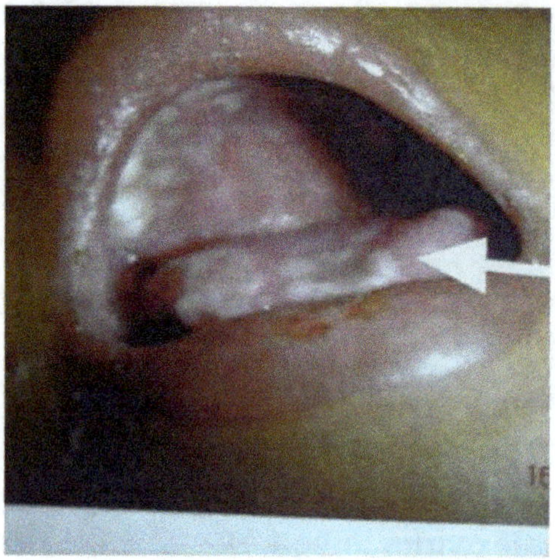

Fig. 9. Primary herpetic gingivostomatitis.

### 4.3 Linear gingival erythema (LGE)

LGE is the most common form of HIV associated periodontal disease in HIV infected children. (Kline 1996, Ramos-Gomez et al 1999). The prevalence of LGE varies widely in different studies, ranging from 0-38%[2]. However, it appears to be more common in cohorts of adolescents aged 13-18 years than in younger children. (Barasch et al 2000; Howell et al 1996).

LGE presents as a fiery red, linear band 2 - 3mm wide on the marginal gingival accompanied by petechiae-like or diffuse red lesions on the attached gingival and oral mucosa. (Figure 10) The erythema may be accompanied by bleeding during brushing and in severe cases by spontaneous bleeding. It is most notable on the buccal surfaces from cuspid to cuspid. Pain is rarely an associated finding in most of these cases. (Ramos-Gomez et al 1999). The degree of erythema is disproportionally intense compared with the amount of plaque that is present on the teeth. (Flaitz & Hicks 1999).

**Treatment**

Appropriate antifungal treatment is recommended because LGE represents an erythematous form of candidiasis. It is important to exclude neutropenia, thrombocytopenia, and plasma cell gingivitis in children with this condition. (Velegraki et al 1999).

There are no known criteria for definitive diagnosis of LGE but it resists conventional plaque removal therapies and oral hygiene measures and this distinguishes it from acute marginal gingivitis. LGE is now described as a candidal infection. Though the microbiology of LGE has not been fully described, C. albicans and C. dubliniensis have been isolated from LGE lesions in both children and adults. (Flaitz & Hicks 2003; Ramos-Gomez et al 1999; Velegraki et al 1999).

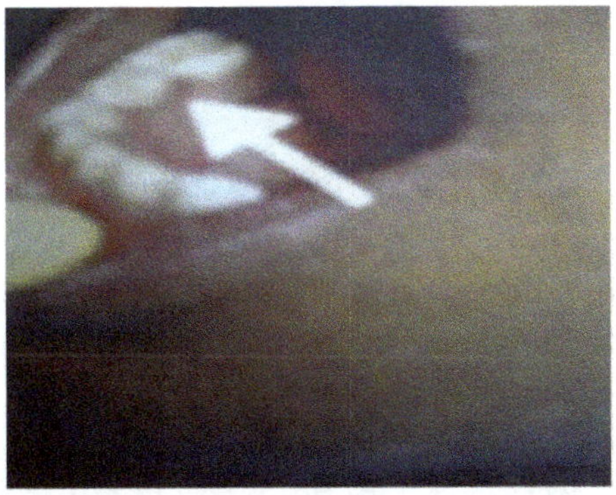

Fig. 10. Linear gingival erythema.

### 4.4 Major salivary gland enlargement

Salivary gland disease in HIV infected children presents as either xerostomia or major salivary gland enlargement. Major salivary gland enlargement refers to lymphocyte mediated salivary gland disease in cases of HIV infection. It may affect the parotid and/or submandibular glands. It was first seen in paediatric HIV infection. It is also called Diffuse Infiltrative Lymphocytosis syndrome or Sjogren syndrome-like disease. (Flaitz & Hicks 2003). (Figure 11).

Major salivary gland enlargement is more common in children than in adults with HIV infection and the prevalence in HIV infected children varies widely in different studies with up to 58% of them being affected. The aetiology of major salivary gland enlargement is unknown but infection with EBV or HIV or the interaction between these two viruses is suspected to be responsible. (Flaitz & Hicks 2003; Fonseca et al., 2000; Katz et al., 1993; Valdez et al., 1994).

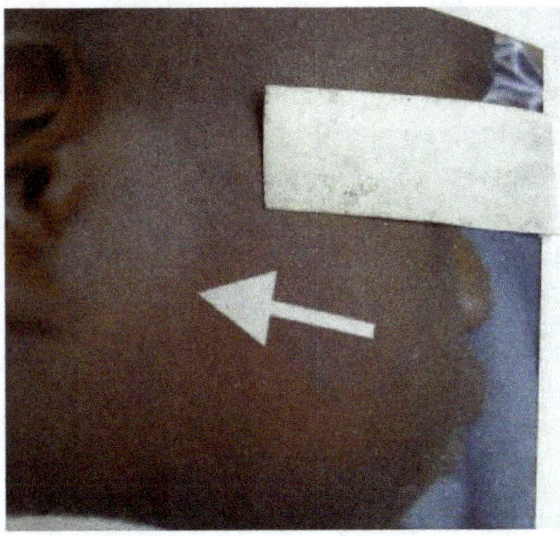

Fig. 11. Parotid gland enlargement.

The parotid gland is most commonly affected with parotid swelling in 10 - 30% of HIV infected children. There is unilateral or bilateral diffuse soft tissue swelling resulting in facial disfigurement. It is sometimes painful, and may be associated with lymphoid interstitial pneumonitis and diffuse lymphadenopathy. There may be concurrent enlargement of the palatine tonsils, resulting in partial airway obstruction, difficulty with swallowing and sleep apnoea. Parotid swelling has been associated with slower progression to AIDS: having a median time to death of 5. 4years as against 3. 4years among patients with oral candidiasis. (Chetty et al., 1999; Flaitz & Hicks 2003; Katz et al., 1993; Ramos-Gomez et al 1999).

There are no established criteria for the definitive diagnosis of salivary gland enlargement (SGE) and the exact pathophysiology remains uncertain. Theories concerning the origin of SGE include lymphoepithelial lesions, cysts involving salivary parenchyma, interglandular lymph nodes, and an inflammatory infiltrate similar to Sjogren's syndrome. Greenspan described the possible relationship between SGE and T-lymphocyte CD8+ cell infiltration in the gland. In addition, genetic loci have been linked to SGE in children, specifically HLADR5 and HLA-DR11, suggesting a genetic predisposition to this condition. (Greenspan & Greenspan 1996; Pinto& De Rossi 2004)

**Treatment**

Salivary gland swelling is usually left untreated because it is usually asymptomatic. However, there are a number of dental management concerns and serious complications in children related to infections of the salivary glands becoming life threatening at a faster rate than in adults. The paediatric dentist should be aware of the possible complications in the paediatric HIV/AIDS population. Often the salivary gland disorders or their potential sequelae can be a predictor of HIV disease progression. Consultation with the child's infectious disease provider, including ordering complete blood counts, should give an indication of the child's immune status. Assessment of salivary function should be performed at the initial dental exam. Subjective complaints of dryness in children are often equivocal, so the clinician should be familiar with examination of the Stensen's and Wharton's ducts to verify flow. Palpation of the major glands and milking of the major glands should be a standard part of the comprehensive head and neck examination of the HIV Positive paediatric patient.

Salivary gland disease can present as benign enlargement with or without xerostomia, xerostomia alone, or parotitis or more ominous conditions such as malignancy. In children, serious complications related to salivary gland infections can become life-threatening at a faster rate than in adults. The clinician should be aware of the etiologic agents that can cause parotitis (bacterial/viral). Knowledge of the child's immune status will often serve as a guide towards diagnosis (i. e., cytomegalovirus or paramyxovirus in immune-compromised children). Thorough examination of salivary ducts can provide valuable information on aetiology-(purulence in saliva, thick mucous saliva) and guide the clinician to adequate treatment. The antibiotic of choice is clindamycin, in a dosage of 8-25mg/kg/day. A therapeutic alternative antibiotic is penicillin, considering the gastrointestinal effects of clindamycin. (Pinto& De Rossi 2004).

### 4.5 Recurrent aphtous ulcers (RAU)

The prevalence of RAU in HIV infected children ranges from 0-7% similar to HIV infected adults. In general RAU tend to recur more frequently in the HIV infected child; and with immunosuppression, major aphthous ulcers are also more likely to develop. (Flaitz & Hicks 2003).

RAU presents as painful ulcers of rapid onset with marked predilection for non keratinised mucosa especially the labial and buccal mucosa, ventral tongue and soft palate. The pharyngeal and oesophageal mucosa may be involved in the most extensive cases. Three clinical varieties have been described based on size, number and duration of lesions present.

### 4.5.1 Minor recurrent aphthous ulcers

This presents as 1-3 shallow, oval or round small ulcers less than 5mm in diameter covered with a pseudo membrane surrounded by an erythematous halo. (Figure 12). They are self limiting and typically heal within 2weeks without scarring. (Flaitz & Hicks 2003; Ramos-Gomez et al 1999).

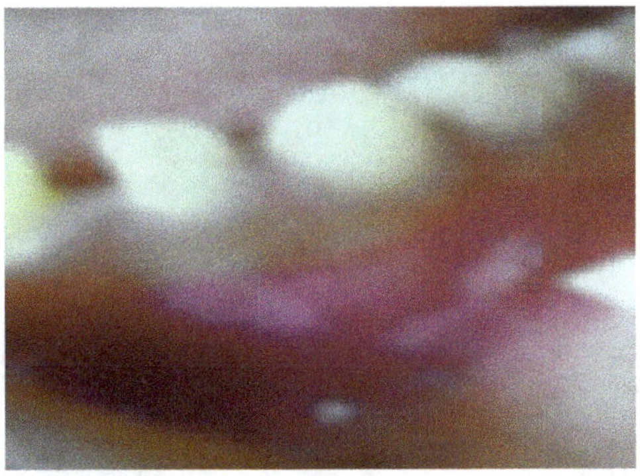

Fig. 12. Minor Aphthous Ulcer.

### 4.5.2 Major recurrent aphthous ulcers

These are oval or round, similar to minor recurrent aphthous ulcers but much larger 1- 2cm in diameter, are fewer in number, and may persist for weeks at a time. They are painful and may interfere with mastication and swallowing. They tend to occur on the soft palate, buccal mucosa, tonsillar area, and tongue. They have well delineated to irregular borders and depressed bases and are often covered by a thick, tenacious, fibrinous exudate. Scaring is a common finding in this condition.

### 4.5.3 Herpetiform recurrent aphthous ulcers

These appear as clusters or crops of tiny recurrent aphthous ulcers, 1 to 2mm in diameter, which may coalesce. They tend to occur in the soft palate, buccal mucosa, tonsillar area, and tongue. Diagnosis is usually clinical, based on the size, site, appearance and duration of the ulcers.

A definitive criterion for all three types of RAU is the response to treatment with steroid agents. Tissue cultures for viral, fungal and mycobacterial organisms and incisional biopsy are necessary for persistent lesions to rule out other causes of ulcers. (Flaitz & Hicks 2003; Ramos-Gomez et al 1999).

### 4.5.4 Treatment

A definitive criterion for all the three types is the response to treatment with steroid agents. Tissue cultures for viral, fungal and mycobacterial organisms and incisional biopsy are necessary for persistent lesions to rule out other causes of ulcers. Topical steroid therapy is the first choice. In severe cases, a short course of prednisolone is indicated. Antifungal agents to prevent oropharyngeal candidiasis are added when steroids are used. These steroids include fluocinomide, clobetasol propionate and dexamethasone elixir. (Ramos-Gomez et al 1999).

## 5. Oral lesions less commonly associated with paediatric HIV infection

### 5.1 HIV associated periodontal diseases

These include:

- Necrotising ulcerative gingivitis (NUG)
- Necrotising ulcerative periodontitis (NUP)
- Necrotising stomatitis (NS)

In children, HIV associated periodontal diseases appear to be associated with both immunodeficiency and malnutrition[4]. HIV infected children from developing countries appear to be more susceptible to necrotising periodontal diseases. A declining immune system with CD4 + cell counts below 200 cells/mm is associated with necrotising ulcerative periodontitis and necrotising stomatitis. (Flaitz & Hicks 2003; Greenspan 1994; Ramos-Gomez et al 1999).

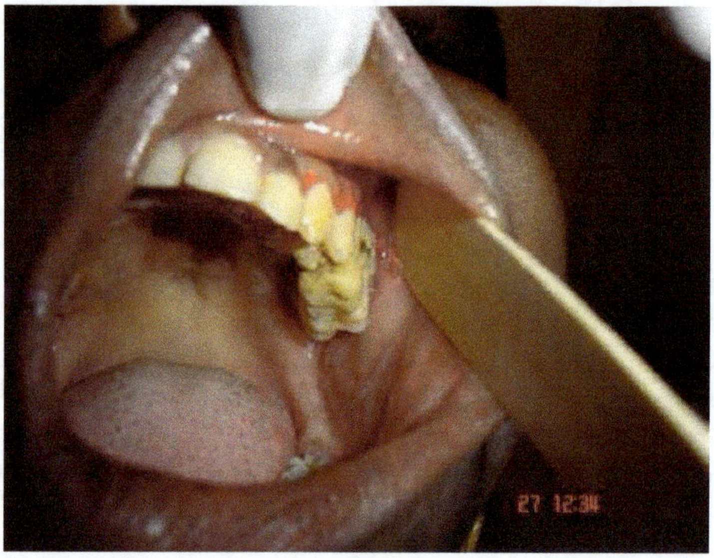

Fig. 13. Necrotising Ulcerative Periodontitis (NUP).

#### 5.1.1 Necrotising ulcerative gingivitis (NUG)

This is uncommon in HIV infected children. It is reported to present with the destruction of one or more interdental papillae accompanied by necrosis, ulceration and/or sloughing. Destruction is limited to the marginal gingival tissues. In the acute stage, the gingival tissues appear fiery red and swollen, and is accompanied by yellowish grey necrotic tissue that bleeds easily. Patients are reported to experience bleeding on brushing, pain and a characteristic halitosis. Symptoms subside gradually over 3 - 4 weeks but recurrences are common.

There may be lymphadenopathy, fever and malaise. Permanent gingival scarring with interdental papillary crater contributes to an increased risk of recurrence. (Flaitz & Hicks 2003). Diagnosis is based on clinical features described above.

#### 5.1.2 Necrotising ulcerative periodontitis (NUP)

NUP has been reported in 0-4% of children. It presents as severe soft tissue necrosis along with destruction of the periodontal attachment and bone over a short period of time. Patients often experience spontaneous gingival bleeding or bleeding when brushing and severe, deep, aching pain in the jawbone. The jawbone may be exposed in the most severe cases. The final stage of NUP is marked by severe gingival recession resulting from rapid bone loss and soft tissue necrosis. (Figures 13 &14) Pocketing may be minimal and tissue destruction may extend across the mucogingival junction. The more extensive disease may contribute to premature exfoliation of primary teeth and aborted development or early loss of primary teeth. (Flaitz & Hicks 2003; Ramos-Gomez et al 1999). Diagnosis of NUP is based on clinical presentations.

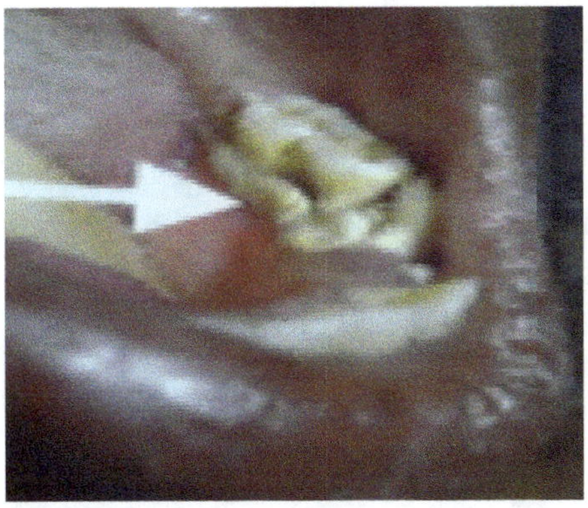

Fig. 14. Necrotising Ulcerative Periodontitis (NUP)

### 5.1.3 Necrotising stomatitis (NS)

This presents as an acute and painful ulceronecrotic lesion on the oral mucosa. The lesion starts from the oral mucosa and may extend to alveolar bone and contiguous soft tissues. The underlying bone may be exposed. Histologic examination reveals the features of non-specific ulceration. No specific microbial organism has been identified as the cause of NS. (Flaitz & Hicks 2003; Ramos-Gomez et al 1999).

### 5.1.4 Treatment for NUG, NUP and NS

**Local treatment**

- Gentle debridement of affected areas to minimize bleeding and pain
- Irrigation with 10%Betadine providone -iodine or 1:4 hydrogen peroxide or Chlorhexidine gluconate (Peridex), 0. 12% to aid debridement.
- Oral hygiene instruction

**Systemic Treatment**

- Metronidazole (Flagyl) 125 mg tablets 8hourly for 7days
- Amoxicillin (Amoxil) 250 mg 8hrly for 7days

If the patient is allergic to penicillin:

- Erythromycin enteric coated 250mg tablet 8hourly for 7 days

The patient should be re-evaluated after one week of treatment and the medication should be repeated if response is not satisfactory.

Supportive therapy: Multivitamins

## 5.2 Viral infections

### 5.2.1 Human Papilloma Virus

Human Papilloma Virus (HPV) induced oral lesions associated with HIV infection include Verucca vulgaris, condyloma acuminatum, focal epithelial hyperplasia, and koilocytic dysplasia which are referred to as oral warts. Oral HPV infections are rare in children. Oral warts present as raised, irregular, flesh coloured lesions.

### 5.2.2 Focal epithelial hyperplasia (Heck's disease)

This is a benign condition associated with HPV types 13 and 32 and is usually seen in children. The lesions appear as multiple, non-tender papules, plaques or nodules with grainy pink mucosal surfaces. The labial, buccal and lateral tongue, mucosa are most often involved, with occasional lesions on the palatal and gingival mucosa. (Figure 15).

**Treatment**

In most cases, conservative excision is treatment of choice. Other methods of treatment include laser ablation, topical podophyllin resin, systemic interferon, and cimetidin. Despite aggressive therapy and multiple treatment modalities, recurrences are common when oral warts are widespread. (Flaitz & Hicks 2003; Howell et al 1996; Ramos-Gomez et al., 1999).

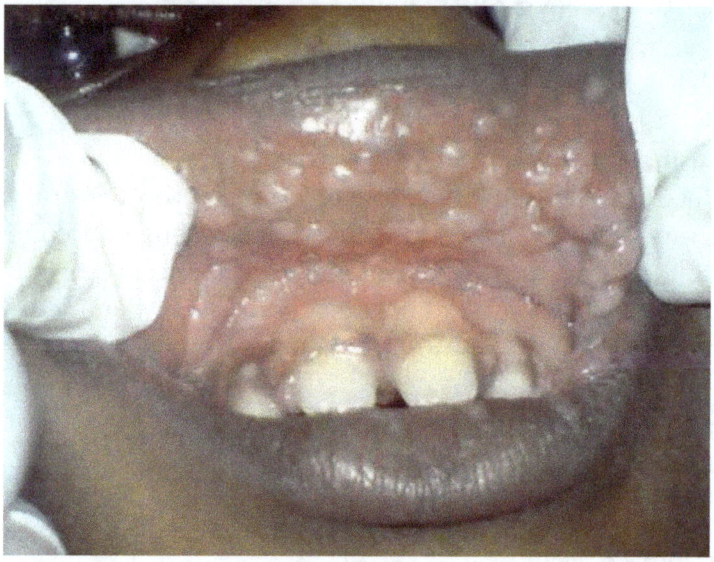

Fig. 15. Focal Epithelial hyperplasia (Heck's disease).

### 5.2.3 Verruca vulgaris

This typically affects the skin, especially the hands and perioral skin. Oral mucosal involvement due to inoculation from these extraoral sites. Intraoral involvement is uncommon and is usually limited to isolated areas of the lip vermillion, labial mucosa and anterior tongue. They present as white, rough, conical or papillary papules or nodules. Treatment is as for Focal Epithelial Hyperplasia above.

### 5.2.4 Condyloma acuminatum

It typically presents as a large sessile, pink nodule with short, blunt surface projections. Multiple lesions may be found that tend to coalesce, forming a discrete, well-delineated enlargement. Diagnosis is usually clinical. Definitive diagnosis can be made by excisional biopsy.

Treatment is as for Focal Epithelial Hyperplasia and oral warts.

### 5.2.5 Cytomegalovirus (CMV)

This presents as a persistent oral ulcer, which may mimic aphthous ulcers, recurrent herpes simplex virus infection, necrotising stomatitis and ulceration not otherwise specified. Occasionally it may present as a brightly erythematous gingivitis. CMV ulcers in the oral cavity usually occur with disseminated CMV disease; therefore the patient should be examined for the systemic disease or other organ involvement including CMV retinitis, colitis, pneumonitis and progressive neurologic disease. Definitive diagnosis can be made through culture and biopsy. (Flaitz et al., 1996; Ramos-Gomez et al., 1999).

### 5.2.6 Varicella Zoster Virus (VZV)

VZV infection can present as Herpes Zoster or Varicella (chicken pox). HIV infected children are at risk for persistent, recurrent, chronic infections with VZV. Children with advanced immunosuppression seem to be at increased risk for recurrent disease and more severe manifestations of VZV. Chronic VZV infection has been described in HIV-infected children and adults with low CD4+ counts. (Gershon et al., 1997; Morris et al., 1996; Ramos-Gomez et al., 1999).

### 5.2.7 Herpes Zoster

The Center for Disease Control and Prevention has classified an HIV-infected child with herpes zoster involving at least 2 distinctive episodes or more than one dermatome as being moderately symptomatic. Herpes Zoster infection results from a reactivation of latent varicella - zoster virus. Fevers, complaints of sensitive teeth, earache or headache as well as pain or paresthesia are prodromal symptoms. A well-delineated unilateral maculo-papular rash that becomes pustular ulcerated follows. Involvement of the second and third branches of the trigeminal nerve produces oral lesions on both keratinised and non keratinsed oral mucosa that extend to the midline. Frequently concurrent vesicles and crusted skin lesions overlie the affected dental quadrant. Most cases heal without complications in children except for facial skin scarring. Definitive diagnosis is by virus antigen typing with laboratory immunologic tests. (Caldwell et al., 1994; Flaitz & Hicks 2003; Ramos-Gomez et al 1999).

### 5.2.8 Molluscum contagiosum

This is a virally induced lesion of the skin, vagina, and rarely, the oral cavity. Lesions are small, discrete, and dome shaped. Their colour ranges from pearly white to skin colour. The lesions may number in the hundreds. Definitive diagnosis is made when molluscum bodies, which are virally transformed epithelial cells are seen, when the core of the lesion is expressed and stained.

(Ramos-Gomez et al 1999).

## 5.3 Xerostomia

Xerostomia is a common symptom of HIV-infected individuals and has many potential causes.

It is more common in HIV infected children than HIV-infected adults. The causes of xerostomia include HIV infection itself, therapeutic antiviral and antimicrobial drugs, prophylactic medications, antiretrovirals (such as didanosine), gamma globulin, or lymphocytic infiltration of the major salivary glands. Clinical features include dry mouth (Figure 16) and severely reduced salivary flow rates. Reduced salivary flow results in a mucosa that is desiccated and is at higher risk for opportunistic infections such as candidiasis and increased caries. Xerostomia may appear with or without parotid swelling. No definitive diagnostic criteria exist for xerostomia. (Flaitz & Hicks 2003; Frezzini et al., 2006; Ramos-Gomez et al 1999).

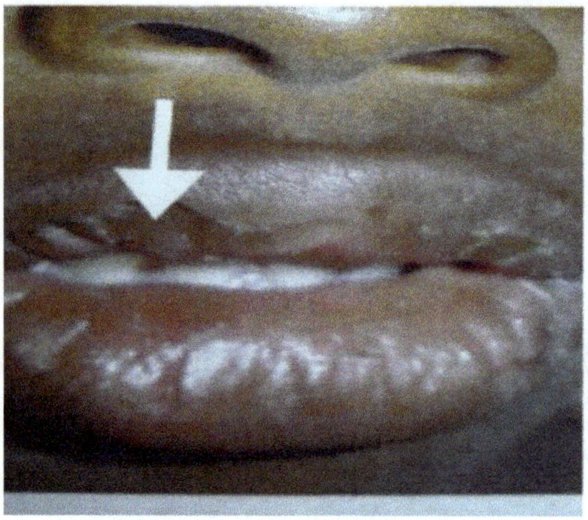

Fig. 16. Dry lips with crusting, resulting from xerostomia.

## 6. Oral lesions strongly associated with HIV infection but rare in children

### 6.1 Kaposi's sarcoma

This is much less common in HIV infected children than adults. The incidence of HIV associated cancers in symptomatic children is less than 2%. However, among HIV infected paediatric population, it is more common in Africa, Latin America and Eastern Europe, where endemic Kaposi's sarcoma is more prevalent in the non-HIV infected population. Human herpes virus - 8 has been identified in all forms of Kaposi's sarcoma. (Flaitz & Hicks 2003; Ramos-Gomez et al 1999; Ranganathan & Hemalatha 2006). Kaposi's sarcoma presents as one or more erythematous, slightly bluish or violaceous macules or swellings with or without ulceration. It is predominantly seen on the palate or gingiva. A definitive criterion is characteristic histologic appearance on biopsy. (William 1993).

### 6.2 Non-Hodgkin's lymphoma

This is far less common in HIV infected children than adults. This presents as a firm, elastic often somewhat reddish or purplish swelling with or without ulceration. The gingiva, palatal mucosa and fauces are more commonly affected. A definitive criterion is the characteristic histological appearance on biopsy, supported by appropriate immuno-cytochemical or molecular biological investigations. (Ramos-Gomez et al 1999; William 1993).

### 6.3 Oral Hairy Leukoplakia (OHL)

This is an opportunistic infection caused by the Epstein-Barr virus (EBV) and is a marker for increasing immunodeficiency. It is a common oral manifestation of HIV infection in adults with a point presence of approximately 20% but it is documented in only 2% of children infected with HIV. It presents as white non-removable lesions with corrugated surface appearing bilaterally on the lateral border of the tongue. These lesions may appear on the ventral and dorsal surfaces of the tongue and more rarely, on the buccal mucosa. Definitive criteria for oral hairy leukoplakia are the presence of Epstein -Barr virus (EBV) in the lesions, to be determined by laboratory histopathology and in-situ DNA hybridization. (Flaitz & Hicks 2003; Morris et al., 1996; Ramos-Gomez et al 1999).

### 6.4 Tuberculosis related ulcers

A combined infection with HIV and mycobacterium tuberculosis is common in LINCs and developing countries. However, secondary and primary tuberculosis lesions of the oral cavity are rare. The lesions present as painless, non-healing ulcerations on the buccal mucosa, hard palate, gingivae and/or tongue. Occasionally, tuberculosis may present with tongue involvement manifesting as macroglossia or a mass in the cheek. In most cases the mucosal lesions are difficult to recognize, but enlarged regional lymph nodes may call attention to the process.

A chest radiograph and a Purified Protein Derivative test with appropriate controls should be obtained. Diagnosis is usually confirmed by identification of acid-fast bacilli in tissue sections or culture. The oral lesions respond to treatment with use of anti-tuberculosis drugs. (Ceballos-Selobrena et al., 1996; Grupta et al., 1997; Hathiram et al., 1997; Haller & Ginsberg 1997; Kolokotronis et al., 1996; Ramesh 1997; Phelan et al., 1997; Ramos-Gomez et al 1999).

## 7. Oral conditions with increased severity in paediatric HIV infection

### 7.1 Gingivitis and periodontitis (increased gingival and plaque indices)

Gingival disease not specifically associated with HIV infection is called conventional gingivitis. Reported prevalence in HIV infected children is 7% and 40%. Clinically, it presents as gingival inflammation in the absence of attachment loss, necrosis or gingival erythematous banding.

(Barasch et al., 2000; Gelbier et al., 2000). An association between the prevalence of gingivitis in HIV infected children and age has been reported. (As low as 6% in less than 1 year olds, 55% in 1year olds, 85% in 2year olds, 87% in 3year olds and 66% in 4year olds). (Ramos et al., 2000).

### 7.2 Over retained primary teeth and delayed eruption of primary and permanent teeth

Delayed eruption of teeth has been reported among children with HIV-infection. Poor general health in some children may be an associated factor. Delayed tooth development has been reported in 31% of paediatric AIDS patients. (Valdez et al 1994). Delayed dental development in paediatric HIV patients has been linked to lower CD4 counts. In the report by Ramos-Gomez et al 2000; it was observed that at age 3, there was an average of two fewer teeth per child among children whose average CD4 count was 200/mm$^3$ than children whose average CD4 count was 800/mm. A study on 173 HIV infected children, delayed eruption was reported in 43% males and 41% females. Accelerated eruption in 11% males and 13% females, while 46% of both males and females have normal eruption pattern. Over retained primary teeth was observed in 25% of the children. (Flaitz et al., 2000).

### 7.3 Dental caries

There is anecdotal evidence of vulnerability of HIV infected children to dental caries. However, some researchers have drawn attention to comparable caries prevalence in infected and non-infected children. Other studies have shown slightly higher prevalence of dental caries in children with HIV. The suggestion that caries development could be directly linked to immunosuppression is yet to be substantiated, although the possibility does exist. Other factors may be responsible for the high caries level in these children, and these include infant feeding practices, the long term use of sugar containing medicines, high consumption of carbohydrate and sugar intake required to prevent or treat any failure to thrive.

A number of studies have reported on the prevalence of dental caries among HIV infected children. (Elderidge & Gallagher 2000; Flaitz et al., 2000; Gelbier et al., 2000; Hicks et al 2000; Obileye et al., 2009, Sowole et al 2009; Tofsky et al 2000; Valdez et al 1994). In a study on dental caries prevalence and dental health behavior in HIV infected children, 63% of the children had past dental caries experience. (Elderidge & Gallagher 2000) This is similar to a previous report by Valdez et al; it was observed that 60% of paediatric AIDS patients had clinical evidence of current or past caries.

In the primary dentition of HIV infected children, the anterior caries (early childhood caries, nursing bottle or baby bottle tooth decay) pattern is common. The pattern of caries observed in this group of children may be as a result of poor oral hygiene practices, inappropriate use of a nursing bottle containing high sucrose liquids at bed time, medications containing high sucrose content, xerostomia induced by medication or HIV infection, the need for high caloric and carbohydrate/sucrose diets, and alterations in saliva viscosity, cytokines, protease inhibitors and immunoglobulin. (Flaitz & Hicks 2003). (Figures 17 & 18)

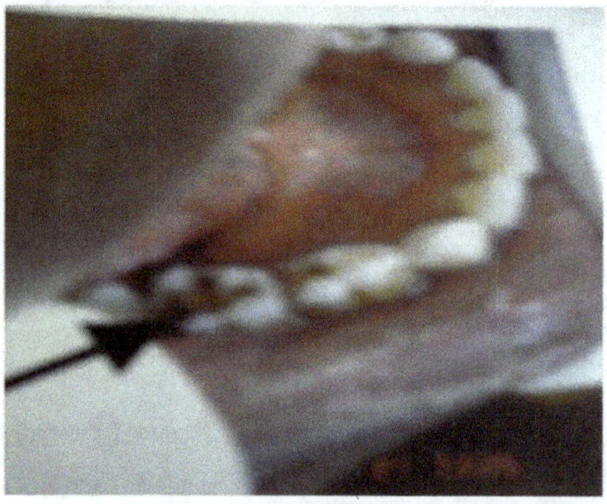

Fig. 17. Dental caries on mandibular primary molars.

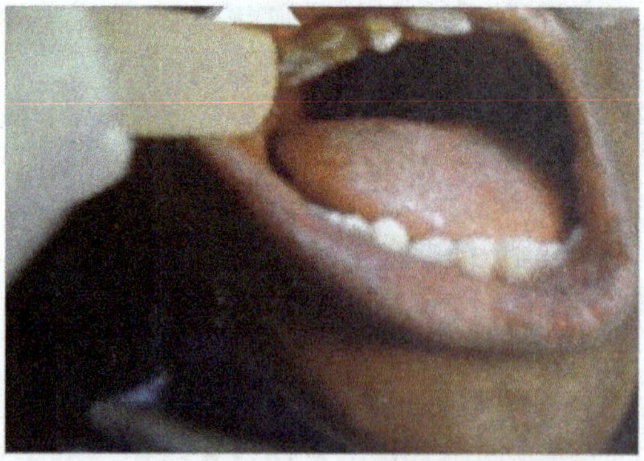

Fig. 18. Dental caries on maxillary primary canines and molars.

Dental caries status in primary dentition of HIV infected children has been reported to be considerably greater than that for the United States paediatric population. (Hicks et al., 2000.) During the 30 month period longitudinal study, there was an almost two fold increase in primary tooth surface caries for the 2-9 year olds. Caries free status in the primary dentition declined from 60% at baseline to 37% at the 30months period. Among 5 to 11 year olds, dmfs and dmft remained relatively stable while the proportion of caries free individuals declined from 72% at baseline to 50% at 18 months. Caries free status decreased with age, lower CD4 percentage and from moderate to severe immunosuppression. (Hicks et al., 2000). A high prevalence of Candida colonization in HIV positive /AIDS children with untreated dental caries has been reported. (Domaneschi et al., 2010). This further reinforces the importance of oral health care in interdisciplinary health unit that manage these patients.
Caries and periodontal disease are among the most common infections known to humans. Both are initiated by oral bacteria and are modulated by the host response. Disease occurs as a result of an imbalance between the provoking bacteria and host response. It is logical to expect, therefore, that alterations of either the associated aetiological factors or the host response to these factors and or agents should result in a change in the clinical presentation of disease. (Fine et al., 2003).

## 8. Conclusions

Oral manifestations are common and prevalent in paediatric HIV infection and have been found to be the earliest indicators of HIV infection. Early intervention in HIV disease is crucial for each individual according to his/her risk and seroconversion status. Comprehensive oral examination should be done at regular intervals especially in LINCs and developing countries where techniques to diagnose, and the drugs to treat HIV infection are not uniformly distributed. The use of oral lesions as predictors of disease progression could be of immense importance. Primary oral health care for HIV infected children should include a careful oral examination at regular intervals to ensure early detection and intervention for pseudomembranous candidiasis and other infections and to prevent more deterioration of the immune system and further opportunistic infections. Preventive oral health care especially where treatment is progression unavailable, can improve a child's overall health. Though these measures cannot stop HIV disease progression, in the absence of medications, improved diagnosis of the oral manifestations can enhance case management, ensure better oral health outcomes, reduce morbidity and improve quality of life of HIV-infected children.

## 9. Acknowledgement

The authors wish to thank the Staff of the Special Paediatric Outpatient Clinic of Lagos University Teaching Hospital and Peadiatric HIV Outpatient Clinic of Massey Children Hospital, Lagos Nigeria for their cooperation and assistance and in particular the parents and children for their consent to participate with the investigations and approval to make use of their clinical photographs.

## 10. References

Abrams EJ. (2000). Opportunistic Infections and Other Clinical Manifestations of HIV Disease in Children. Pediatr Clin North Am 47: 95 -96

Agbelusi GA, Wright AA (2005). Oral lesions as Indicators of HIV Infection among Routine Dental patients in Lagos, Nigeria. Oral Dis 11:370-373.

Ammann AJ. (2004). Overview of Paediatric HIV Disease. In The AIDS Knowledge Base: A Textbook on HIV Disease Cohen PT, Sande MA, Volberding PA et al.,8. 11-8. 17, 2nd Edition, University of California

Ammann AJ. (2006). Handbook of Pediatric HIV Care 2nd Edition. Eds Zeicher SL, Read JS. Cambridge University Press New York NY, 2006. ISBN-10:0521529069

Arendorf (1998). Bredekamp B, Cloete CAC, Sauer G. (1998). Oral Manifestations in 600 South African Patients, J Oral Pathol Med. 27: 176-179

Barasch A., Salford MM., Catalantto FA., Fine DH & Katz RV. (2000). Oral soft tissue manifestations in HIV-positive vs. HIV-negative children from an inner city population; a two-year observational study. Pediatr Dent. May-Jun;22 (3): 215-20

Barone R, Ficarra G, Gaglioti D, Orsi A, Mazzotta F. (1990) Prevalence of Oral Lesions among HIV-infected Intravenous Drug Abusers and Other Groups. Oral Surg Oral Med Oral Pathol 69: 169-173.

Barnett T, Whiteside A. (2006) *AIDS* in the twenty-first century: *Disease and Globalization*. 2nd edition. New York: Palgrave Macmillan; 2006. 416

Brown DM, Jabra-Rizk MA, Falker WA, Baqui AAMA, Meiler TF. (2000). Identification of Candida dubliniensis in a Study of HIV-Seropositive Pediatric Dental Patients. Pediatr Dent 2000; 22: 234 - 238

Centres for Disease Control and Prevention. (1993) Classification System for HIV Infection and Expanded Surveillance Case Definition for AIDS among Adolescents and Adults. *MMWR* 41:1-19.

Caldwell MB, Oxtoby MJ, Simond RJ, et al. (1994) Revised Classification System for Human Immunodeficiency Virus Infection in Children Less Than 13 Years of Age. *MMWR* 43: 1 - 10

Ceballos-Salobrena A, Agurre-Urizar JM, Bagan-Sebastian JV. (1996). Oral Manifestations Associated with Human Immunodeficiency Virus Infection in a Spanish Population. *J Oral Pathol Med* 1996; 25: 523 - 526.

Chadwick & Yogev, 1995;

Chetty R, Vaithilingum M, Thejpal R. (1999). Epstein Barr Virus Status and the Histopathological Changes of Parotid Gland Lymphoid Infiltrates in HIV-Positive Children. *Pathology* 1999; 31: 413 - 417

Chiou CC, Groll AH, Gonzalez CE, et al. Esophageal Candidiasis in Paediatric Acquired Immunodeficiency Syndrome. Clinical Manifestations and Risk Factors. Pediatr Infect Dis J 2000; 19: 729 - 734

Coogan MM, Greenspan J, Challacombe SJ. Oral lesions in infection with human immunodeficiency virus. Bull World Health Organ. 2005; 83:700-6.

De Cock, KM., Fowler, MG., Mercier E., de Vincenzi, I., Saba, J., Hoff, E., et al. (2000) Prevention of mother-to-child HIV transmission in resource-poor countries: translating research into policy and practice. *JAMA*. 2000; 283 (1175–1182).

Domaneschi C, Masserente D, De Freitas R, De Souza Marques H, Paula C, Migliari D, Antunes J (2010). Oral Clonozation by Candida species in AIDS pediatric patients. Oral Dis 2010; Nov 29 doi 1111/j. 1601-0825. 2010. 01765. x.

Elderidge K, Gallagher JE. Dental Caries Prevalence and Dental Health Behaviour in HIV Infected Children. Int J Pediatr Dent 2000; 10: 19 -26

Fine DH, Nelson EM, Schoen D, Barasch A. (2003). Clinical implications of the oral manifestations of HIV infection in children *Dent Clin N Am* 2003; 47: 159-174

Flaitz C, Nichols CM, Hicks MJ. (1996). Herpes viridea-associated Persistent Mucocutaneous Ulcers in Acquired Immunodeficiency Syndrome: A Clinicopatholgic Study. *Oral Surg Oral Med Oral Pathol Oral Radiol Endod* 1996; 81: 433 - 441.

Flaitz CM, Hicks MJ. (1999). Oral Candidiasis in Children with Immune Suppression: Clinical Appearance and Therapeutic Considerations. J Dent Child 1999; 66 (May - Jun): 161 - 166.

Flaitz CM, Wullbrandt B, Sexton J, et al. (2000). Prevalence of Orodental Findings in HIV Infected Romanian Children. Pediatr Dent 2000; 23: 44 - 50

Flaitz CM, Hicks MJ. (2003) Oral Manifestations in Paediatric HIV Infection. In: Shearer WT, Hanson IC, eds. Medical Management of AIDS in Children. USA: Elsevier Science, 2003: 248 - 269

Fonseca R, Cardoso AS, Pomarico I. (2000) Frequency of Oral Manifestation in Children Infected with Human Immunodeficiency Virus. Quintessence Int 2000; 31: 419 - 422.

Fowler MG, Simonds RJ, Roongpisuthipong A. (2000). Update on perinatal HIV transmission. Pediatr Clin North Am 2000; 47: 21-37

Frezzini, C. Leao, JC. Cedro, M. Porter, S. (2006). Aspects of HIV Disease Relevant to Dentistry in the 21st Century. *Dent Update*, 2006; 33:276-286

Gray G, McIntyre J. (1999) International AIDS Society Newsletter 1999; 178: 368-74

Gelbier M, Lucas VS, Zervou NE, Roberts GJ, Novelli V. (2000)A Preliminary Investigation of Dental Disease in Children HIV Infection. Int J Pediatr Dent 2000; 10: 13 - 18.

Gershon AA, Mervish N, LaRussa P, et al (1997). Varicella zoster Virus Infection in Children with Underlying Human Immunodeficiency Virus Infection. J Infect Dis 1997; 176: 1496 - 1500

Giaquinto C, Penazzato M, Rosso R, Bernardi S, Rampon O, Nasta P, Ammassari A, Antinori G et al., (2010). Italian Paediatric HIV Infection Working Group. Italian consensus statement on paediatric HIV infection. *Infection*. 2010; 38(4):301-19

Glick M (2005). Orofacial disorders in children with HIV disease. *Dent. Clin North Am.* 2005 Jan; 49(1): 259-71, x-xi

Greene WC (2007). A history of AIDS: looking back to see ahead. *Eur J Immunol.* 2007; 37:S94-102.

Greenspan D, Schiodt M, Greenspan JS, Pindborg JJ. AIDS and the Mouth, Diagnosis and Management of Oral Lesions. Copenhagen: Munksgaard; 1990

Greenspan D, Greenspan JS. (1993) Oral Manifestations of Human Immunodeficiency Virus Infection. *Dent Clin North Am* 1993; 37 (Jan): 21 - 23.

Greenspan D. (1994) Treatment of Oral Candidiasis in HIV Infection. *Oral Surg Oral Med Oral Pathol* 1994; 78: 211-215.

Greenspan,JS, Greenspan D. (1995). Oral manifestations of HIV infection. Proceedings of the Second International workshop on the Oral manifestations of HIV infection. *Quintessence,* Carol Stream IL, 1995.

Grupta A, Shinde KJ, Bhardway I. (1997). Primary Lingual Tuberculosis: A Case Report. *J Laryngol Otol* 1997; 112: 86 - 87

Haller JO, Ginsberg KJ. (1997) Tuberculosis in Children with Acquired Immunodeficiency Syndrome. *Pediatr Radiol* 1997; 27: 186 - 188

Hathiram BT, Grewal DS, Irani DK, Tankwal PM, Patanker M. (1997). Tuberculoma of the Cheek: A Case Report. *J Larygngol Otol* 1997; 111: 872 - 873

Hicks MJ, Flaitz CM, Bruce Carter A, et al. (2000). Dental Caries in HIV Infected Children: A Longitudinal Study. *Pediatr Dent* 2000; 22: 359 - 364

Howell RB, Jandinski J, Palumbo P, Shey Z, Houpt MI. (1996) Oral Soft Tissue Manifestations and CD4 Lymphocyte Counts in HIV-Infected Children. *Pediatr Dent*. 1996; 18:114-116.

Katz MH, Mastrucci MT, Leggott PJ, Westenhouse J, Greenspan JS & Scott GB. (1993). Prognostic significance of oral lesions in children with perinatally acquired human immunodeficiency virus infection. *Am J Dis Child* 1993 Jan; 147(1): 45-8.

Kline MW. Oral Manifestations of Pediatric Human Immunodeficiency Virus Infection: A Review of the Literature. Pediatr 1996; 97 (Mar): 380 - 388.

Kolokotronis A, Antoniadis D, Trigonidis G, Papanagiotou P. (1996) Oral Tuberculosis. *Oral Dis* 1996; 2: 242 - 243

Lamster IB, Begg MD, Mitchell Lewis D et al., (1994) Oral manifestations of HIV Infection in Homosexual Men and Intravenous Drug Users. Study Design and Relationship of Epidemiologic, Clinical and Immunologic parameters to Oral Lesions. *Oral Surg Oral MedOral Pathol* 1994; 78:163-174

Leao JC, Ribeiro CM, Carvalho AA, Frezzini C, Porter S. (2009) Oral complications of HIV disease Clinics (Sao Paulo) 2009; 64(5) : 459-70.

Magalhaes MG, Bueno DF, Serra E, Gonclaves R. (2001) Oral manifestations of HOIV positive children. *J Clin Pediatr Dent* 2001; 25(2): 103-106

Massarente, DB. Domaneschi, C. Marques, HH. Andrade, SB. Goursand, D & Antunes, JL. (2011). Oral health-related quality of life of paediatric patients with AIDS. *BMC Oral Health*. 2011; 5; 11:2.

Morris CR, Araba-Owoyele L, Spector SA, et al. (1996). Disease Patterns and Survival After Acquired Immunodeficiency Syndrome Diagnosis in Human Immunodeficiency Virus Infected Children. *Pediatr Infect Dis J* 1996; 15: 321

Naidoo S, Chikte U (2004). Orofacial manifestations in paediatric HIV: a comparative study of institutionalized and hospital outpatients. *Oral Dis* 2004;10: 13-18

National AIDS and STD Control Program Federal Ministry of Health and Social Services in Collaboration with Nigeria Medical Association. Handbook of HIV Infection and AIDS for Health Workers. 2nd Edition Nigeria 1992.

Newell, ML., Coovadia, H., Cortina Borja, M., Rollins, N., Gaillard, P., Dabis, F. (2004). Mortality of infected and uninfected infants born to HIV-infected mothers in Africa: a pooled analysis. *Lancet*. (2004) 364:1236–1243

Olaniyi TO, Sunday P (2005). Oral manifestations of HIV infection in 36 Nigerian children. *J Clin Pediatr Dent* 2005; 30(1): 89-92

Obileye MF. (2006) Oral Manifestations of HIV/AIDS and response to Management in HIV positive children attending two dedicated paediatric HIV Outpatient clinics in Lagos State (Dissertation) Lagos, Nigeria: National Postgraduate Medical College of Nigeria, 2006

Obileye, MO., Agbelusi, GA., Orenuga OO & Temiye EO. (2009). Dental Caries Status of HIV infected Nigerian Children. *Nig. Qtr. J. Hosp Med*. 2009; 19 (4):

Oleske J, Minnefor A, Cooper R Jr et al., (1983) Immune deficiency syndrome in children. *J Am Med Assoc* 1983; 249: 2345-49.

Olumide YM (2002) A Self Instructional Textbook of Acquired Immune Deficiency Syndrome HIV/AIDS for Medical Students, Resident Doctors and Medical Practitioners. 1st edition Nigeria Longman, 2002

Onunu AN, Obuekwe N (2002) HIV Related Oral Diseases in Benin City, Nigeria. *West Afr J Med* 2002; 21(Jan/Mar): 9-11

Orne-Glieman Becquet R, Ekouevi DK, Leroy V, Perez F, Dabis F. (2008) Children and HIV/AIDS: From research to policy and action in resource-limited settings. *AIDS.* 2008; 23: 22 (7):797-805

Petersen PE. (2003). The World Oral Health Report 2003: continuous improvement of oral health in the 21st Century – the approach of the WHO Global Oral Health Programme. *Community Dent Oral Epidemiol* 2003; 31(Suppl. 1): 3–24

Petersen PE. (2004). Strengthening the prevention of HIV/AIDS-related oral disease: a global approach. *Community Dent Oral Epidemiol* 2004; 32: 399-401

Phelan JA, Jimenez V, Tompkins DC. (1997) Tuberculosis. *Dent Clin North Am* 1997; 40: 327 - 341.

Pinto A, De Rossi SS. (2004) Salivary Gland Disease in pediatric HIV Patients: An Update. *J Dent Child* 2004; 71(1): 33-37

Ramesh V. (1997) Tuberculoma of the Tongue Presenting as Macroglossia. *Cutis* 1997; 60: 201 - 202.

Ramos -Gomez FJ, Hilton JF, Canchola AJ, Greenspan D, Greenspan JS & Maldonado YA (1996). Risk factors for HIV-related Orofacial soft tissue manifestations in children. *Pediatr Dent.* 1996; 18(2): 121-6

Ramos-Gomez FJ, Greenspan D, Greenspan JS. Orofacial manifestations and management of HIV-infected children. In: Oral and Maxillofacial Surgery in Children and Adolescents. Kaban. LB. Ed. Philadelphia, WB Saunders Co. Pp 37-47

Ramos-Gomez FJ (1997) Oral aspects of HIV infections in children. *Oral Diseases* 1997; 3 (Suppl 1): S31-S35

Ramos-Gomez FJ, Flaitz C, Catapano P, Murray P, Milnes AR, Dorenbaum A & Collaborative Workgroup on Oral manifestations of Paediatric HIV infection, Oral Aids Centre, University of California, San Francisco. (1999). Classification, Diagnostic Criteria, and Treatment Recommendations for Orofacial Manifestations in HIV–infected Pediatric Patients. *J. Clin Pediatr Dent* 1999; 23: 85 - 96.

Ramos–Gomez FJ, Petru A, Hilton JF, Canchola AJ, Wara D, Greenspan JS. (2000). Oral Manifestations and Dental Status in Paediatric HIV Infection. *Int J Paediatr Dent* 2000; 10: 3 – 11

Ranganathan K, Hemalatha R (2006). Oral lesions in HIV infection in developing countries: an overview. *Adv Dent. Res.* 2006; 19: 63-8

Rosemberg, ZD. Faucias, L (1994) Immunopathology and Pathogenesis of HIV Infection in pediatric AIDS. In: *The Challenge of HIV Infection in Infants, children and adolescents* (2nd Ed.), Pizzo AP, Wilfort CM, eds. pp. (115-127), Williams & Wilkin, Baltimore.

Sauer G, Bredekamp A, Arendorf TM (1995) Proceedings of the 29th Scientific Congress of the International Association of Dental Research. Cape Town 1995: Abstract No. 85.

Schimdt-Westhausen A, Grunewald T, Reichart PA, Pohle HD. (1997) Oral Manifestations in 70 German HIV Infected Women 1997; 3 (Suppl 1):S28-S30

Scully C (1997) The HIV global pandemic: the development and emerging implications. *Oral Diseases* 1997; 3 (Suppl 1): 51-6. l

Soares, LF., de Araújo Castro, GFB, de Souza IPR & Pinheiro M. (2004). Pediatric HIV-related oral manifestations - a five-year retrospective study· *Braz. Oral Res*, 2004; 18(1):

Sowole CA, Orenuga OO, Chikte SA (2009). Access to oral health care and treatment needs of HIV positive paediatric patients *Brazilian Oral Research and Integrated Pediatric Clinic.* 2009 9(2): 141-146, maio/ago

Sullivan (2003). Prevention of Mother - to- Child Transmission of HIV—What Next? J *AIDS* 2003; 34: S67-72.

Swendeman D, Ingram BL, Rotheram-Borus MJ. (2009) Common elements in self-management of HIV and other chronic illnesses: an integrative framework. *AIDS Care.* 2009; 21(10):1321-34.

Tofsky N, Nelson EM, Lopez RN, Catalanotto FA, Fine DH, Katz RV. Dental Caries in HIV-Infected Children versus Household Peers: Two-Year Findings. *Pediatr Dent* 2000; 22: 207

Ukpebor M, Braimoh OB. (2007). HIV/AIDS; Oral Complications and Challenges, The Nigerian Experience. *Benin Journal of Postgraduate Medicine* 2007; 9(1):44-54

UNAIDS Joint United Nations Programme on HIV/AIDS (UNAIDS). *Report on the Global AIDS Epidemic* (2002). Geneva: *UNAIDS*, 2002

UNAIDS Joint United Nations Programme on HIV/AIDS (UNAIDS). *Report on the Global AIDS Epidemic* (2004). Geneva: *UNAIDS*, 2004.

UNAIDS/WHO (2005) *Report on the Global AIDS Epidemic* 2005. Geneva

UNAIDS. *AIDS* (2006). *Epidemic Update - Special report on HIV/AIDS - December 2006.* Geneva: UNAIDS; 2006.

UNAIDS (2009) *Report on the Global AIDS Epidemic Update* 2009. Geneva

Velegraki A, Nicolatou O, Theodoridou A, et al. Paediatric AIDS - Related Linear Gingival Erythema: A Form Erythematous of Candidiasis? *J Oral Pathol Med* 1999; 28: 178 - 182.

William DM (1993). In: EC - Clearing House on Oral Problems Related to HIV Infection of the Immunodeficiency Virus: Classification and Diagnostic Criteria for Oral Lesions in HIV Infection. *J Oral Pathol Med* 1993; 22: 289 - 291.

World Health Organization. (2003) Global Health-Sector Strategy for HIV/AIDS 2003-2007. Geneva: *WHO*, 2003.

World Health Organization (2003) *The World Health Report,* Shaping the Future. Geneva: WHO, 2003

Working Group on Mother To Child Transmission of HIV. Rates of mother- to- child transmission of HIV-1 in Africa, America and Europe: Results from 13 perinatal studies. *Journal of Acquired Immune Deficiency Syndrome and Human Retrovirology* 1995; 8: 506-510

Wright AA. (2003) A Study of Oral Manifestations of HIV/AIDS and Response to Management at the General Hospital Lagos, Nigeria (Dissertation) Lagos, Nigeria: National Postgraduate Medical College of Nigeria, 2003;48

Yengopal V, Bhayat A, Coogan M. (2011). Pediatric Oral HIV Research in the Developing World. *Adv Dent Res.* 2011; 23(1): 61-6.

Zijenah LS, Katzenstein DA (2002). Immunopathogenesis of AIDS In: *AIDS in Africa.*, Essex M, Mboup S, Phyllis J, Richard K, Marlick G, Tiou SD. Pp 35,Khuser Academic /Plenum Publishers, New York.

# 12

# Re-Emergence of HIV Infection and Syphilis among Men who have Sex with Men

Maria Antonella Di Benedetto, Nino Romano and Alberto Firenze
*Dipartimento di Scienze per la Promozione della Salute, University of Palermo
Italy*

## 1. Introduction

Sexual activity has been shown to be the primary mode of transmission for several important viral and bacterial infections among men who have sex with men (MSM) throughout the world and therefore sexually transmitted infections (STIs) are still one of major public health problem worldwide. Since the earliest days of the human immunodeficiency virus (HIV) epidemic MSM have been profoundly affected by the disease; by the time the first AIDS cases were reported in the early 1980s, HIV had already spread widely among homosexual and drug-user communities. In western Europe, has been estimated that HIV incidence peaked around 1983 among MSM and in 1987-88 among injecting drug users, with 120.000 homosexual/bisexual men infected by 1985, and 144.000 injecting drug users infected by 1989 (Downs et al., 2000). MSM account for a substantial proportion of HIV infections and compose a "bridging group" for transmission to heterosexuals because of the high frequency of reported bisexuality. Widescale behavioural modification in response to the emerging HIV/AIDS pandemic saw dramatic reductions in the incidence of many acute STIs in the late 1980s (WHO, 2007). However, these have not been maintained and many states are now observing increases in rates of diagnosed STIs; then the proportion of homosexual men reporting "unsafe sex", often measured as unprotected anal intercourse (UAI) with casual partners, has increased since the mid-1990s (Prestage et al., 2005). In western Europe, among MSM, HIV diagnoses increased in 2002 (22%, from 2757 in 2001 to 3371 in 2002) after a slow decline in the previous years. Increased high risk sexual behaviour and migration of HIV-infected people from sub-Saharan Africa have contributed to the rise in the incidence of STIs since 2000 (Hamers & Downs, 2004). On the other hand, antiretroviral treatment, which lowers the viral load, may reduce the likelihood that an HIV infected person infect a partner during unprotected sexual intercourse. Mathematical modelling suggests that the effect of antiretroviral treatment on lowering transmission at the population level could be offset by an increase, even modest, in risk behaviour, and the net effect of these opposing forces on HIV incidence has been much debated (Katz et al., 2002).

This HIV infection increase, in some industrialized countries, has also coincided with several reported outbreaks of syphilis among the MSM population (Couturier et al., 2004); in particular, oral sex between men appears to have been important in the transmission of syphilis in outbreaks reported overseas, probably because among MSM unprotected oral sex is considered a safe practice. Data of literature report that syphilis transmission attributed to oral sex has been estimated between 20 and 46% (Peterman & Furness, 2007). Syphilis remains a global problem despite the existence of simple and validated screening tests; moreover, it has been described as strongly associated with prevalent HIV infection among MSM thereby playing an important role in the increase of this infection in a susceptible population. The interaction between HIV infection and syphilis is of great interest for the epidemiological and clinical implications that apply to both heterosexuals and MSM (Peterman & Furness, 2007). The World Health Organization (WHO) estimates 12 million new syphilis cases worldwide annually, of which 140.000 in western Europe where the infection has re-emerged both in homosexual men, in particular in HIV-positive gay men, and in heterosexuals (WHO, 2001; Simms et al., 2005; Xu et al., 2011). An increase of cases among MSM has been found in Italy (Istituto Nazionale di Statistica [ISTAT], 2005), Sweden (Velicko et al., 2004), Scotland (Wallace et al., 2005) and in Germany (Marcus & Hamouda, 2004), suggesting that syphilis is now endemic in the MSM population in parts of Western Europe. In the USA, the scenario is similar because an increase in syphilis cases among MSM occurred between 2000 and 2005, characterised by high rates of HIV co-infection and high-risk sexual behaviour (Fenton et al., 2008). As infection is frequently asymptomatic, annual serological screening for syphilis is to recommend in this group of men. Syphilis offers a classic example of the re-emergence of an easily diagnosed and readily treatable STD.

In this report we review the recent epidemiology of HIV infection and syphilis among MSM in the developed and developing world and discuss potential reasons for the emerging trends and their implications for prevention and control.

## 2. HIV /AIDS

HIV infects defense/immune system cells such as CD4+ T cells, macrophages and dendritic cells. After infection HIV uses CD4+ cells as host to make copies and infect other cells, this leads to the reduction of CD4+ cells and immune system totally collapse. The development from HIV to AIDS is checked by decline of CD4+ cells. Two types of HIV has been characterized, HIV-1 and HIV-2. HIV-1 is the most virulent and pathogenic strain; the HIV-2 epidemic remains limited, both in terms of prevalence and with respect to geographic spread because, worldwide, the predominant virus is HIV-1. The relatively uncommon HIV-2 type is concentrated in West Africa (Senegal, Ivory Coast, Guinea Bissau) and other countries characterized by a considerable immigration of people coming from West Africa. The HIV-1 is further divided into 3 groups: 1. group M (main) ; 2. group O (outlier) ; 3. group N (non M - non O). These groups have been identified in there envelop region. The major HIV pandemic is caused by HIV-1 group M strains; groups O and N of HIV-1 are rare and limited to Cameroon in Central Africa (McCutchan, 2006). Group O accounts for less than 10% of HIV-1 infections in Cameroon and has spread little beyond these confines ; only a handful of group N infections have been identified. Within HIV-1 group M, nine subtypes are recognized namely subtypes A, B, C, D, F, G, H, J and K, that represent lineages of HIV and have different geographic location. Many of the HIV-1 group M subtypes are rare and remain at low prevalence. In contrast, subtype B is widespread globally, dominating epidemics in the Americas, Western Europe, and Australia. Subtype C accounts for more than 50% of all infections worldwide, concentrated in Southern and East Africa, and in India; subtype D strains are found principally in East Africa, and to a lesser extent in West Africa. In some parts of the world less information is available about HIV diversity, particularly North Africa, the Middle East, and parts of Central Asia (McCutchan, 2006).

The study and monitoring of the genetic evolution of the HIV-1 represent an essential strategy for controlling the global HIV-1 epidemic and for developing efficient preventive and therapeutic strategies.

### 2.1 The current scenario in developed countries

The HIV epidemic is resurging in gay communities in developed world. As a consequence, a number of European countries have conducted behavioural surveys among MSM to monitor HIV and STIs risk in this population ; behavioural surveillance provides important information for planning and evaluating prevention interventions (Elford et al., 2009). In Canada (Public Health Agency of Canada, 2007), the United States (CDC, 2007) and Australia (National Centre in HIV Epidemiology and Clinical Research, 2007) MSM represent the risk group diagnosed most frequently with HIV infection. In particular, in the United States, the MSM population accounted for the majority of new HIV infections in 2006. This re-emergence has led some commentators to suggest that HIV prevention in MSM is faltering so president Obama's released National HIV/AIDS Strategy calls for more emphasis on addressing the HIV prevention and care needs of MSM (The White House Office of National AIDS Policy, 2010).

#### 2.1.1 European Union and European Free Trade Association countries

The number of newly diagnosed HIV cases reported among men who have sex with men (MSM) has recently increased throughout European Union (EU) and European Free Trade Association (EFTA) countries. The predominant mode of transmission for HIV infection in EU and EFTA countries is sex between men. In 2006, 7693 newly diagnosed HIV infections among MSM were reported (56.7 per million men aged 15-64 years). In most of the European countries with data for 2000-2006, the number of new HIV diagnoses increased by 86%, the median age at HIV diagnosis remained unchanged (36 years), whereas the proportion of MSM presenting with an AIDS-defining illness at the time of HIV diagnosis declined from 25% in 2000 to 10% in 2006. Basically there is a decrease of cases of AIDS and death in the presence of an increase of HIV infection. (Likatavicius et al., 2008). In general, reported HIV prevalence ranged between 8% and 68% among MSM with sexually transmitted infections, between 10% and 18% among those recruited in community settings, but remained <10% in central Europe and Ireland. Whereas the decreasing rates of AIDS diagnoses and AIDS deaths reflect relatively good access to therapy, the increasing numbers of new HIV diagnoses and relatively high prevalence of HIV among MSM suggest the need for Europe-wide HIV prevention among MSM. Currently, the prevalence of HIV among homosexual and bisexual men is 10–20% in most western European countries; prevalence is usually higher in large cities than elsewhere ( Hamers & Downs, 2004). In the below report, there are summarized the results of serological investigations carried out in several European countries, which show the pattern of increasing HIV incidence in these last years. In Madrid, in a study among homosexual and bisexual men who repeatedly attended voluntary HIV testing centres, HIV incidence decreased from 4.7 per 100 person-years in 1988 to 1.1 in 1995, but then increased to 2.2 in 2000. More recently, incidence studies based on the serological testing algorithm for recent HIV seroconversion (STARHS) have been done among homosexual and bisexual men attending sexually transmitted infection clinics in the Netherlands and the UK (Hamers & Downs, 2004). In Amsterdam, an overall incidence of 3.0 infections per 100 person-years during 1991–2001 was noted, with a significant increase over time. The increase was evident in men older than 34 years but not in younger men. In the UK, the overall annual incidence was 2.4% (3.1% in London, 1.0% elsewhere) with no significant trends in HIV incidence during 1995–2001. However, more recent data showed an increasing trend to 3.5% in 2002 (Hamers & Downs, 2004). Belgium is currently experiencing an alarming upward trend among MSM in the number of new HIV diagnoses that, in the past decade, increased by 228% ( from 101 cases diagnosed in 1999 to 332 cases in 2008). The majority of new HIV infections were diagnosed among Belgians citizens (72%), followed by other European nationalities, sub-Saharan Africa and other/unknown nationality ( Sasse & Defraye, 2009).

In Slovenia, of a total of 48 newly diagnosed HIV infection cases reported for 2008 (23.5/million population), 34 cases, representing more than two thirds, were MSM. Since 1999, the annual reported rate of newly diagnosed HIV cases in MSM raised from 2.5 to 16.7 per million men 15-64 years old, an increase of more than six times. The overall increase in the number of newly diagnosed HIV cases in Slovenia during recent years has been due almost exclusively to the increase in new diagnoses among MSM (Klavs et al., 2009).

Increases in risky sexual behaviour in a population in which HIV is already highly prevalent, coupled with increases in sexually transmitted infections that enhance the risk of HIV transmission, have the potential to lead to an expansion of HIV transmission among homosexual and bisexual men (Hamers & Downs, 2004).

### 2.1.2 United States / Canada

On June, 5, 1981, MMWR published a report of *Pneumocystis carinii* pneumonia in five previously healthy young men in Los Angeles. These cases were later recognized as the first reported cases of AIDS in the United States; since that time, this disease has become one of the greatest public health in the world. HIV infection and AIDS have claimed the lives of more than 22 million persons worldwide, including more than 500.000 persons in USA (CDC, 2006). Prevention interventions have contributed to a steady decline (from an estimated 8.048 in 2001 to 5.962 in 2004) in new HIV/AIDS diagnoses (CDC, 2005) but despite these successes, several challenges remain. In the United States, in contrast to other risk groups for which HIV/AIDS diagnoses have decreased, cases among MSM increased 8,6% from 2001 up to 72% in 2006 (CDC, 2008a). Among MSM with new infections, 46% were white, 35% were black, and 19% were Hispanic. Among MSM aged 13-29 years, the number of new HIV infections in blacks (5.220) was 1.6 times the number in whites (3.330) and 2.3 times the number in Hispanics (2.300). Among black and Hispanic MSM, most new infections were in persons aged 13-29, whereas, among white MSM, most new infections were in persons aged 30-39 years (CDC, 2008b). In Milwaukee county has been reported a 144% increase during 2000-2008 in black homosexual men aged 15-29 years. Interestingly, an increase in syphilis diagnoses among young black MSM in Milwaukee preceded the increase in HIV diagnoses, which suggests that changes in risk behavior or sexual networks might explain the increase (CDC, 2011).

The Centers for Disease Control and Prevention have documented a dramatic increase in the rates of sexually transmitted diseases among men who have sex with men (MSM) living in major urban centres across the country over the past 10 years (CDC, 2004). The MSM currently represent the group with the largest number of new HIV infections in the USA and its incidence have been increasing consistently since the early 1990s. Based upon national surveillance at sexually transmitted disease clinics, median positivity rates for gonorrhoea and chlamydia are higher among HIV-infected MSM than among HIV-uninfected or unknown status MSM. Syphilis seroreactivity rates are up to four times greater among HIV-infected MSM than HIV-uninfected or unknown status MSM (http:www.cdc.gov/STD/stats06/msm.htm as cited in Mayer et al., 2010). This trend of higher comparative rates of incident sexually transmitted infection (STI) among HIV-infected MSM is also evident in community samples both nationally (Whittington, 2002, as cited in Mayer et al., 2010 ) and internationally (Dodds, 2007, & Dougan, 2007, as cited in Mayer et al., 2010). Consistent with high rates of STI among HIV-infected MSM, some studies suggest that rates of high-risk sexual behaviors (i.e. anal intercourse without a condom) may be up to three times higher among HIV-infected MSM compared with HIV-uninfected MSM (Mayer et al., 2010).

In Canada at the end of 2005, an estimated 58.000 people were living with HIV infection which represents an increase of about 16% from the 2002 estimate of 50.000. In terms of exposure category, prevalent infections in 2005 were comprised of 29.600 MSM (51%), 9.860 IDU (17%), 8.620 heterosexual/non-endemic (15%), 7.050 heterosexual/endemic (12%), 2.250 MSM-IDU (4%), and 400 attributed to other exposure (<1%). The largest absolute increase was among the MSM exposure category with 3.400 more prevalent infections since 2002 (13% increase) (Boulos et al., 2006). This trend among MSM and MSM-IDU is been associated with increases in risky sexual behavior. The causes of this increase are complex and may include decision-making based on false assumptions about a partner's HIV status, dissatisfaction and difficulties with condom use, feelings of marginalization, depression and the choice to not use condoms as a gesture of commitment to a partner. The scenario is different among Aboriginal persons because the distribution of new cases of HIV in 2005 was 53% IDU versus 10% MSM and 3% MSM-IDU; this highlights the uniqueness of the HIV epidemic among Aboriginal Canadians and underscores the complexity of Canada's HIV epidemic (Boulos et al., 2006). Moreover, an estimated 16.900 persons HIV positives (26% of total prevalent infections) were unaware of their HIV-infected status and this proportion varied from an estimated 19% of HIV-infected MSM, to 25% of HIV-infected people who inject drugs, and 35% of HIV-infected heterosexuals (Yang et al., 2010).

### 2.1.3 Australia

Since 2000 the annual number of new diagnoses of HIV in Australia has increased by 38%. Gay men continue to be the most affected, accounting for 64% of people who were newly diagnosed as having HIV infection in 2004-2008, and 82% of the infections that were determined to have been acquired no more than a year before they were diagnosed (de Wit et al., 2010). Recent trends in new HIV diagnoses differ across Australian jurisdictions (Figure 1), the region with the highest number of HIV diagnoses each year is the state of New South Wales (NSW) with approximately 70% of these cases attributed to homosexual transmission (de Wit et al., 2010). While the population rate of HIV diagnosis doubled in Victoria between 1999 and 2006, increased markedly in South Australia and Western Australia in that period and steadily increased in Queensland since 1999, in NSW over the past decade the rate has remained relatively stable (Guy et al., 2007, as cited in de Wit et al., 2010). Historically, NSW has had the highest HIV infection rate; the apparent stability of the current HIV epidemic in gay men in NSW may reflect testing patterns, HIV status knowledge and disclosure and the well-reasoned use of risk-reduction strategies that this enables. A mathematical model has been used in conjunction with HIV/AIDS data from the Australian National HIV/AIDS

Registry to estimate numbers and ages of Australian men who have sex with men living with HIV infection from 1980 to 2005 (Murray et al., 2009). The average age of HIV-infected Australian MSM is estimated to exceed 44 years of age by the year 2010 and has increased by 1 year of age for each two calendar years since the mid-1980s. HIV-infected MSM over 60 years of age have been increasing in number by 12% per year since 1995. A consequence of successful therapy with subsequent ageing of those infected has meant that from 2001 estimated deaths from other causes exceed AIDS deaths in Australia (Murray et al., 2009). Australian guidelines recommend annual testing for HIV and sexually transmitted infections (STIs) for all men who have sex with men (MSM) and 3-6 monthly testing for those at higher risk as defined by behavioural criteria; a recent study (Guy et al., 2010) showed that there is poor adherence to national guidelines that recommend regular re-testing of MSM for STIs, particularly among those at higher risk who require more frequent testing.

Clinical strategies are urgently needed to encourage more frequent HIV/STI testing among MSM, especially in the higher risk subgroup.

### 2.2 The current scenario in developing / transitional countries

MSM in developing/transitional countries have a several-fold higher odds of HIV infection compared to the general population, with an 18-fold higher risk in Asia (Baral et al., 2007, as cited in Solomon et al., 2010). MSM in Africa are a highly vulnerable population at risk for HIV infection, in spite of this, the Africa region has documented limited HIV and STDs data on MSM, largely due to stigmatization of homosexual behaviour in the population (Smith et al., 2009). After Asia and sub-Saharan Africa, the region most impacted by HIV infection is Latin America where high rates HIV prevalence have been documented among MSM with no evidence of significant decrease (Halperin et al., 2009).

#### 2.2.1 India

There are more than 39.5 million people living with HIV worldwide, more than 2.5 million live in India where sexual transmission is the predominant mode of HIV transmission and is estimated to be the major risk for about 86% of those infected (National AIDS Control Organization, 2006, as cited in Solomon et al., 2010). The overall HIV prevalence in India is 0.36% ; the high reported HIV prevalence among some high-risk groups such as female sex workers (FSW) and men who have sex with men (above 5%), puts the country in the classification of concentrated epidemic. Protecting India's large population of FSW and MSM from infection is a critical priority and it is also an effective way to protect the remaining population from infection (UNAIDS, 2009, as cited in Gutierrez et al., 2010). A study carried out in Mumbai (formerly known as Bombay) found high rates of unprotected sex, bisexuality and HIV among urban Indian MSM (Kumta et al., 2010); another study conducted in Andhra Pradesh (AP) also found that MSM reported high rates of unprotected anal sex with other men and women. Andhra Pradesh (total population of 76.2 million) is among the six states in India with the highest HIV prevalence; about 10% of all AIDS cases in India are in AP (Dandona et al., 2005).

In India, the first evidence of HIV was described among sex workers in Tamil Nadu (TN) (Simoes et al., 1987, as cited in Solomon et al., 2010), then spreading to monogamous housewives via their husbands (Gangakhedkar et al., 1997, & Newmann et al., 2000, as cited in Solomon et al., 2010). Since heterosexual transmission was the primary driver of HIV in India, most prevention programs have targeted these individuals; recent evidence suggests that the HIV epidemic is declining among these populations (Arora et al., 2008, & Kumar et al., 2006, as cited in Solomon et al., 2010). By contrast, MSM remain the only high-risk population in India where HIV prevalence is increasing (National AIDS Control Organization, 2007, as cited in Solomon et al., 2010). There are an estimated 2.35 million sexually active MSM in India (National AIDS Control Organization, 2006, as cited in Solomon et al., 2010) ; historically, MSM in India have been a hidden population because of Section 377 of the Indian Penal Code which criminalizes anal intercourse and Indian culture's requirement of opposite sex marriage (Herget, 2006, as cited in Solomon et al., 2010). Consequently, few studies of HIV epidemiology among MSM in India exist. Most derive from urban sexually transmitted infection (STIs) clinics and few have characterized MSM in rural/semi-urban areas. In a landmark decision on July 2, 2009, the Delhi High Court repealed Section 377 (Nilajana, 2009, as cited in Solomon et al., 2010). While this allows more freedoms for MSM, it is likely that stigma and discrimination will continue and may even increase as MSM become more visible in Indian society. A study conducted across 18 different cities (classified in six urban sites, six semi-urban, six rural) in the south Indian state of Tamil Nadu showed HIV and syphilis prevalence of 9 and 8% respectively among not married MSM and of 14 and 11% among married MSM; HIV infections were not restricted to the large metropolitan cities because several semi-urban and rural settings also had HIV-infected MSM (Solomon et al., 2010).

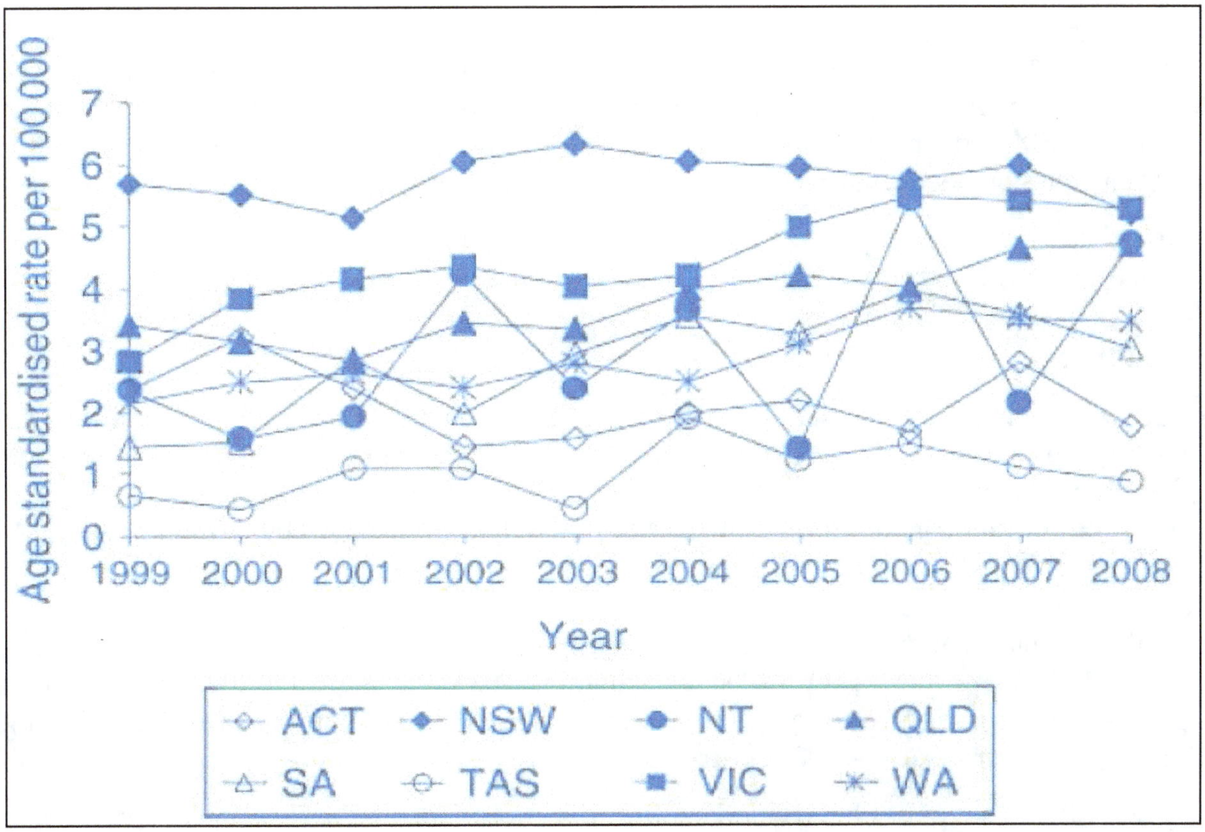


Fig. 1. Newly diagnosed HIV infection, 1999–2008, by year and state and territory, Australia. (Source: de Wit et al., 2010)

### 2.2.2 Sub-Saharan Africa

In sub-Saharan Africa the scenario is similar to that of India because research on MSM was neglected for a long time; most African countries do not include MSM in their HIV surveillance systems. Criminalisation of male-to-male sex, social denial and difficulty in reaching this population were the explanations given for the weak involvement of researchers in this area (Dahoma et al., 2011). However, recently, the assumption that this population could be significantly vulnerable to HIV and STIs has encouraged a growing number of epidemiological studies. Although heterosexual contact remains the main mode of HIV transmission in sub-Saharan Africa, HIV prevalence there has been described to be higher within MSM population than in the general population. In the first epidemiological study conducted on MSM in Senegal, HIV prevalence was 21.5% compared with less than 1% for the general Senegalese population. The high frequency of sexual contact with women reported by this study's participants also suggests that a sexual bridge between MSM and women could contribute to the expansion of the HIV epidemic (Wade et al., 2005). High levels of HIV infection also were reported among MSM in Zanzibar where a survey conducted from April through June 2007 among 509 MSM participants showed HIV prevalence of 12.3% (65/509) (Dahoma et al., 2011). Moreover, the study showed high levels of bisexual activity (70.8% of participants) which in combination with high risk sexual behaviour (i.e. inconsistent condom use) raise concerns about the potential bridging role of MSM in transmitting HIV infection into the general population ( Dahoma et al., 2011). In Nigeria results from a survey conducted in Lagos, Kano and Cross River states during 2007 showed that MSM are highly affected by HIV and that condom use in anal sex is low in commercial and non-commercial partnerships. HIV is more established among MSM in Lagos, there were wide variations in HIV prevalence with estimates ranging from 17.4%, to 9.3% and 1.1% in Lagos, Kano and Cross River respectively (Merrigan et al., 2011). Moreover, as previously observed in other African countries, significant proportions of Nigerian MSM had unprotected sex with female partners indicating a potential bridge for HIV transmission between MSM and the general population (Merrigan et al., 2011).

These data suggest that prevention interventions should be systematically implemented within the high-risk group of MSM in the African context.

### 2.2.3 China

In China, men who have sex with men have now become one of the priority populations for prevention and control of HIV pandemic because MSM transmission of HIV is a critical and growing public health problem. The estimated number of people living with HIV in China has also increased markedly from 400.000 in 2007 to 740.000 in 2009. Among new HIV infections reported in China, the proportion of MSM transmission has risen dramatically. According to pooled prevalence estimates from meta-analyses (Chow et al., 2011), the overall national HIV prevalence among MSM in China has increased from 1.3% during 2003-2004 to 2.4% during 2005-2006 and then to 4.7% during 2007-2008; moreover, a significantly positive correlation was observed between HIV and syphilis prevalence among Chinese MSM during 2003–2008 countrywide.

With substantial increases in HIV and syphilis infection, Chow et al. (2011) also observed an increase in prevalent HIV-syphilis co-infections (1.4% during 2005-2006 to 2.7% during 2007-2008) (Figure 2). In 2009, 32.5% of 48.000 new HIV infections was attributed to male homosexual exposure, which is almost triple the reported level in 2007 (12.2% of 50.000 new cases) (UNGASS, 2010, as cited in Chow et al., 2011). In Shenyang city, the capital of Liaoning Province in northeast China, MSM transmission accounted for 39.6% of new infections in 2009. Epidemiological studies from 2006 suggested that HIV infection among MSM in Shenyang was increasing rapidly, with an HIV incidence density of 5.4/100 person-years (Xu et al., 2010). A 3-year prospective open cohort follow-up survey (from 2007 to 2009) that recruited a total of 1282 MSM (229 in 2007, 598 in 2008 and 455 in 2009) revealed a significant increase in incidence density of HIV from 4.7/100 person-years to 10.2 /100 person years (Table 1). Furthermore, due to a higher transmission probability of HIV associated with penile-anal intercourse and levels of risk related behaviour, Chinese MSM have an approximately 45-fold higher risk of acquiring HIV than other males in the general population (Zhang et al., 2011).

| *Type of recruited MSM cohorts* | *Infection rate* | *Incidence density (95% CI)* |
|---|---|---|
| Recruited cohort in 2007 | 5.7 % | 4.7/100 person-years |
| Recruited cohort in 2008 | 6.2 % | 6.1/100 person-years |
| Recruited cohort in 2009 | 8.1 % | 10.2/100 person-years |

Table 1. China. Shenyang city : new infection rates and incidence density of HIV. (Source: Zhang et al., 2011)

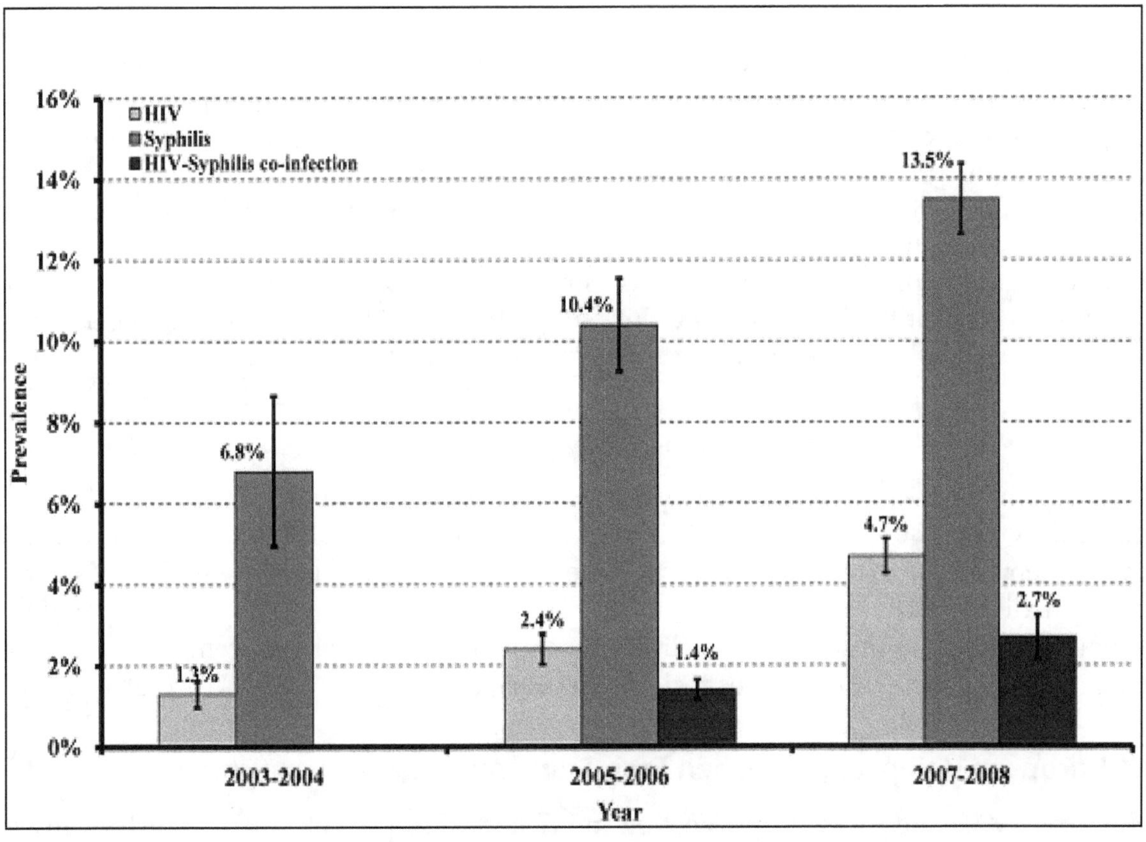


Fig. 2. China : estimated prevalence of HIV, syphilis infection and HIV-syphilis co-infection among men who have sex with men during 2003–2008. (Source : Chow et al., 2011)

## 3. Treponema pallidum / Syphilis

Syphilis. The name of this widespread and ancient disease is familiar to health care providers worldwide, it was coined by the Italian physician Girolamo Fracastoro in his tale of the shepherd Syphilus, who contracted the disease after insulting the pagan Sun god.

Syphilis is a genital ulcerative disease caused by the spirochaete *Treponema pallidum* subsp. *pallidum* (Fenton et al., 2008), identified in 1905 by Schaudinn & Hoffmann (Waugh, 2005, as cited in Fenton et al., 2008). The disease is treatable with standard antibiotics (Pao et al., 2002, as cited in Fenton et al., 2008), but in the absence of therapy, gives rise to four sequencial clinical stages commonly known as primary, secondary, latent (divided into early and late stages) and tertiary syphilis (Table 2) (Botham et al., 2006). In the initial stages, the infection is highly transmissible and often presents as ulcerative genital lesions. Secondary syphilis results from the multiplication and dissemination of Treponemes throughout the body. The most common manifestation is a disseminated mucocutaneous rash.

The secondary stage occurs up to 6 months after the healing of the primary lesion and lasts for several weeks or months and may reoccur in approximately 25% of untreated patients (Stamm, 1998, as cited in Fenton et al., 2008). The oral cavity is the most common extra-genital site of infection; oral chancres are observed in about 4–12% of patients with primary syphilis and occur at the site of penetration of the organism into the mucosa. Anatomical sites commonly affected are especially the tongue, gingiva, soft palate and lips (Ficarra & Carlos, 2009) (Figure 3). The tertiary or late stage of syphilis is rarely seen today in the era of effective and prevalent antibiotic therapy. Treponemes invade the central nervous or cardiovascular systems, eyes, skin, and other internal organs, producing damage as a result of their invasive properties and inflammation (Fenton et al., 2008). With minor differences, syphilis generally presents similarly in HIV-positive and HIV-negative patients. In primary syphilis, HIV-infected patients may present with more than one chancre (up to 70% of patients) and with larger and deeper lesions. About a quarter of HIV-infected patients present with concomitant lesions of both primary and secondary stages of syphilis at the time of diagnosis. Approximately one-third of patients with early syphilis have invasion of Treponemes in the cerebrospinal fluid (CSF), regardless of their HIV status. However, by contrast with HIV-uninfected patients, most of the new cases of clinical neurosyphilis in HIV-infected individuals are identified early at the initial presentation, suggesting that HIV infection may be associated with an increased risk of developing neurological complications (Zetola & Klausner, 2007).

### 3.1 The current scenario in developed countries

Rates of syphilis in many developed cities worldwide reached their lowest recorded levels towards the end of the 1990s. Since 1997, however, outbreaks of syphilis among men who have sex with men have been reported in North America and Europe, and those with HIV infection have been disproportionately affected (CDC, 2002). Australia has two distinct patterns of infectious syphilis: a substantially declining occurrence in Indigenous remote communities and an increasing incidence in males residing in urban and regional areas (Ward et al., 2011).

#### 3.1.1 European Union and European Free Trade Association countries

In the early 1990s rates of syphilis infection in Western Europe (WE) were at historically low levels, these decreases were accompanied by marked reductions in the incidence of congenital syphilis and tertiary disease. But **syphilis has re-emerged in western Europe**

**since 2000** and a large increase and outbreaks affecting major urban centres in Europe, mainly in MSM, have been reported (Figure 4) (Sullivan et al., 2009). **Changes in sexual behaviour have facilitated the spread of syphilis especially among men who have sex with men and improved surveillance systems and case detection have lead to an increase in the reported numbers of cases.** The first of several outbreaks of syphilis in MSM was observed in Hamburg (Germany) in 1996/1997, and syphilis incidence began to increase nationwide in 2001 (Marcus & Hamouda, 2005); in Germany, for syphilis cases in MSM, 7% in the year 2002 were classified as re-infections.

| INFECTIOUS | NON-INFECTIOUS |
|---|---|
| **Primary**<br>One or more ano-genital or oral ulcers (chancres) are present, which may vary considerably in appearance. Serological tests are reactive.<br>**Secondary**<br>Skin spots or rashes are present, particularly on the trunk, palms and soles,often with generalised lymphadenopathy. The primary chancre may still be present. Non-treponemal (RPR, VDRL) titre 1:4.<br>**Latent**<br>No symptoms of syphilis are present, but treponemal (TPPA, FTA-Abs) tests are reactive and the non-treponemal (RPR, VDRL) tests have increased two titres.<br>**Early latent**<br>Disease acquired within the past two years. | **Late latent**<br>Disease acquired more than two years ago or at an unknown time.<br>**Neurosyphilis**<br>Syphilis of any stage with clinical symptoms of neurosyphilis or raised CSF protein or WCC in the absence of other known causes of these abnormalities.<br>**Tertiary**<br>Characteristic abnormalities of the cardiovascular, skin, bone or other systems.<br>**Congenital syphilis**<br>A condition affecting an infant whose mother had untreated or inadequately treated syphilis at delivery. |

Table 2. Classification of syphilis. (Source: Botham et al., 2006 )

This proportion increased to 16% in 2004, in seven cities (Frankfurt, Cologne, Berlin, Mannheim, Munich, Leipniz, Hamburg) with > 100.000 population, with the highest incidence of syphilis in 2004 (>10/100.000), 25% of reported cases in MSM were classified as re-infections. This datum indicates an intense circulation of syphilis in restricted subgroups of MSM in the largest cities (Marcus & Hamouda, 2005). In Denmark an outbreak of syphilis began in 2003 and continued in 2004. Data from the national surveillance system showed that most cases are in men who have sex with men, and that a large proportion of these patients are also HIV positive. The majority of cases were reported from Copenhagen municipality; the outbreak did not seem to be affecting the age group under 20 years. Probably, most of the MSM found with both syphilis and HIV were already HIV positive when they acquired syphilis infection (Cowan, 2004). In the United Kingdom, between 1997 and 2002, diagnoses of primary, secondary, and early latent syphilis made at genitourinary medicine clinics increased by 213% in heterosexual males, 1412% in men who have sex with men (MSM), and 22% in females. These increases were initially observed in larger cities and then progressed to suburban and rural settings (Simms et al., 2005). In 2004, among MSM/bisexual men an alarming increase of 212% as regards 2003 has been observed in

Scotland; most of the diagnoses (91%) were made in the Glasgow and Edinburgh clinics ( Figure 5) (Wallace et al., 2005). The Swedish Surveillance system of syphilis is population-based. All health care specialists have the responsibility to notify diagnosed syphilis directly to the national surveillance system SmiNet. Also all laboratories diagnosing syphilis have the responsibility to notify to the SmiNet. From the data obtained through the surveillance system seems that the major contributor to the recent rise in syphilis cases in Sweden is infections among MSM (Figure 6) (Velicko et al., 2008). Among MSM who acquired a syphilis infection in Sweden in recent years, the majority acquired it in big cities, especially Stockholm (up to 96% of all reported cases among MSM); syphilis incidence among MSM was 20-28 times that of males in general in Sweden.

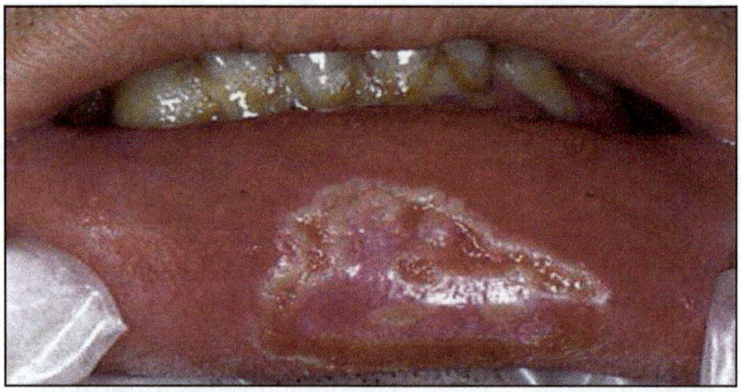

Fig. 3. Secondary oral syphilis: mucous patches covered by *grayish, white* pseudomembranes of the lower vestibular mucosa. (Source : Ficarra & Carlos, 2009).

It can be assumed that MSM to a larger extent choose to live in big cities since they assure more anonymity and less stigmatisation for MSM (Velicko et al., 2008). In contrast to WE countries, in Central and Eastern Europe between 1998 and 2007 there was a general decline in the number of reported syphilis cases (Savage et al., 2009). During the same period the sex ratio was relatively stable at around 1:1, with the exception of Slovenia where the male: female ratio rose to almost 5:1 in 2007 and 39% of male cases were reported to be MSM (Savage et al., 2009). Recent increases in overall early syphilis reported rates in Slovenia (in 2008 increase of 130% compared with 2007), with great majority of cases occurring in men (94%) and among cases in men a substantial proportion of cases among men known to have sex with men (44%) and among those almost one in three with a foreign MSM partner within three months preceding syphilis diagnosis, suggest recent increase in unsafe sexual behaviour among MSM and sexual mixing of Slovenian MSM with MSM abroad (Klavs et al., 2009). Most worrying, two in three early syphilis cases reported in 2008 among MSM were men with known HIV infection, indicating unsafe sexual behaviour among HIV-positive MSM aware of their infection. In the Czech Republic, most cases of syphilis, total of 18.000 were diagnosed after the World War II during the mass screening of the population aged 15 to 40 years in 1951. In the following years, the incidence of syphilis decreased considerably; the absolute number of reported syphilis cases has increased rapidly during the 1990s as a result of geopolitical and socioeconomic changes (Kuklova et al., 2011). The syphilis rate has risen eightfold from 1.6 per 100.000 inhabitants in 1990 to 13.5 per 100.000 inhabitants in 2001 due to high proportion of syphilis cases among immigrants coming mainly from the Ukraine, Moldavia, the Russian Federation and Georgia. After reaching a peak in 2001, the incidence of syphilis has been decreasing but, after 2006, the incidence has increased again. Men, in particular MSM, prevail over women among the infected persons (Kuklova et al., 2011).

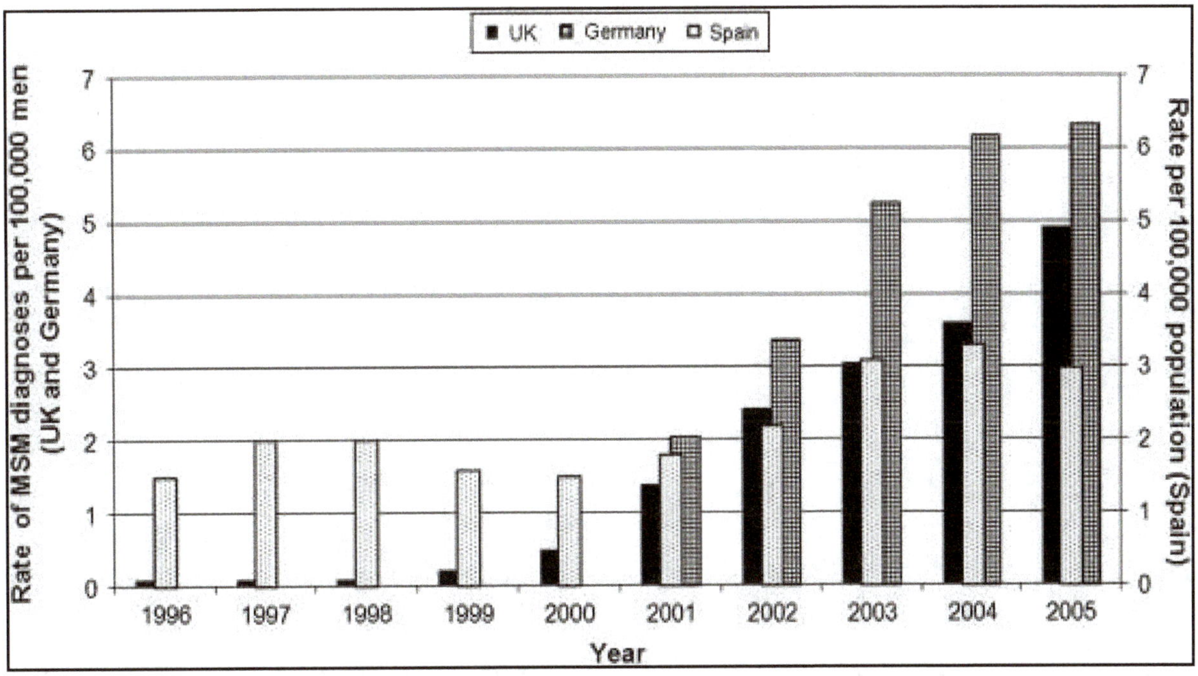


Fig. 4. Primary and secondary syphilis rates in United Kingdom and Germany (rate of diagnoses among MSM per 100,000 men) and Spain (rate per 100,000 population), 1996-2005. (Source: Sullivan et al., 2009).

### 3.1.2 United States / Canada

Although syphilis is uncommon in much of the US population, several groups are disproportionately affected, including African Americans, Hispanics, and men who have sex with men (MSM).

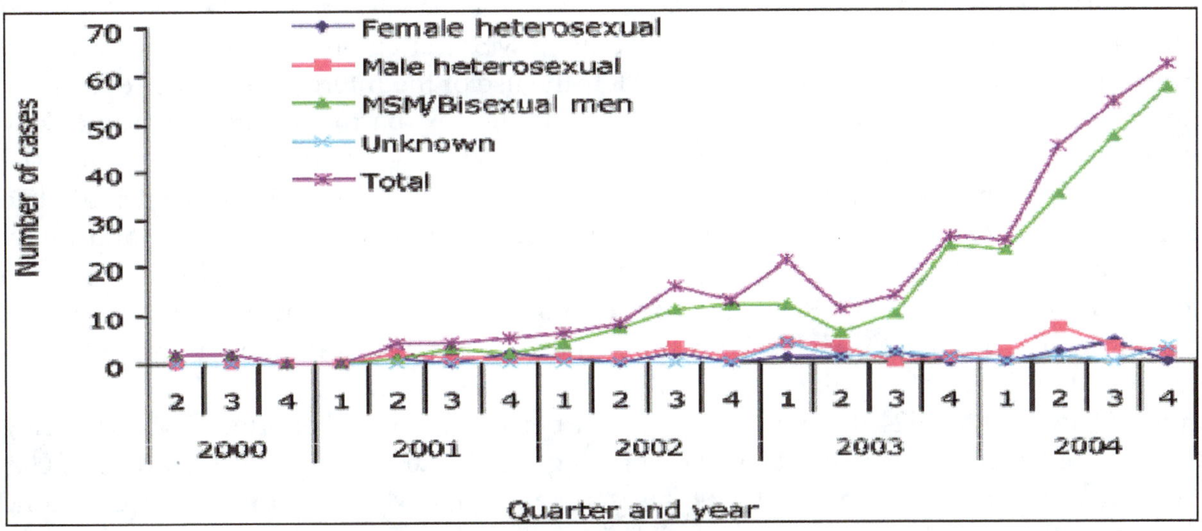


Fig. 5. Number of cases of infectious syphilis diagnosed at STI clinics in Scotland by sexual orientation and quarterly totals, 2000-2004. The majority of cases were diagnosed at sexually transmitted infections (STIs) clinics in Edinburgh (45%) and Glasgow (42%). ( Source : Wallace et al., 2005)

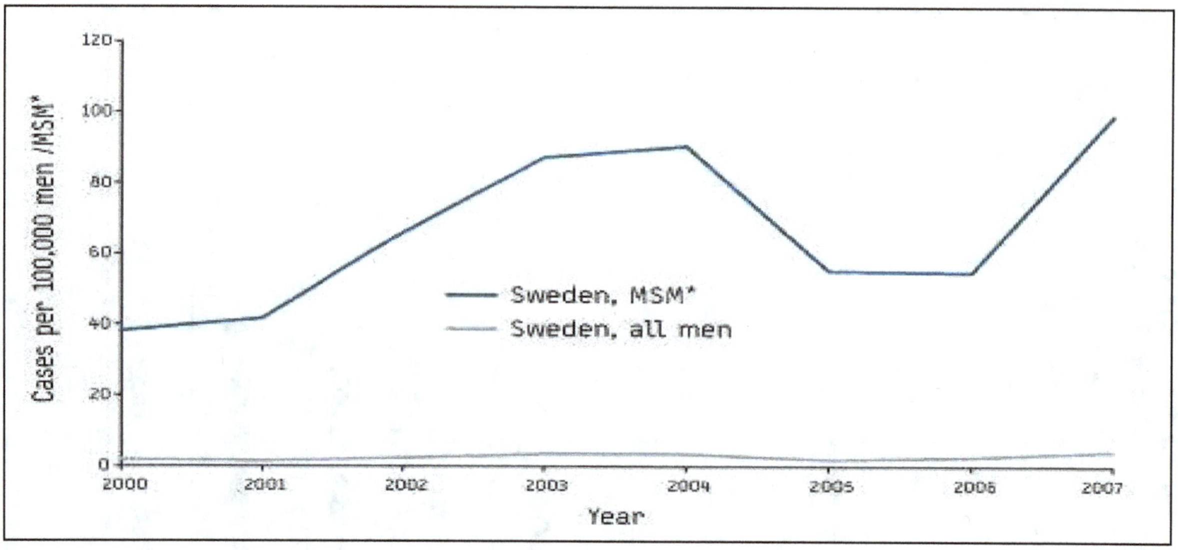


Fig. 6. Estimated syphilis incidence among MSM and observed syphilis incidence among all males, notified cases in Sweden, 2000-2007. (Source: Velicko et al., 2008)

After steady decreases for >1 decade, rates of syphilis in the United States reached their lowest point during 2000, when the rate of primary and secondary syphilis was 2.1 cases per 100,000 persons. By 2005, the rate of primary and secondary syphilis increased to 3.0 cases per 100,000 persons, representing an increase from 5976 to 8724 cases, of which 86% occurred in men. This increase in the rate ratio of male to female patients (from 1.2 in 1996 to 5.7 in 2005) was a reflection of the disproportionate burden of disease among MSM, who accounted for ~65% of all persons with primary and secondary syphilis (Zetola & Klausner, 2007). Large metropolitan communities of MSM have been particularly affected by concurrent epidemics of syphilis and HIV infection; genital ulcers bleed frequently during sexual intercourse, resulting in potential increases in HIV infectiousness. In California more of 60% of MSM with syphilis are HIV infected, and it is estimated that, in major cities, 20-50% of MSM with syphilis have also HIV infection. The increase in the rate of syphilis and other sexually transmitted diseases (STDs) among MSM suggests a decrease in safer sex practices. In this regard, the success of HAART, the use of the Internet to meet sex partners, the increased frequency of serosorting (i.e., finding sex partners with the same HIV serostatus), and the increase in recreational drug use, both illicit (e.g., crystal methamphetamine) and prescribed (e.g., sildenafil citrate), have all likely contributed to increases in the rate of syphilis. In addition, the idea that oral sex is "safer" sex and rarely associated with HIV transmission may explain the role of oral sex in syphilis transmission (Zetola & Klausner, 2007). Recently, considering the high incidence of asymptomatic syphilis in HIV positive MSM, has been stressed the importance of frequent routine syphilis testing in this group of population. In USA, syphilis cases occurring among MSM increased from 441 in 2000 to 4424 in 2003; the estimated percentage of all reported cases occurring among MSM in 2003 was 62% (Table 3) (Heffelfinger et al., 2007). During 2000 through 2003, there was an estimated increase of 2298 cases among white MSM; in contrast, cases among heterosexual men and women decreased 50% (from 5532 to 2753) between 2000 and 2003.

In Canada, a review of infectious syphilis cases carried out in Ottawa, from 2001-2006, showed that rates of syphilis have risen more than tenfold (Leber et al., 2008) and that the majority of cases (83.5%) occurring among men who have sex with men. These individuals differed from the general MSM population residing in Ottawa in their being older, more likely to be HIV positive, and more sexually promiscuous; inconsistent condom use by MSM engaged in either oral or anal sex was pervasive. Visceral manifestations of syphilis, including neurosyphilis, were more common in persons co-infected with HIV. Multiple sexual partners, unprotected oral sex, and increased age among MSM were the predominant risk factors contributing to this syphilis epidemic (Leber et al., 2008). Co-infection with HIV modified the clinical presentation of syphilis, necessitating a more intensive diagnostic and therapeutic approach. The interconnection of urban sexual networks has likely contributed to the dynamics of local syphilis transmission and suggests that effective interventions will require a coordinated national approach (Leber et al., 2008).

| Year | Total No. of cases | Cases among men | Cases among women | Male-Female Case ratio | Cases among MSM | Cases among heterosexual men and women [a] |
|---|---|---|---|---|---|---|
| 2000 | 5973 | 3528 | 2445 | 1.44 | 441 | 5532 |
| 2001 | 6100 | 4132 | 1968 | 2.10 | 1653 | 4447 |
| 2002 | 6862 | 5268 | 1594 | 3.30 | 3257 | 3605 |
| 2003 | 7177 | 5959 | 1218 | 4.89 | 4424 | 2753 |
| a. Calculated by subtracting estimated cases among MSM from the total number of cases. | | | | | | |

Table 3. Numbers of Primary and Secondary Syphilis Cases Among Different Groups, Along With Male–Female Case Ratios: United States, 2000–2003. (Source: Heffelfinger et al., 2007).

### 3.1.3 Australia

Syphilis appeared to be well controlled in large urban centres in Australia during the 1990s, probably as a result of HIV prevention efforts; an overall decrease in syphilis rate was seen until 2001. Since 2001, enhanced syphilis surveillance has been undertaken in south-eastern Sydney for all new laboratory syphilis notifications. The New South Wales (NSW) surveillance classifications for newly diagnosed adult cases are showed in Table 2. However, in 2002 the overall rates of syphilis increased by 14.1%, possibly related to public health activities such as active testing for STIs at selected sex-on-premise venues (Victoria), a targeted syphilis campaign coinciding with the Gay Games in Sidney in 2002 (New South Wales), and the establishment of a syphilis registry (Queensland) (Yohannes et al., 2004, as cited in Botham et al., 2006). In particular, inner Sidney has recently experienced a rapid increase in infectious syphilis, similar to other developed cities with large gay male populations. During 2001-04, 1275 syphilis notifications were received ; of these notifications 1112 were classified as 361 infectious syphilis, 221 non-infectious syphilis and 530 treated syphilis. The majority of infectious syphilis diagnoses were made in the earlier primary or secondary stages. The enhanced syphilis surveillance program showed infectious syphilis is affecting a defined population in Sidney: men (31:1 male-to-female ratio for 2004), English speaking and Australian born (Botham et al., 2006). The male-to-female ratio for 2004 of 31:1 strongly suggests transmission between men (Botham et al., 2006). The public health response to this epidemic has included work by the Sexually Transmitted Infections in Gay Men Action Group (STIGMA). This group was formed in 2000 and initiated the project for enhanced syphilis surveillance and also developed and disseminated guidelines entitled *Sexually Transmitted Infection Testing Guidelines for Men who have Sex with Men*. These guidelines recommend annual syphilis serology for all men who have had sex with another man in the previous year; this recommendation, promoted to clinicians and the gay community, may have contributed to the overall increase in syphilis notifications. Data of literature (Jin et al., 2009) showed that in Sidney STIs peak among MSM occurred in the 35-44 year age group, suggesting a decline in sexual "safety" among older gay men, and that syphilis incidence was almost 10-fold higher in HIV-positive than in HIV-negative MSM and it was not related to a CD4 count below 350 μL ; UAI with HIV positive partners was of particular importance in the transmission of syphilis. Within Australia, syphilis has also increased largely in gay men in the Queensland and Victoria (Bourke & Schmidt, 2009).

### 3.2 The current scenario in developing/transitional countries

Infectious diseases continue to cause an enormous burden of death and disability in developing countries; a relevant role is represented from sexually transmitted infections. Even if the last years have seen a re-emergence of international interest in the role of MSM in STDs epidemics globally, data on their incidence and prevalence, in particular of syphilis, are still poor in most of the developing countries. This is most evident in sub-Saharan Africa, north Africa and the Caribbean, where stigma around homosexuality is still considered appalling. However, even in Asia and Latin America, studies conducted usually lack a clear understanding of these populations and their diverse behaviours (Càceres et al., 2008).

#### 3.2.1 India

Reports from sexually transmitted disease clinics and single health care institutions in India suggest an increase in genital ulcerative sexually transmitted infections such as syphilis. The little information available on rates of syphilis in India show an incidence rate of 5.4 per 100 person years in a sexually transmitted disease clinic in India from 1993-2000 and prevalence rates as high as 21.9% amongst a convenience sample of long-distance truck drivers in 2000 (Gawande et al., 2000, & Reynolds et al., 2006, as cited in Schneider et al., 2010). A recent study (Schneider et al., 2010) carried out in Andhra Pradesh in the general population (6.235 men and 6.382 women study participants) showed prevalence rates of 2.08% for men and 1.42% for woman; nearly one in four persons surveyed that were seropositive for syphilis were also HIV infected. 85 men, that declared to have sex with men > 6 months ago, showed a syphilis prevalence of 2.4% while other 47, that declared own homosexuality within last 6 months, showed a prevalence of 6.4%. The strong association between syphilis and HIV seroprevalence in this population-based study suggests that acceleration of direct linkages between syphilis testing and HIV counselling and testing would be useful in enhancing the control of STIs and HIV in India; particular attention should be paid to homosexuals men of India that have one of the highest rates of HIV prevalence amongst groups at high risk of sexual transmission of HIV.

#### 3.2.2 Sub Saharan Africa

In 1999, WHO estimated that were 4 million cases of syphilis among adults in sub-Saharan Africa. In Africa syphilis is endemic and the incidence is high also among pregnant woman; this is a worrying fact because maternal syphilis has a severe impact on pregnancy outcome and there are significant challengens to implementing syphilis screening programmes in sub-Saharan Africa (Watson-Jones et al., 2005). Many prevalence studies have been conducted in the general population but unfortunately, data on the prevalence of syphilis in MSM are scanty, likely because of stigma and discrimination against homosexuality. Some studies conducted among blood donors have shown a variable prevalence among different sub - Saharan geographical areas : in Burkina-Faso a study (Nagalo et al., 2011) showed that seroprevalence of syphilis (3.96%) was lower than the prevalence of among blood donors in Tanzania (4.6% among HIV negative, 12.1% among HIV positive) (Matee et al., 2006) but higher than the 1.1% observed in Nigeria (Buseri et al., 2009), where recently no syphilis was detected among 879 examined MSM (Merrigan et al., 2011) suggesting a lower prevalence of syphilis in Nigerian population compared to other African populations. A recent study carried out in Ghana in a sample of 1366 prison inmates, including 403 homosexuals men, revealed seroprevalence syphilis rates of 13.7 % and 23.3% in heterosexual and homosexual respectively and syphilis seropositivity was significantly associated with HIV seropositivity (Adjei et al., 2008). These results confirm data previously reported and emphasize the need for preventive interventions in areas such as prisons that are known to be high-risk environments for the spread of bloodborne and sexually transmitted infections.

### 3.2.3 China

Syphilis was nearly eradicated in China in 1964 (Cohen et al., 1996, as cited in Chow et al., 2011) but recently it has returned to become one of the top five most reported notifiable diseases. Has been documented a 30-fold increase in syphilis diagnoses from 0.2 cases per 100.000 individuals in 1989 to 6.5 cases per 100.000 individuals in 1999 and a further 3-fold increase over the following decade to 22 cases per 100.000 individuals in 2008 (Tucker et al., 2010, as cited in Chow et al., 2011). Cross-sectional studies have found a high prevalence of syphilis among men who have sex with men in China. Sample representativeness remains one of the challenges in effective STDs surveillance and prevention targeting men who have sex with men worldwide. Although convenience samples are widely used in studies of MSM, previous studies suggested that these samples might not be representative of the broader MSM population. This issue becomes even more critical in many developing countries where needed resources for conducting probability sampling are limited. A study carried out in Beijing during 2009 among four MSM samples using different recruitment methods showed rates of Syphilis infection of 21.8%, 36.2%, 11.8%, and 13.8%; rates of inconsistent condom use were 57%, 52%, 58%, and 38%. Significant differences were found in various socio-demographic characteristics (e.g., age, migration history, education, income, and places of employment) and risk behaviours (e.g., age at first sex, number of sex partners, involvement in commercial sex, and substance use) among samples recruited by different sampling methods (peer outreach, informal social network, Internet, and venue-based) (Guo et al., 2011). Other recent studies (Xu et al., 2011; Zhang et al., 2011) carried out in Shenyang city (in 2009) and Liaoning (from April 2008 to January 2009) showed a syphilis prevalence of 14.9% and 5% respectively. These variable results of seroprevalence confirm the importance of using multiple sampling methods to reach MSM from diverse backgrounds and in different social segments and to improve the representativeness of the MSM samples when the use of probability sampling approach is not feasible.

## 4. Conclusion

Men who have sex with men, among all races and ethnicities, remain at great risk for HIV infection and syphilis; behavioural prevention remains central to reduce their transmission and can be the key to this process. Sex is life, but we have to be conscious of the fact that safe sex is the first premise. Sexually transmitted diseases (STDs) are among the first ten causes of unpleasant diseases in young adult males in developing countries and the second major cause of unpleasant diseases in young adult women worldwide. In general, STDs are epidemics and present enormous health and economic consequences. The surest way to avoid transmission of sexually transmitted diseases, including syphilis, is to abstain from sexual contact or to be in a long-term mutually monogamous relationship with a partner who has been tested and is known to be uninfected. Avoiding alcohol and drug use may also help prevent transmission of syphilis because these activities may lead to risky sexual behavior (Zetola & Klausner), (Mayer et al. 2010). It is important that sex partners talk to each other about their HIV status and history of other STDs so that preventive action can be taken. An adequate screening for re-emerging STDs should be done on a routine basis in every part of the world, in particular among highly vulnerable subjects at risk for HIV and syphilis as homosexual men; individuals unaware of their infection are a priority for being tested and diagnosed to enable them to take advantage of care services and receive counselling to prevent further spread of HIV and *T. pallidum*. Partner selection based on perceived serostatus could be used as a strategy for risk reduction among MSM but it strategy has some limits since those most recently infected may be most infectious and least likely to know of their status, reliance on partner's awareness and disclosure of their own serostatus may be a risky strategy. Individuals who are infected with STDs are 5-10 times more likely than uninfected individuals to acquire or to transmit HIV through sexual contact. The breaking of the genital tract or trauma of the rectal mucosa creates a portal of entry for HIV, and HIV positive individuals co-infected with other STDs, especially ulcerative infections such as syphilis, are more likely to shed HIV in their genital secretions. The most effective method available for protection against STDs and HIV is the correct and consistent use of condom that is increasing everywhere except in developing countries. In particular, high risk sexual behaviours reported in Africa and in India among MSM and high levels of bisexual activity are of grave concern. Most worrisome is that condom use messages for preventing HIV and STDs do not appear to have penetrated this population given the low proportion of MSM using condom ; three most often repeated reasons for not using condoms with regular partners include non availability, feeling the partner is safe and feeling that condoms do not give sexual pleasure (Kumta et al., 2010). Interestingly, a study carried out in the south-eastern part of India (Andhra Pradesh) showed that one of the primary reasons for low condom usage was that many married MSM did not disclose their sexual orientation to their wives and therefore struggled to explain the necessity of condom use (Gutierrez et al., 2010). This datum suggests that in some parts of the developing world prevention work is handicapped unless it addresses broader issues surrounding sexual identity, stigma and discrimination. Internet is commonly used by MSM to find sexual partners. The net is a relatively safe space where sexuality can be addressed in a frank and honest way because the web allows anonymity and confidentially. In a context where homosexuality is penalised, blackmail and police harassment are common and the media are homophobic, internet may be a way to support and inform men who have sex with men about HIV/STDs and other issues which men ask about (Pebody, 2010). For example, in

Romania, Kovacs used a sexual networking site to build a support network of HIV positive MSM (an extremely marginalised and, until then, invisible group in Romania). In another example, in Thailand, Mplus Organisation works with various groups including men selling sex, transgender people and MSM; the organisation lets their existing contacts know that staff will be present on various social networking sites and MSM Messenger at specific times, where they are available to interact and answer questions (Pebody, 2010). These data suggest that Internet is a double edged sword because on the one hand promotes sexual encounters and promiscuity, on the other hand can help prevent the spread of HIV and other sexually transmitted infections such as syphilis. Interestingly, during a recent syphilis outbreak that involved 7 MSM in San Francisco who met in an online chat, electronic notification of the cluster was provided to hundreds of chat room users. Despite very limited contact information, the Department of Public Health was able to notify and treat 42% of the named sex partners (Klausner et al., 2000). The major challenge for the future is to reduce the rates of new infections in a context of increasingly diverse and complex prevention responses. A key requisite for this development is the occurrence of transformations that tackle homophobic violence and ensure the respect for the human rights of gay men, transgenders and other MSM.

In conclusion, more research is need to further clarify which strategies (i.e. reducing unprotected anal sex, condom distribution, having oral sex instead of anal sex, reducing number of partners, avoiding serodiscordant partners, strategic positioning or reducing anal sex even with condom use) are most effective in reducing sexually transmitted infections transmission among MSM, the messages most effective in promoting preventive behaviours, and the methods and settings in which these messages can be most effectively delivered.

## 5. References

Adjei, A.A., Armah, H.B., Gbagbo, F., Ampofo, W.K., Boamah, I., Adu-Gyamfi, C., Asare, I., Hesse, I.F. & Mensah, G. (2008). *Correlates of HIV, HBV, HCV and syphilis infections among prison inmates and officers in Ghana: A national multicenter study.* BMC Infect Dis, 8:33.

Botham, S.J., Ressler, K.A., Bourne, C. & Ferson, M.J. (2006). *Epidemic infectious syphilis in inner Sydney--strengthening enhanced surveillance.* Aust N Z J Public Health, 30(6):529-33.

Boulos, D., Yan, P., Schanzer, D., Remis, R.S. & Archibald, C.P. (2006). *Estimates of HIV prevalence and incidence in Canada, 2005.* Can Commun Dis Rep 32(15):165-74

Bourke, S. & Schmidt, T. (2009). *Sexually transmissible infections - Old enemies and a new friend.* Aust Fam Phisician, 38(6):373.

Buseri, F.I., Muhibi, M.A. & Jeremiah, Z.A. (2009). *Sero-epidemiology of transfusion-transmissible infectious diseases among blood donors in Osogbo, south-west Nigeria.* Blood Transfus, 7(4):293-9.

Cáceres, C.F., Konda, K., Segura, E.R. & Lyerla, R. (2008). *Epidemiology of male same-sex behaviour and associated sexual health indicators in low- and middle-income countries: 2003-2007 estimates.* Sex Transm Infect, 84 Suppl 1:i49-i56.

CDC. (2002). *Primary and secondary syphilis among men who have sex with men- New York city, 2001.* MMWR, 51 : 853-6

CDC. (2004). *Trends in primary and secondary syphilis and HIV infections in men who have sex with men – San Francisco and Los Angeles, California, 1998-2002*. MMWR, 53 : 575-78

CDC).(2005). *HIV/AIDS surveillance report, 2004*. Available from http://www.cdc.gov/hiv/stats/hasrlink.htm

CDC. (2006). *Twenty-five years of HIV/AIDS- United States, 1981-2006*. MMWR, 55 (21): 585-89

CDC. (2007). *HIV/AIDS Surveillance Report 2006*. Atlanta (GA) : U.S. Department of Health and Human Services, CDC and Prevention 181- 46

CDC. (2008a). *Trends in HIV/AIDS diagnoses among men who have sex with men*. MMWR, 57:681-86

CDC. (2008b). *Subpopulation estimates from the HIV incidence surveillance System- United States 2006*. MMWR, 57: 985-89

CDC. (2011). *Increase in newly diagnosed HIV infections among young black men who have sex with men- Milwaukee County, Wisconsin, 1999-2008*. MMWR, 60:99-102

Chow, E.P., Wilson, D.P. & Zhang, L. (2011). *HIV and Syphilis Co-Infection Increasing among Men Who Have Sex with Men in China: A Systematic Review and Meta-Analysis*. 6(8):e22768. PLos One, Epub 2011 Aug 15.

Couturier, E., Michel, A., Janier, M., Dupin, N. & Semaille, C. *Syphilis surveillance in France, 2000-2003*. Euro Surveill. 2004 ; 9 (12) : pii = 493

Cowan, S. (2004).*Syphilis in Denmark-Outbreak among MSM in Copenhagen, 2003-2004*. Euro Surveill, 9 (12) :25-7.

Dahoma, M., Johnston, L.G., Holman, A., Miller, L.A., Mussa, M., Othman, A., Khatib, A., Issa, R., Kendall, C. & Kim, A.A. (2011). *HIV and related risk behaviour among men who have sex with men in Zanzibar, Tanzania: results of a behavioural surveillance survey*. AIDS Behav, 15(1):186-92.

Dandona, L., Dandona, R., Gutierrez, J.P., Kumar, G.A., McPherson, S. & Bertozzi, S.M. (2005). *Sex behaviour of men who have sex with men and risk of HIV in Andhra Pradesh, India*. AIDS, 19(6):611-9.

de Wit, J.B., Prestage, G.P. & Duffin, I.R. (2010). *Gay men: current challenges and emerging approaches in HIV prevention*. N S W Public Health Bull, 21(3-4):65-68.

Downs, A.M., Heisterkamp, S.H., Ravà, L., Houweling, H., Jager, J.C. & Hamers,.F.F. ( 2000). *Back-calculation by birth cohort, incorporating age- specific disease progression, pre-AIDS mortality and change in European AIDS case definition. European Union Concerted Action on Multinational AIDS Scenarios*. AIDS; 14(14):2179-89.

Elford, J., Jeannin, A., Spencer, B., Gervasoni, J.P., van de Laar, M.J. & Dubois-Arber, F. (2009). *HIV and STI behavioural surveillance among men who have sex with men in Europe*. Euro Surveill, 14(47). pii: 19414

Fenton, K.A., Breban, R., Vardavas, R., Okano, J.T., Martin, T., Aral, S.& Blower, S. (2008). *Infectious syphilis in high-income settings in the 21st century*. Lancet Infect Dis 8 (4) :244-53

Ficarra, G. & Carlos, R. (2009). *Syphilis: the renaissance of an old disease with oral implications*. Head Neck Pathol, 3(3):195-206.

Guo, Y., Li, X., Fang, X., Lin, X., Song, Y., Jiang, S. & Stanton, B. (2011). *A comparison of four sampling methods among men having sex with men in China: implications for HIV/STD surveillance and prevention*. AIDS Care, Epub ahead of print

Gutierrez, J.P., McPherson, S., Fakoya, A., Matheou, A. & Bertozzi, S.M. (2010). *Community-based prevention leads to an increase in condom use and a reduction in sexually transmitted infections (STIs) among men who have sex with men (MSM) and female sex workers (FSW): the Frontiers Prevention Project (FPP) evaluation results.* BMC Public Health, 18; 10:497

Guy, R., Goller, J.L., Spelman, T., El-Hayek, C., Gold, J., Lim, M., Leslie, D., Tee, B.K., Roth, N., Anderson, J., Fairley, C.K., Kaldor, J. & Hellard, M. (2010). *Does the frequency of HIV and STI testing among men who have sex with men in primary care adhere with Australian guidelines?* Sex Transm Infect, 86(5): 371-6.

Halperin, D.T., de Moya, E.A., Pérez-Then, E., Pappas, G. & Garcia Calleja, J.M. (2009). *Understanding the HIV epidemic in the Dominican Republic: a prevention success story in the Caribbean?* J Acquir Immune Defic Sindr, 51 Suppl 1: S52-9.

Hamers, F.F. & Downs, A.M. (2004).*The changing face of the HIV epidemic in western Europe: what are the implications for public health policies?* Lancet ; 364(9428):83-94.

Heffelfinger, J.D., Swint, E.B., Berman, S.M. & Weinstock, H.S. (2007). *Trends in primary and secondary syphilis among men who have sex with men in the United States.* Am J Public Health, 97(6): 1076-83.

Istituto Nazionale di Statistica (ISTAT). (2005). Notification of Infectious Diseases in Italy-year 2002-Informazioni 2005; 2 : 9-15

Jin, F., Prestage, G.P., Zablotska, I., Rawstorne, P., Imrie, J., Kippax, S.C., Donovan, B., Templeton, D.J., Kaldor, J.M. & Grulich, A.E. (2009). *High incidence of syphilis in HIV-positive homosexual men: data from two community-based cohort studies.* Sex Health, 6(4): 281-4.

Katz, M.H., Schwarcz, S.K., Kellogg, T.A., Klausner, J.D., Dilley, J.W., Gibson, S. & McFarland, W. (2002). *Impact of highly active antiretroviral treatment on HIV seroincidence among men who have sex with men: San Francisco.* Am J Public Health, 92(3): 388-94.

Klausner, J.D., Wolf, W., Fischer-Ponce, L., Zolt, I. & Katz, M.H. (2000). *Tracing a syphilis outbreak through cyberspace.* JAMA, 284(4): 447-9.

Klavs, I., Bergant, N., Kastelic, Z. & Kustec, T. (2009). *Disproportionate and increasing burden of HIV infection among men who have sex with men in Slovenia: surveillance data for 1999-2008.* Euro Surveill, 14 (47):pii=19419

Kuklová, I., Velcevský, P. & Kojanová, M. (2011). *Syphilis among STD clinic patients in Prague in 2009.* Cent Eur J Public Health, 19(2): 84-90.

Kumta, S., Lurie, M., Weitzen, S., Jerajani, H., Gogate, A., Row-kavi, A., Anand, V., Makadon, H. & Mayer, K.H.(2010). *Bisexuality, sexual risk taking, and HIV prevalence among men who have sex with men accessing voluntary counseling and testing services in Mumbai, India.* J Acquir Immune Defic Syndr, 53(2):227-33.

Leber, A., MacPherson, P. & Lee, B.C. (2008). *Epidemiology of infectious syphilis in Ottawa. Recurring themes revisited.* Can J Public Health, 99(5):401-5..

Likatavicius, G., Klavs, I., Devaux, I., Alix,J. & Nardone, A.(2008). *An increase in newly diagnosed HIV cases reported among men who have sex with men in Europe, 2000-6: implications for a European public health strategy.* Sex Transm Infect, 84(6):499-505.

Marcus, U. & Hamouda, O. (2005). *Syphilis in Germany, 2004: diagnoses increasing, particularly in smaller cities and rural areas.* Euro Surveill, 10(7):E050728.3.

Matee, M.I., Magesa, P.M. & Lyamuya, E.F. (2006). *Seroprevalence of human immunodeficiency virus, hepatitis B and C viruses and syphilis infections among blood donors at the Muhimbili National Hospital in Dar es Salaam, Tanzania.* BMC Public Health, 6:21.

Mayer, K.H., O'Cleirigh, C., Skeer, M., Covahey, C., Leidolf, E., Vanderwarker, R. & Safren, S.A. (2010). *Which HIV- infected men who have sex with men in care are engaging in risky sex and acquiring sexually transmitted infections: findings from a Boston community health centre.* Sex Transm Infect, 86(1):66-70.

McCutchan, F.E. 2006. *Global epidemiology of HIV.* J Med Virol, 78 Suppl 1:S7-S12.

Merrigan, M., Azeez, A., Afolabi, B., Chabikuli, O.N., Onyekwena, O., Eluwa, G., Aiyenigba, B., Kawu, I., Ogungbemi, K. & Hamelmann, C. (2011). *HIV prevalence and risk behaviours among men having sex with men in Nigeria.* Sex Transm Infect, 87(1):65-70

Murray, J.M., McDonald, A.M. & Law, M.G. (2009). *Rapidly ageing HIV epidemic among men who have sex with men in Australia.* Sex Health, 6(1): 83- 86

Nagalo, M.B., Sanou, M., Bisseye, C., Kaboré, M.I., Nebie, Y.K., Kienou, K., Kiba, A., Dahourou, H., Ouattara, S., Zongo, J.D. & Simporé, J. (2011). *Seroprevalence of human immunodeficiency virus, hepatitis B and C viruses and syphilis among blood donors in Koudougou (Burkina Faso) in 2009.* Blood Transfus, 4(1):1-6. doi: 10.2450/2011.0112-10.

National Centre in HIV Epidemiology and Clinical Research. (2007). HIV/AIDS, Viral Hepatitis and Sexually Transmissible Infections in Australia Annual Surveillance Report 2007. National Centre in HIV Epidemiology and Clinical Research, The University of New South Wales. Sidney, NSW. Camberra: Australian Institute of Health and Welfare.

Pebody, R. (2010). *Internet proving a key way to reach men who have sex with men in Africa, Asia and beyond.* Available from http://aidsmap.com/page/1447379/

Peterman, T.A. & Furness, B.W. (2007). *The resurgence of syphilis among men who have sex with men.* Curr Opin Infect Dis, 20(1):54-9.

Prestage, G., Mao, L., Fogarty, A., Van de Ven, P., Kippax, S., Crawford, J., Rawstorne, P., Kaldor, J., Jin, F. & Grulich, A. (2005). *How has the sexual behaviour of gay men changed since the onset of AIDS: 1986-2003.* Aust NZJ Public Health, 29:530-35

Public Health Agency of Canada. (2007). *HIV/AIDS Epi Updates, November 2007, surveillance and Risk Assessment Division,* Centre for Infectious Disease Prevention and Control, Public Health Agency of Canada.

Sasse, A. & Defraye, A. (2009). *HIV infections and STI co-infections in men who have sex with men in Belgium: sustained increase in HIV diagnoses.* Euro Surveill, 14 (47) : pii=19420

Savage, E.J., Hughes, G., Ison, C. & Lowndes, C.M. European Surveillance of Sexually Transmitted Infections network. (2009). *Syphilis and gonorrhoea in men who have sex with men: a European overview.* Euro Surveill, 14 (47) pii: 19417.

Schneider, J.A., Lakshmi, V., Dandona,R., Kumar, G.A., Sudha, T. & Dandona, L. (2010). *Population-based seroprevalence of HSV-2 and syphilis in Andhra Pradesh state of India.* BMC Infect Dis, 10:59.

Simms, I., Fenton, K.A., Ashton, M., Turner, K.M., Crawley-Boevey, E.E., Gorton, R., Thomas, D.R., Lynch, A., Winter, A., Fisher, M.J., Lighton, L., Maguire, H.C. & Solomou, M. (2005). *The re-emergence of syphilis in the United Kingdom: the new epidemic phases.* Sex Transm Infect, 32 : 220-26

Smith, A.D., Tapsoba, P., Peshu, N., Sanders, E.J. & Jaffe, H.W. (2009). *Men who have sex with men and HIV/AIDS in sub-Saharan Africa.* Lancet, 374 (9687) : 416-223

Solomon, S.S., Srikrishnan, A.K., Sifakis, F., Mehta, S.H., Vasudevan, C.K., Balakrishnan, P., Mayer, K.H., Solomon, S. & Celentano, D.D. (2010). *The emerging HIV epidemic among men who have sex with men in Tamil Nadu, India: geographic diffusion and bisexual concurrency.* AIDS Behav, 14(5):1001-10..

Sullivan, P.S., Hamouda, O., Delpech, V., Geduld, J.E., Prejean, J., Semaille, C., Kaldor, J., Folch, C., Op de Coul, E., Marcus, U., Hughes, G., Archibald, C.P., Cazein, F., McDonald, A., Casabona, J., van Sighem,A. & Fenton, K.A. (2009). *Re-emergence of the HIV epidemic among men who have sex with men in North America, Western Europe, and Australia, 1996-2005.* Ann Epidemiol, 19(6):423-31

The White House Office of National AIDS Policy. National HIV/AIDS Strategy for the United States. Available from http//www.whitehouse.gov/administration/eop/onap/. Accessed on December 15, 2010

Velicko, I., Arneborn, M. & Blaxult, A. (2008). *Syphilis epidemiology in Sweden: re-emergence since 2000 primarily due to spread among men who have sex with men.* Euro Surveill, 13(50). pii: 19063

Wade, A.S., Kane, C.T., Diallo, P.A., Diop, A.K., Gueye, K., Mboup, S., Ndoye, I. & Lagarde, E. (2005). *HIV infection and sexually transmitted infections among men who have sex with men in Senegal.* AIDS, 19(18):2133-40.

Wallace, L., Winter, A. & Goldberg, D. (2005). *Increase in reported syphilis infections in Scotland in 2004.* Euro Surveill, 10 (30) : pii 2758

Ward, J.S., Guy, R.J., Akre, S.P., Middleton, M.G., Giele, C.M., Su, J.Y., Davis, C.A., Wand, H., Knox, J.B., Fagan, P.S., Donovan, B., Kaldor, J.M. & Russell, D.B. (2011). *Epidemiology of syphilis in Australia: moving toward elimination of infectious syphilis from remote Aboriginal and Torres Strait Islander communities?* Med J Aust, 194(10):525-9.

Watson-Jones, D., Oliff, M., Terris-Prestholt, F., Changalucha, J., Gumodoka, B., Mayaud, P., Semakafu, A.M., Kumaranayake, L., Gavyole, A., Mabey, D. & Hayes, R. (2005). *Antenatal syphilis screening in sub-Saharan Africa: lessons learned from Tanzania.* Trop Med Int Health, 10(9):934-43.

World Health Organization. (2001). *Global prevalence and incidence of selected curable sexually transmitted infections.* Available from http// www.who.int/hiv/pub/sti/who_hiv_aids_2001.02.pdf

World Health Organization. (2007). *Sexually transmitted infections.* Fact sheet N°110. Available from http://www.who.int/mediacentre/factsheets/fs110/en/

Xu, J.J., Reilly, K.H., Lu, C.M., Ma, N., Zhang, M., Chu, Z.X., Wang, J.J., Yun, K. & Shang, H. (2011). *A cross sectional study of HIV and syphilis infections among male students who have sex with men (MSM) in northeast China: implications for implementing HIV screening and intervention programs.* BMC Public Health, 11: 287

Yang, Q., Boulos, D., Yan, P., Zhang, F., Remis, R.S., Schanzer, D. & Archibald, C.P. (2010). *Estimates of the number of prevalent and incident human immunodeficiency virus (HIV) infections in Canada, 2008.* Can J Public Health, 01(6):486-90.

Zetola, N.M. & Klausner, J.D. (2007). *Syphilis and HIV infection: an update.* Clin Infect Dis, 44(9):1222-8.

Zhang, M., Chu, Z., Wang, H., Xu, J., Lu, C. & Shang, H. (2011). *A Rapidly Increasing Incidence of HIV and Syphilis Among Men Who Have Sex with Men in a Major City of China.* AIDS Res Hum Retroviruses, Epub ahead of print.

# Permissions

All chapters in this book were first published in HIVIEHAATSIAC, by InTech Open; hereby published with permission under the Creative Commons Attribution License or equivalent. Every chapter published in this book has been scrutinized by our experts. Their significance has been extensively debated. The topics covered herein carry significant findings which will fuel the growth of the discipline. They may even be implemented as practical applications or may be referred to as a beginning point for another development.

The contributors of this book come from diverse backgrounds, making this book a truly international effort. This book will bring forth new frontiers with its revolutionizing research information and detailed analysis of the nascent developments around the world.

We would like to thank all the contributing authors for lending their expertise to make the book truly unique. They have played a crucial role in the development of this book. Without their invaluable contributions this book wouldn't have been possible. They have made vital efforts to compile up to date information on the varied aspects of this subject to make this book a valuable addition to the collection of many professionals and students.

This book was conceptualized with the vision of imparting up-to-date information and advanced data in this field. To ensure the same, a matchless editorial board was set up. Every individual on the board went through rigorous rounds of assessment to prove their worth. After which they invested a large part of their time researching and compiling the most relevant data for our readers.

The editorial board has been involved in producing this book since its inception. They have spent rigorous hours researching and exploring the diverse topics which have resulted in the successful publishing of this book. They have passed on their knowledge of decades through this book. To expedite this challenging task, the publisher supported the team at every step. A small team of assistant editors was also appointed to further simplify the editing procedure and attain best results for the readers.

Apart from the editorial board, the designing team has also invested a significant amount of their time in understanding the subject and creating the most relevant covers. They scrutinized every image to scout for the most suitable representation of the subject and create an appropriate cover for the book.

The publishing team has been an ardent support to the editorial, designing and production team. Their endless efforts to recruit the best for this project, has resulted in the accomplishment of this book. They are a veteran in the field of academics and their pool of knowledge is as vast as their experience in printing. Their expertise and guidance has proved useful at every step. Their uncompromising quality standards have made this book an exceptional effort. Their encouragement from time to time has been an inspiration for everyone.

The publisher and the editorial board hope that this book will prove to be a valuable piece of knowledge for researchers, students, practitioners and scholars across the globe.

# List of Contributors

**Vani Subbarao**
Madwaleni Hospital, Elliotdale, Eastern Cape, South Africa

**David Lowe**
Clinical Infectious Disease Research Initiative, Institute of Infectious Diseases and Molecular Medicine, University of Cape Town, South Africa
Wellcome Trust Centre for Research in Clinical Tropical Medicine, Department of Medicine, Imperial College London, UK

**Reza Aghamohammadzadeh**
British Heart Foundation Clinical Research Fellow, UK
NIHR Manchester Biomedical Research Centre Clinical Research Fellow, UK

**Robert J. Wilkinson**
Clinical Infectious Disease Research Initiative, Institute of Infectious Diseases and Molecular Medicine, University of Cape Town, South Africa
Wellcome Trust Centre for Research in Clinical Tropical Medicine, Department of Medicine, Imperial College London, UK
Division of Mycobacterial Research, MRC National Institute for Medical Research, The Ridgeway, Mill Hill, London UK

**Jan Siewe, Kourosh Zarghooni and Rolf Sobottke**
Department for Orthopaedic and Trauma Surgery, University of Cologne, Germany

**Nicole F. Bernard et al.**
Research Institute of the McGill University Health Centre
Division of Experimental Medicine, McGill University, Clinique du Quartier
Division of Clinical Immunology and Allergy, McGill University Health Centre, Toronto, Ontario
Centre de Recherche du Centre Hospitalier de l'Université de Montréa Montréal, Québec, Canada

**Elaheh Aghdassi**
The University Health Network, Toronto, Canada

**Olga Perovic**
National Institute for Communicable Diseases, a Division of the National Health Laboratory Service
University of Witwatersrand South Africa

**Ashika Singh**
National Institute for Communicable Diseases, a Division of the National Health Laboratory Service

**Muhwa J. Chakaya**
Chief Research Officer, Centre for Respiratory Diseases Research, Kenya Medical Research Institute, Kenya

**Christophoros Kosmidis, Georgios Anthimidis and Kalliopi Vasiliadou**
Interbalkan European Medical Center, Department of Surgery, Thessaloniki Greece

**E.F. Silva**
Federal University of São Paulo - São Paulo, Brazil

**Katrin Hahn**
Universitätsklinikum Charité Campus Mitte, Klinik für Neurologie, Berlin

**Ingo Husstedt**
Universitätsklinikum Münster, Klinik und Poliklinik für Neurologie, Münster Germany

**Stefano Coaccioli**
Dept of Internal Medicine and Rheumatology, Perugia University Medical School, "Santa Maria" General Hospital, Terni, Italy

**Omolola Orenuga and Gbemisola Agbelusi**
Faculty of Dentistry, College of Medicine, University of Lagos, Lagos, Nigeria

**Mutiat Obileye**
Dental Clinics, Lagos State University Teaching Hospital, Ikeja, Nigeria

**Christiana Sowole**
Dental Public Health, Chatham, United Kingdom

**Maria Antonella Di Benedetto, Nino Romano and Alberto Firenze**
Dipartimento di Scienze per la Promozione della Salute, University of Palermo, Italy

# Index

## O



## P



## R



## S



## T



## V

www.ingramcontent.com/pod-product-compliance
Lightning Source LLC
LaVergne TN
LVHW081027210926
848485LV00004B/965
*9781639873067*